D1611889

In Vitro Mutagenesis Protocols

Methods in Molecular Biology™

John M. Walker, SERIES EDITOR

60. **Protein NMR Protocols**, edited by *David G. Reid, 1996*
59. **Protein Purification Protocols**, edited by *Shawn Doonan, 1996*
58. **Basic DNA and RNA Protocols**, edited by *Adrian J. Harwood, 1996*
57. **In Vitro Mutagenesis Protocols**, edited by *Michael K. Trower, 1996*
56. **Crystallographic Methods and Protocols**, edited by *Christopher Jones, Barbara Mulloy, and Mark Sanderson, 1996*
55. **Plant Cell Electroporation and Electrofusion Protocols**, edited by *Jac A. Nickoloff, 1995*
54. **YAC Protocols**, edited by *David Markie, 1995*
53. **Yeast Protocols**: *Methods in Cell and Molecular Biology*, edited by *Ivor H. Evans, 1996*
52. **Capillary Electrophoresis**: *Principles, Instrumentation, and Applications*, edited by *Kevin D. Altria, 1996*
51. **Antibody Engineering Protocols**, edited by *Sudhir Paul, 1995*
50. **Species Diagnostics Protocols**: *PCR and Other Nucleic Acid Methods*, edited by *Justin P. Clapp, 1996*
49. **Plant Gene Transfer and Expression Protocols**, edited by *Heddwyn Jones, 1995*
48. **Animal Cell Electroporation and Electrofusion Protocols**, edited by *Jac A. Nickoloff, 1995*
47. **Electroporation Protocols for Microorganisms**, edited by *Jac A. Nickoloff, 1995*
46. **Diagnostic Bacteriology Protocols**, edited by *Jenny Howard and David M. Whitcombe, 1995*
45. **Monoclonal Antibody Protocols**, edited by *William C. Davis, 1995*
44. **Agrobacterium Protocols**, edited by *Kevan M. A. Gartland and Michael R. Davey, 1995*
43. **In Vitro Toxicity Testing Protocols**, edited by *Sheila O'Hare and Chris K. Atterwill, 1995*
42. **ELISA**: *Theory and Practice*, by *John R. Crowther, 1995*
41. **Signal Transduction Protocols**, edited by *David A. Kendall and Stephen J. Hill, 1995*
40. **Protein Stability and Folding**: *Theory and Practice*, edited by *Bret A. Shirley, 1995*
39. **Baculovirus Expression Protocols**, edited by *Christopher D. Richardson, 1995*
38. **Cryopreservation and Freeze-Drying Protocols**, edited by *John G. Day and Mark R. McLellan, 1995*
37. **In Vitro Transcription and Translation Protocols**, edited by *Martin J. Tymms, 1995*
36. **Peptide Analysis Protocols**, edited by *Ben M. Dunn and Michael W. Pennington, 1994*
35. **Peptide Synthesis Protocols**, edited by *Michael W. Pennington and Ben M. Dunn, 1994*
34. **Immunocytochemical Methods and Protocols**, edited by *Lorette C. Javois, 1994*
33. **In Situ Hybridization Protocols**, edited by *K. H. Andy Choo, 1994*
32. **Basic Protein and Peptide Protocols**, edited by *John M. Walker, 1994*

31. **Protocols for Gene Analysis**, edited by *Adrian J. Harwood, 1994*
30. **DNA–Protein Interactions**, edited by *G. Geoff Kneale, 1994*
29. **Chromosome Analysis Protocols**, edited by *John R. Gosden, 1994*
28. **Protocols for Nucleic Acid Analysis by Nonradioactive Probes**, edited by *Peter G. Isaac, 1994*
27. **Biomembrane Protocols**: *II. Architecture and Function*, edited by *John M. Graham and Joan A. Higgins, 1994*
26. **Protocols for Oligonucleotide Conjugates**: *Synthesis and Analytical Techniques*, edited by *Sudhir Agrawal, 1994*
25. **Computer Analysis of Sequence Data**: *Part II*, edited by *Annette M. Griffin and Hugh G. Griffin, 1994*
24. **Computer Analysis of Sequence Data**: *Part I*, edited by *Annette M. Griffin and Hugh G. Griffin, 1994*
23. **DNA Sequencing Protocols**, edited by *Hugh G. Griffin and Annette M. Griffin, 1993*
22. **Microscopy, Optical Spectroscopy, and Macroscopic Techniques**, edited by *Christopher Jones, Barbara Mulloy, and Adrian H. Thomas, 1993*
21. **Protocols in Molecular Parasitology**, edited by *John E. Hyde, 1993*
20. **Protocols for Oligonucleotides and Analogs**: *Synthesis and Properties*, edited by *Sudhir Agrawal, 1993*
19. **Biomembrane Protocols**: *I. Isolation and Analysis*, edited by *John M. Graham and Joan A. Higgins, 1993*
18. **Transgenesis Techniques**: *Principles and Protocols*, edited by *David Murphy and David A. Carter, 1993*
17. **Spectroscopic Methods and Analyses**: *NMR, Mass Spectrometry, and Metalloprotein Techniques*, edited by *Christopher Jones, Barbara Mulloy, and Adrian H. Thomas, 1993*
16. **Enzymes of Molecular Biology**, edited by *Michael M. Burrell, 1993*
15. **PCR Protocols**: *Current Methods and Applications*, edited by *Bruce A. White, 1993*
14. **Glycoprotein Analysis in Biomedicine**, edited by *Elizabeth F. Hounsell, 1993*
13. **Protocols in Molecular Neurobiology**, edited by *Alan Longstaff and Patricia Revest, 1992*
12. **Pulsed-Field Gel Electrophoresis**: *Protocols, Methods, and Theories*, edited by *Margit Burmeister and Levy Ulanovsky, 1992*
11. **Practical Protein Chromatography**, edited by *Andrew Kenney and Susan Fowell, 1992*
10. **Immunochemical Protocols**, edited by *Margaret M. Manson, 1992*
9. **Protocols in Human Molecular Genetics**, edited by *Christopher G. Mathew, 1991*
8. **Practical Molecular Virology**: *Viral Vectors for Gene Expression*, edited by *Mary K. L. Collins, 1991*
7. **Gene Transfer and Expression Protocols**, edited by *Edward J. Murray, 1991*
6. **Plant Cell and Tissue Culture**, edited by *Jeffrey W. Pollard and John M. Walker, 1990*
5. **Animal Cell Culture**, edited by *Jeffrey W. Pollard and John M. Walker, 1990*

Methods in Molecular Biology™ • 57

In Vitro Mutagenesis Protocols

Edited by

Michael K. Trower

Glaxo Research and Development Ltd., Glaxo-Wellcome
Medicines Research Centre, Stevenage, Hertfordshire, UK

Humana Press Totowa, New Jersey

Dedication

To my wife, Diana,
and my children, Isabella, Florence, and Sebastian

Preface

In Vitro Mutagenesis Protocols is about mutagenesis. Not mutagenesis in which living cells are exposed to cocktails of chemicals or doses of damaging radiation, but rather a more refined approach in which specific DNA sequences are targeted for alteration in vitro as designated by the investigator. This facility has been brought about by the advent of recombinant DNA technology, the arrival of which has provided extraordinarily powerful tools for the manipulation of DNA. Such tools have empowered us with the capability to readily engineer defined-target DNA sequences, providing unprecedented opportunities to study gene regulation and to probe structure/function relationships in proteins. This technology has also enabled us to revise DNA sequences for other purposes such as vector construction.

In Vitro Mutagenesis Protocols was designed to bring together a wide and varied array of specific mutagenesis protocols for both site-directed and random mutagenesis into a single-source volume. The book is informally divided into two parts, the first on protocols for site-directed mutagenesis, incorporating a number of methods based on strand selection, amber stop codon suppression, gapped-duplex formation, solid-phase technology, triple-helix formation, the ligase chain reaction, and a host of polymerase chain reaction-based procedures including splicing by overlap extension and the megaprimer technique. The second is devoted to random mutagenic approaches encompassing protocols, many in combination with the polymerase chain reaction, based on degenerate oligonucleotides, cassette mutagenesis, linker-scanning mutagenesis, chemical mutagenesis, nested-deletion mutagenesis, the infidelity of *Taq* DNA polymerase, and a DNA repair mechanism-deficient strain of *Escherichia coli*. In my role as editor I have striven to ensure that the chapters are understandable to the informed nonspecialist molecular biologist and that each protocol details extensive practical information to ensure that already competent scientists can utilize the methodology described at their own laboratory benches.

The revolutionary impact that in vitro mutagenesis has made in our understanding of the biological universe cannot be understated. This technology will continue to play a critical role in research laboratories around the world, whether it is for identifying altered protein properties and activities crucial to the development of the biotechnology industry or for unraveling the biological roles of the wealth of genes of unknown function currently being isolated from the human genome and those of other model organisms. It is clear that the need for efficient, rapid, and practical in vitro mutagenesis protocols has never been greater. It is therefore my fervent hope and wish that the time, effort, and sacrifices taken in creating this volume of protocols will be rewarded through satisfying the thirst of those scientists eager to drink from this particular fountain of knowledge!

Michael K. Trower

Contents

Preface .... *v*

Contributors .... *xi*

Ch. 1. Site-Directed Mutagenesis Using Positive Antibiotic Selection,
      Richard N. Bohnsack *1*

Ch. 2. In Vitro Site-Directed Mutagenesis Using the Unique Restriction
      Site Elimination (USE) Method,
      Li Zhu *13*

Ch. 3. Site-Directed Mutagenesis Using Double-Stranded Plasmid DNA
      Templates,
      Jeffrey Braman, Carol Papworth, and Alan Greener *31*

Ch. 4. Site-Directed Mutagenesis Using a Uracil-Containing Phagemid
      Template,
      Christian Hagemeier *45*

Ch. 5. Oligonucleotide-Directed Mutagenesis Using an Improved
      Phosphorothioate Approach,
      Susan J. Dale and Ian R. Felix *55*

Ch. 6. Analysis of Point Mutations by Use of Amber Stop Codon
      Suppression,
      Scott A. Lesley *65*

Ch. 7. A Simple Method for Site-Directed Mutagenesis
      with Double-Stranded Plasmid DNA,
      Derhsing Lai and Sidney Pestka *75*

Ch. 8. Double-Stranded DNA Site-Directed Mutagenesis,
      Stéphane Viville *87*

Ch. 9. Solid-Phase In Vitro Mutagenesis Using a Plasmid DNA Template,
      Roy Edward *97*

Ch. 10. Targeted Mutagenesis Mediated by the Triple Helix Formation,
      Peter M. Glazer, Gan Wang, Pamela A. Havre,
      and Edward J. Gunther *109*

Ch. 11. A Universal Nested Deletion Method Using an Arbitrary Primer
      and Elimination of a Unique Restriction Site,
      Li Zhu and Ann E. Holtz *119*

Ch. 12. Ordered Deletions Using Exonuclease III,
      Denise Clark and Steven Henikoff *139*

vii

Ch. 13. Ligase Chain Reaction for Site-Directed In Vitro Mutagenesis,
         Gerard J. A. Rouwendal, Emil J. H. Wolbert, Lute-Harm Zwiers,
         and Jan Springer 149
Ch. 14. PCR-Based Site-Directed Mutagenesis,
         Atsushi Shimada 157
Ch. 15. In Vitro Recombination and Mutagenesis by Overlap
         Extension PCR,
         Robert J. Pougulis, Abbe N. Vallejo, and Larry R. Pease 167
Ch. 16. Site-Directed Mutagenesis Using Overlap Extension PCR,
         Ashok Aiyar, Yan Xiang, and Jonathan Leis 177
Ch. 17. Modification of the Overlap Extension Method for Extensive
         Mutagenesis on the Same Template,
         Ivan Mikaelian and Alain Sergeant 193
Ch. 18. Site-Directed Mutagenesis In Vitro by Megaprimer PCR,
         Sailen Barik 203
Ch. 19. Using PCR for Rapid Site-Specific Mutagenesis in Large Plasmids,
         Brynmor A. Watkins and Marvin S. Reitz, Jr. 217
Ch. 20. PCR-Assisted Mutagenesis for Site-Directed Insertion/Deletion
         of Large DNA Segments,
         Daniel C. Tessier and David Y. Thomas 229
Ch. 21. Site-Directed Mutagenesis Using a Rapid PCR-Based Method,
         Gina L. Costa, John C. Bauer, Barbara McGowan, Mila Angert,
         and Michael P. Weiner 239
Ch. 22. A Simple Method to Introduce Internal Deletions or Mutations
         into Any Position of a Target DNA Sequence,
         Marjana Tomic-Canic, Françoise Bernerd,
         and Miroslav Blumenberg 249
Ch. 23. A Simple Method for Site-Specific Mutagenesis that Leaves
         the Rest of the Template Unaltered,
         Marjana Tomic-Canic, Ivana Sunjevaric,
         and Miroslav Blumenberg 259
Ch. 24. Multiple Site-Directed Mutagenesis,
         Kolari S. Bhat 269
Ch. 25. Construction of Linker-Scanning Mutations by Oligonucleotide
         Ligation,
         Grace M. Hobson, Patricia P. Harlow,
         and Pamela A. Benfield 279
Ch. 26. Construction of Linker-Scanning Mutations Using PCR,
         Patricia P. Harlow, Grace M. Hobson,
         and Pamela A. Benfield 287
Ch. 27. Use of Codon Cassette Mutagenesis for Saturation Mutagenesis,
         Deena M. Kegler-Ebo, Glenda W. Polack, and Daniel DiMaio 297

Contents

Ch. 28. Saturation Mutagenesis by Mutagenic Oligonucleotide-Directed
    PCR Amplification (Mod-PCR),
    Lillian W. Chiang *311*
Ch. 29. Random Mutagenesis of Short Target DNA Sequences via PCR
    with Degenerate Oligonucleotides,
    Frank Kirchhoff and Ronald C. Desrosiers *323*
Ch. 30. Random Sequence Mutagenesis for the Generation
    of Active Enzymes,
    Margaret E. Black and Lawrence A. Loeb *335*
Ch. 31. Random Mutagenesis by Using Mixtures of dNTP and dITP in PCR,
    Oscar P. Kuipers *351*
Ch. 32. PCR-Mediated Chemical Mutagenesis,
    Donald J. Roufa *357*
Ch. 33. Oligonucleotide-Directed Random Mutagenesis Using the
    Phosphorothioate Method,
    Susan J. Dale and Maxine Belfield *369*
Ch. 34. An Efficient Random Mutagenesis Technique Using an *E. coli*
    Mutator Strain,
    Alan Greener, Marie Callahan, and Bruce Jerpseth *375*
Index *387*

Contributors

MILA ANGERT • *Stratagene Inc., La Jolla, CA*

ASHOK AIYAR • *Department of Biochemistry, School of Medicine, Case Western Reserve University, Cleveland, OH*

SAILEN BARIK • *Department of Biochemistry and Molecular Biology, School of Medicine, University of South Alabama, Mobile, AL*

JOHN C. BAUER • *Stratagene Inc., La Jolla, CA*

MAXINE BELFIELD • *Amersham International, Buckinghamshire, UK*

PAMELA A. BENFIELD • *Research and Development, DuPont Merck, Wilmington, DE*

FRANÇOISE BERNERD • *L'Oréal Laboratories, Clichy, France*

KOLARI S. BHAT • *Department of Cell Biology, Vanderbilt University, Nashville, TN*

MARGARET E. BLACK • *Department of Pathology, School of Medicine, University of Washington, Seattle, WA*

MIROSLAV BLUMENBERG • *Department of Dermatology, New York University Medical Center, New York, NY*

RICHARD N. BOHNSACK • *Department of Biochemistry, Medical College of Wisconsin, Milwaukee, WI*

JEFFREY BRAMAN • *Stratagene Inc., La Jolla, CA*

MARIE CALLAHAN • *Stratagene Inc., La Jolla, CA*

LILLIAN W. CHIANG • *Department of Neurobiology, Stanford University School of Medicine, Stanford, CA*

DENISE CLARK • *Fred Hutchinson Cancer Research Center, Howard Hughes Medical Institute, Seattle, WA*

GINA L. COSTA • *Stratagene Inc., La Jolla, CA*

SUSAN J. DALE • *Amersham International, Buckinghamshire, UK*

RONALD C. DESROSIERS • *New England Regional Primate Research Center, Harvard Medical School, Southboro, MA*

DANIEL DIMAIO • *Department of Genetics, Yale University School of Medicine, New Haven, CT*

xi

Roy Edward • *Dynal Ltd., Wirral, UK*

Ian R. Felix • *Amersham International, Buckinghamshire, UK*

Peter M. Glazer • *Department of Therapeutic Radiology, Yale University School of Medicine, New Haven, CT*

Alan Greener • *Stratagene Inc., La Jolla, CA*

Edward J. Gunther • *Department of Therapeutic Radiology, Yale University School of Medicine, New Haven, CT*

Christian Hagemeier • *Laboratory of Molecular Biology, Department of Pediatrics, Humboldt University, Berlin, Germany*

Patricia P. Harlow • *Research and Development, DuPont Merck, Wilmington, DE*

Pamela A. Havre • *Department of Therapeutic Radiology, Yale University School of Medicine, New Haven, CT*

Steven Henikoff • *Fred Hutchinson Cancer Research Center, Howard Hughes Medical Institute, Seattle, WA*

Grace M. Hobson • *Research and Development, DuPont Merck, Wilmington, DE*

Ann E. Holtz • *Clontech Laboratories, Palo Alto, CA*

Bruce Jerpseth • *Stratagene Inc., La Jolla, CA*

Deena M. Kegler-Ebo • *Department of Genetics, Yale University School of Medicine, New Haven, CT*

Frank Kirchhoff • *Virology Institute, Erlangen-Nurnberg University, Erlangen, Germany*

Oscar P. Kuipers • *Netherlands Institute for Dairy Research, Ede, The Netherlands*

Derhsing Lai • *Department of Molecular Genetics and Microbiology, University of Medicine and Dentistry of New Jersey-Robert Wood Johnson Medical School, Piscataway, NJ*

Jonathan Leis • *Department of Biochemistry, School of Medicine, Case Western Reserve University, Cleveland, OH*

Scott A. Lesley • *Promega Corp., Madison, WI*

Lawrence A. Loeb • *Department of Pathology, School of Medicine, University of Washington, Seattle, WA*

Barbara McGowan • *Stratagene Inc., La Jolla, CA*

Ivan Mikaelian • *MRC-LMB, Cambridge, UK*

Carol Papworth • *Stratagene Inc., La Jolla, CA*

Contributors   *xiii*

L<small>ARRY</small> R. P<small>EASE</small> • *Department of Immunology, Mayo Clinic, Rochester, MN*
S<small>IDNEY</small> P<small>ESTKA</small> • *Department of Molecular Genetics and Microbiology, University of Medicine and Dentistry of New Jersey-Robert Wood Johnson Medical School, Piscataway, NJ*
G<small>LENDA</small> W. P<small>OLACK</small> • *Department of Genetics, Yale University School of Medicine, New Haven, CT*
R<small>OBERT</small> J. P<small>OUGULIS</small> • *Department of Immunology, Mayo Clinic, Rochester, MN*
M<small>ARVIN</small> S. R<small>EITZ</small>, J<small>R</small> • *Laboratory of Tumor Cell Biology, National Cancer Institute, National Institutes of Health, Bethesda, MD*
D<small>ONALD</small> J. R<small>OUFA</small> • *Center for Basic Cancer Research, Division of Biology, Kansas State University, Manhattan, KS*
G<small>ERARD</small> J. A. R<small>OUWENDAL</small> • *Agrotechnological Research Institute, Wageningen, The Netherlands*
A<small>LAIN</small> S<small>ERGEANT</small> • *Ecole Normale Superieure de Lyon, France*
A<small>TSUSHI</small> S<small>HIMADA</small> • *Department of Molecular Pathology, Takara Shuzo Co., Shiga, Japan*
J<small>AN</small> S<small>PRINGER</small> • *Agrotechnological Research Institute, Wageningen, The Netherlands*
I<small>VANA</small> S<small>UNJEVARIC</small> • *Department of Genetics and Development, Columbia University, New York, NY*
D<small>ANIEL</small> C. T<small>ESSIER</small> • *National Research Council of Canada, Biotechnology Research Institute, Montreal, Quebec, Canada*
D<small>AVID</small> Y. T<small>HOMAS</small> • *National Research Council of Canada, Biotechnology Research Institute, Montreal, Quebec, Canada*
M<small>ARJANA</small> T<small>OMIC</small>-C<small>ANIC</small> • *Department of Dermatology, New York University Medical Center, New York, NY*
A<small>BBE</small> N. V<small>ALLEJO</small> • *Department of Immunology, Mayo Clinic, Rochester, MN*
S<small>TÉPHANE</small> V<small>IVILLE</small> • *Institute for Genetic and Molecular and Cellular Biology, Louis Pasteur University, Strasboug, France*
G<small>AN</small> W<small>ANG</small> • *Department of Therapeutic Radiology, Yale University School of Medicine, New Haven, CT*
B<small>RYNMOR</small> A. W<small>ATKINS</small> • *Laboratory of Tumor Cell Biology, National Cancer Institute, National Institutes of Health, Bethesda, MD*
M<small>ICHAEL</small> P. W<small>EINER</small> • *Glaxo Inc., NC*

EMIL J. H. WOLBERT • *Agrotechnological Research Institute, Wageningen, The Netherlands*
YAN XIANG • *Department of Biochemistry, School of Medicine, Case Western Reserve University, Cleveland, OH*
LI ZHU • *Clontech Laboratories, Palo Alto, CA*
LUTE-HARM ZWIERS • *Agrotechnological Research Institute, Wageningen, The Netherlands*

CHAPTER 1

Site-Directed Mutagenesis Using Positive Antibiotic Selection

Richard N. Bohnsack

1. Introduction

A number protocols have been established for site-directed mutagenesis based on the work of Smith *(1)* and Hutchinson et al. *(2)* that use hybridization of a mismatched oligonucleotide to a DNA template followed by second-strand synthesis by a DNA polymerase. These techniques provide efficient means for incorporating and selecting for the desired mutation *(3–5)*. Oligonucleotide hybridization techniques use single-stranded DNA, usually derived from M13 phagemid vectors, which is hybridized to a mutagenic oligonucleotide. Second-strand synthesis is primed by the mutagenic oligonucleotide to provide a heteroduplex containing the desired mutation. If no selection method for mutants is employed, the theoretical yield of mutants using this procedure is 50% (owing to the semiconservative mode of DNA replication). In practice, however, the yield of mutants may be much lower. This is assumed to be owing to such factors as incomplete in vitro DNA polymerization, primer displacement by the DNA polymerase used to synthesis the second strand, and in vivo host-directed mismatch repair mechanisms that favor the repair of the nonmethylated newly synthesized mutant strand *(6)*. Several improvements have been developed that increase the efficiency of mutagenesis to the point where greater than 90% of recovered clones incorporate the desired point mutation. The Altered Sites II Mutagenesis Systems use antibiotic resistance to select for the mutant strand to provide a reliable procedure for highly efficient site-directed mutagenesis.

From: *Methods in Molecular Biology, Vol. 57: In Vitro Mutagenesis Protocols*
Edited by: M. K. Trower Humana Press Inc., Totowa, NJ

Figure 1 is a schematic outline of the Altered Sites II protocol. The mutagenic oligonucleotide and an oligonucleotide that restores antibiotic resistance to the phagemid, the antibiotic repair oligonucleotide, are simultaneously annealed to the template DNA, either ssDNA *(5)* or alkaline-denatured dsDNA. Synthesis and ligation of the mutant strand by T4 DNA polymerase and T4 DNA ligase links the two oligonucleotides. The mutant plasmids are replicated in a mismatch repair deficient *Escherichia coli mutS* strain, either ES1301 *(7,8)* or BMH 71-18 *(6)*, following clonal segregation in a second host such as JM109. In addition to the repair oligonucleotide and the mutagenic oligonucleotide, a third oligonucleotide can be incorporated in the annealing and synthesis reactions that inactivates the alternate antibiotic resistance. The alternate repair and inactivation of the antibiotic resistance genes in the Altered Sites II vectors allows multiple rounds of mutagenesis to be performed without the need for additional subcloning steps.

Figure 2 is a plasmid map for the pALTER-1 vector that is included with the Altered-Sites II system *(5)*. The pALTER-1 vector contains a multiple cloning site flanked by opposing SP6 and T7 RNA polymerase promoters, inserted into the DNA encoding the lacZ α-peptide. Cloning of a DNA insert into the multiple cloning site results in inactivation of the α-peptide. The vector contains the gene sequences for ampicillin and tetracycline resistance. The plasmid provided has a frameshift in the ampillicin gene that is repaired in the first round of mutagenesis. Propagation of the plasmid and recombinants is performed under tetracycline resistance. The pALTER-1 vector also contains the f1 origin of replication, which allows for the production of ssDNA on infection with the helper phage R408 or M13KO7 *(9–11)*. Two other vectors are available, pALTER-*Ex*1 and pALTER-*Ex*2. The pALTER-*Ex*1 is identical to pALTER-1 but contains a novel multiple cloning site with an expression cassette *(12)*. The pALTER-*Ex*2 vector has the same multiple cloning site, expression cassette, and f1 origin as pALTER-*Ex*1, but has a ColE1-compatible P15a origin of replication and gene sequences for tetracycline and chloramphenicol resistance *(12)*.

Protocols for the preparation of template DNA and competent cells are given in the Materials section. Design of the mutagenic oligonucleotide is discussed in Note 1, ref. *13*, and Chapters 11 and 15 of ref. *14*.

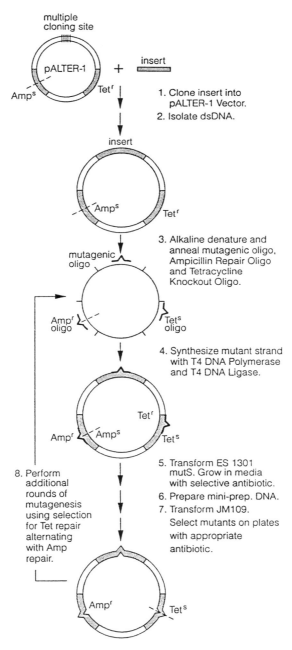

Fig. 1. Schematic diagram of the Altered Sites II in vitro mutagenesis procedure using the pALTER-1 vector as an example.

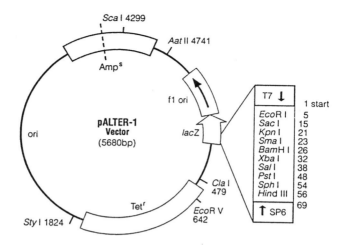

Fig. 2. pALTER-1 vector circle map.

2. Materials
2.1. Reagents for Preparation of ssDNA and Plasmid Miniprep DNA Templates

1. Helper phage (Either R408 or M13K07).
2. $3.75M$ Ammonium acetate in 20% polyethylene glycol (mol wt = 8000).
3. Chloroform:isoamyl alcohol (24:1).
4. TE-Saturated phenol:chloroform:isoamyl alcohol (25:24:1).
5. $5M$ NaCl stock.
6. Resuspension buffer: 25 mM Tris-HCl, pH 8.0, 10 mM EDTA, and 50 mM glucose.
7. Lysis buffer: 0.2M NaOH, 1% SDS. Prepare fresh.
8. Neutralization solution: 3.5M potassium acetate, pH 4.8.
9. DNase-free RNase A (100 mg/mL)

2.2. Reagents for Denaturation of dsDNA Template

1. $2M$ NaOH, 2 mM EDTA.
2. $2M$ Ammonium acetate, pH 4.6.
3. 70 and 100% Ethanol.
4. TE buffer: 10 mM Tris-HCl, pH 8.0, 1 mM EDTA.

2.3. Regents for the Annealing Reaction and Mutant Strand Synthesis

1. Oligonucleotides (*see* Table 1 and Note 1).
2. 10X Annealing buffer: 200 mM Tris-HCl, pH 7.5, 100 mM MgCl$_2$, 500 mM NaCl.

Table 1
Repair and Knockout Oligonucleotide to be Used in Annealing Reactions[a]

Plasmid	Selection	Repair oligo	Knockout oligo
pALTER-1 and pALTER-*Ex*1	Amp^sTet^r to Amp^rTet^s First round	Amp repair	Tet knockout
pALTER-1 and pALTER-*Ex*1	Amp^rTet^s to Amp^sTet^r Second round	Tet repair	Amp knockout
pALTER-*Ex*2	Cm^sTet^r to Cm^rTet^s First round	Cm repair	Tet knockout
pALTER-*Ex*2	Cm^rTet^s to Cm^sTet^r Second round	Tet repair	Cm knockout

[a]Abbreviations: Amp^r, ampicillin resistant; amp^s, ampicillin sensitive; Cm^r, chloramphenicol resistant; Cm^s, chloramphenicol sensitive; Tet^r, tetracycline resistant; Tet^s, tetracycline sensitive.

3. 10X Synthesis buffer: 100 mM Tris-HCl, pH 7.5, 5 mM dNTPs, 10 mM ATP, 20 mM DTT.
4. T4 DNA polymerase (10 U/μL).
5. T4 DNA ligase (20 U/μL).

2.4. Reagents for Preparation of Competent Cells and Transformation

1. Solution A: 30 mM potassium acetate, 100 mM RbCl, 10 mM CaCl$_2$, 50 mM MnCl$_2$, and 15% (w/v) glycerol; adjust to pH 5.8 with acetic acid. Filter-sterilize prior to use.
2. Solution B: 10 mM MOPS, 75 mM CaCl$_2$, 10 mM RbCl, and 15% (w/v) glycerol; adjust to a final pH of 6.8 with KOH. Filter-sterilize prior to use.
3. *E. coli* strains ES1301 *mutS* and JM109 (Promega, Madison, WI).

3. Methods

3.1. Preparation of Template

Templates may be either single-stranded phagmid DNA or double-stranded plasmid DNA (*see* Note 2)

3.1.1. Preparation of Single-Stranded DNA Template

1. Prepare an overnight culture of cells containing recombinant phagmid DNA by picking a single antibiotic resistant colony from a fresh plate. Inoculate 3 mL of LB broth containing the appropriate antibiotic and shake at 37°C.
2. The next morning, inoculate 50 mL of LB broth with 1 mL of the overnight culture. Shake vigorously at 37°C for 30 min in a 250-mL flask.

3. Infect the culture with helper phage at a multiplicity of infection (MOI) of 10. Continue shaking for 6 h. The volume of phage to be added to arrive at an MOI of approx 10–20 can be calculated by assuming that the cell concentration of the starting culture ranges from 5×10^7 to 1×10^8 cells/mL. An MOI of 10 requires 5×10^8 to 1×10^9 phage/mL.

4. Harvest the supernatant by pelleting the cells at 12,000g for 15 min. Transfer the supernatant into a fresh tube and centrifuge at 12,000g for 15 min to remove any remaining cells.

5. Precipitate the phage by adding 0.25 volumes of 3.75M ammonium acetate in 20% polyethylene glycol (mol wt 8000) to the supernatant. Allow solution to stand on ice for 30 min then centrifuge at 12,000g for 15 min. Thoroughly drain the supernatant.

6. Resuspend the pellet in 1 mL of TE buffer, pH 8.0, and transfer 500 µL of the sample to each of two microcentrifuge tubes.

7. To each tube, add 500 µL of chloroform:isoamyl alcohol (24:1) to lyse the phage, vortex for 1 min. Separate phases by centrifuging for 2 min in a microcentrifuge. Transfer the upper aqueous phases to fresh microcentrifuge tubes.

8. Add an equal volume of TE-saturated phenol:chloroform:isoamyl alcohol (25:24:1) to each tube, vortex 1 min, and centrifuge as in step 7.

9. Transfer the aqueous phases to fresh tubes and repeat the phenol extraction as in step 8. Repeat the extraction until there is no material visible at the interface of the two phases. Transfer the aqueous phases to fresh microcentrifuge tubes and add NaCl to a final concentration of 0.25M (0.05 vol of a 5M NaCl stock). Add 2 vol of 100% ethanol and incubate on ice for 30 min. Precipitate ssDNA by centrifuging at top speed in a microcentrifuge for 15 min. Carefully rinse the pellet with 1 mL of 70% ethanol and dry the pellet under vacuum. Resuspend the pellet in a small volume of H_2O and estimate the concentration of DNA (*see* Note 3). The ssDNA is ready for use in the annealing reaction (*see* Section 3.3.).

3.1.2. Plasmid Miniprep Procedure

1. Place 1.5 mL of an overnight culture into a microcentrifuge tube and centrifuge at 12,000g for 2 min. The remaining overnight culture can be stored at 4°C.

2. Remove the medium by aspiration, leaving the bacterial pellet as dry as possible.

3. Resuspend the pellet by vortexing in 100 µL of ice-cold resuspension buffer.

4. Add 200 µL of lysis buffer. Mix by inversion. Do not vortex. Incubate on ice for 5 min.

5. Add 150 µL of ice-cold neutralization solution. Mix by inversion and incubate on ice for 5 min.
6. Centrifuge at 12,000*g* for 5 min.
7. Transfer the supernatant to a fresh tube, avoiding the white precipitate.
8. Add 1 vol of TE-saturated phenol:chloroform:isoamyl alcohol (25:24:1). Vortex for 1 min and centrifuge at 12,000*g* for 2 min.
9. Transfer the upper aqueous phase to an fresh tube and add 1 volume of chloroform:isoamyl alcohol (24:1). Vortex for 1 min and centrifuge as in step 8.
10. Transfer the upper aqueous phase to a fresh tube and add 2.5 vol of 100% ethanol. Mix and incubate on dry ice for 30 min.
11. Centrifuge at 12,000*g* for 15 min. Rinse the pellet with cold 70% ethanol and dry the pellet under vacuum.
12. Dissolve the pellet in 50 µL of sterile deionized H_2O. Add 0.5 µL of DNase-free RNase A.
13. The concentration of plasmid DNA can be estimated by electrophoresis on an agarose gel.

3.2. Denaturation of Double-Stranded DNA Template

Double-stranded DNA must be alkaline denatured prior to use in the mutagenesis protocol.

1. Set up the following alkaline denaturation reaction. This generates enough DNA for one mutagenesis reaction: dsDNA template, 0.05 pmol (approx 0.2 µg); 2*M* NaOH, 2 m*M* EDTA, 2 µL; sterile deionized H_2O to 20 µL final volume.
2. Incubate for 5 min at room temperature.
3. Add 2 µL of 2*M* ammonium acetate, pH 4.6, and 75 µL of 100% ethanol.
4. Incubate for 30 min at −70°C.
5. Precipitate the DNA by centrifugation at top speed in a microcentrifuge for 15 min.
6. Drain and wash the pellet with 200 µL of 70% ethanol. Centrifuge again as in step 5. Dry pellet under vacuum.
7. Dissolve pellet in 10 µL of TE buffer and proceed immediately to the annealing reaction (*see* Section 3.3.).

3.3. Annealing Reaction and Mutant Strand Synthesis

In the following example, both the antibiotic repair and knockout oligonucleotides are included in the reaction mixture. It is not necessary to include the antibiotic knockout oligonucleotide in the mutagenesis if a second round of mutagenesis is not desired.

1. Prepare the mutagenesis annealing reaction as described in the following using the appropriate antibiotic repair and knockout oligonucleotides (*see* Table 1 and Notes 1 and 4): 0.05 pmol dsDNA or ssDNA mutagenesis template (200 ng dsDNA, 100 ng ssDNA), 1 µL (0.25 pmol) antibiotic repair oligonucleotide (2.2 ng/µL), 1 µL (0.25 pmol) antibiotic knockout oligonucleotide (2.2 ng/µL), 1.25 pmol mutagenic oligonucleotide (phosphorylated), 2 µL annealing 10X buffer, sterile deionized H_2O to a final volume of 20 µL.
2. Heat the annealing reactions to 75°C for 5 min and allow them to cool slowly to room temperature. Slow cooling minimizes nonspecific annealing of the oligonucleotides. Cooling at a rate of approx 1°C/min to 45°C followed by more rapid cooling to room temperature (22°C) is recommended.
3. Place the annealing reactions on ice and add the following: 3 µL synthesis 10X buffer, 1 µL T4 DNA polymerase, 1 µL T4 DNA ligase, 5 µL (final vol 30 µL) sterile deionized H_2O.
4. Incubate the reaction at 37°C for 90 min.

The mutagenesis reaction is then transformed into competent cells of the *E. coli* strain ES1301 *mutS* (*see* Section 3.5. and Note 5).

3.4. Preparation of Competent Cells

The following is the rubidium chloride method of Hanahan *(15)* and may be used to prepare compentent cells of both ES1301 *mutS* and JM109.

1. Inoculate 5 mL of LB medium with 10 µL of a glycerol stock of either ES1301 *mutS* or JM109 cells. Incubate at 37°C overnight.
2. Inoculate 50 mL of LB medium with 0.5 mL of the overnight bacterial culture.
3. Grow cells until the OD_{600} reaches 0.4–0.6 (approx 2–3 h at 37°C).
4. Centrifuge cells for 5 min at 5000g, 4°C, in a sterile disposable tube.
5. Decant the supernatant and resuspend the cells in 1 mL of solution A. Bring the volume up to 20 mL with solution A.
6. Incubate cells on ice for 5 min then pellet the cells as described in step 4.
7. Decant the supernatant and resuspend the cells in 2 mL of ice-cold solution B. Incubate on ice for 15–60 min.
8. Freeze the cells on crushed dry ice in 0.2-mL aliquots. Competent cells prepared by this method can be stored at −70°C for 5–6 wk.

3.5. Transformation into ES1301 **mutS** *Strain*

1. Thaw competent ES1301 *mutS* cells (*see* Section 3.4.) on ice. Add 15 µL of the mutagenesis reaction to 100 µL of competent cells and mix gently.
2. Incubate cells on ice for 30 min.

3. Heat shock the cells at 42°C for 90 s after the incubation on ice to improve the transformation efficiency.
4. Add 4 mL of LB medium without antibiotic and incubate for 1 h at 37°C with shaking.
5. After 1 h, add selective antibiotic to the culture. Final concentrations should be 125 µg/mL ampicillin, 10 µg/mL tetracycline, or 20 µg/mL chloramphenicol depending on the vector and antibiotic repair oligonucleotide used in the mutagenesis reaction.
6. Incubate culture overnight at 37°C with shaking.
7. Isolate plasmid DNA by alkaline lysis procedure as outlined in Section 3.1.2.

3.6. Transformation into JM109 Strain and Clonal Segregation

1. Thaw JM109 competent cells (*see* Section 3.4.) on ice. Add 0.05–0.1 µg of plasmid DNA prepared from the overnight culture of ES1301 *mutS* cells and mix briefly.
2. Let the cells stand on ice for 30 min.
3. Heat shock for 90 s at 42°C.
4. Add 2 mL LB medium and incubate at 37°C for 1 h to allow the cells to recover.
5. Aliquot the culture into two microcentrifuge tubes and centrifuge for 1 min in a microcentrifuge.
6. Decant the supernatant and resuspend the cell pellets in 50 µL of LB medium.
7. Plate the cells in each tube on an LB plate containing the appropriate selective antibiotic.

The Altered Sites II protocol generally produces 60–90% mutants, so colonies may be screened by direct sequencing. Assuming greater than 60% mutants are obtained, screening five colonies will give a greater than 95% chance of finding the mutation. The SP6 and T7 sequencing primers can be used for sequencing if the mutation is within 200–300 bp from the end of the DNA insert. Often it is convenient to incorporate a unique restriction site into the mutagenic oligonucleotide without altering the amino acid sequence. These sites can be used to screen for plasmids that have incorporated the mutagenic oligonucleotide.

When using this technique for doing multiple rounds of mutagenesis, it is convenient to screen simultaneously for antibiotic sensitive isolates. Simply inoculate each isolate into two tubes of media, one containing each antibiotic; antibiotic clones will be identified easily. Antibiotic sensitive isolates can also be identified by replicate plating in a grid format.

Single colonies can be picked and used to inoculate two plates containing selective antibiotic in sequence.

4. Notes

1. The mutagenic oligonucleotide must be complimentary to the ssDNA strand produced by the mutagenesis vectors in the presence of helper phage. This is true for double-stranded mutagenesis as well, since the mutagenic oligonucleotide must hybridize to the same strand as the antibiotic repair oligonucleotide for the coupling to be effective.

   The stability of the complex between the oligonucleotide and the template is determined by the base composition of the oligonucleotide and the conditions under which it is annealed. In general, a 17–20 base oligonucleotide with the mismatch located in the center will be sufficient for single base mutations. This gives 8–10 perfectly matched nucleotides on either side of the mismatch. For mutations involving two or more mismatches, oligonucleotides 25 bases or longer are needed to allow for 12–15 perfectly matched bases on either side of the mismatch. Larger deletions may require an oligonucleotide having 20–30 matches on either side of the mismatched region.

2. Mutagenesis can be performed using either dsDNA or ssDNA templates. The double-strand procedure is faster and does not require the prior preparation of ssDNA. The single-strand procedure maybe useful, however, when trying to maximize the total number of transformants, such as for generating mutant libraries. Double-stranded DNA must be alkaline denatured before use in the mutagenesis reaction. Poor quality dsDNA inhibits second-strand synthesis during mutagenesis, therefore, it is recommended that sequencing quality DNA be used for the mutagenesis reaction.

3. Differences in yields of ssDNA have been observed to be dependent on the particular combination of host, vector, and helper phage. Generally, higher yields have been observed using the Altered Sites II vectors in combination with R408 helper phage and the JM109 train.

4. The annealing conditions required may vary with the composition of the oligonucleotide. AT-rich complexes tend to be less stable than GC-rich complexes and may require a lower annealing temperature to be stabilized. Routinely, oligonucleotides can be annealed to a DNA template by heating to 75°C for 5 min followed by slow cooling to room temperature. For more detailed discussions of oligonucleotide design and annealing conditions, *see* refs. *13* and *14*. The amount of oligonucleotides used in the annealing reaction may vary, depending on the size and amount of DNA template. A 25:1 oligonucleotide:template molar ratio for the mutagenic oligonucleotide and a 5:1 oligonucleotide:template molar ratio for the antibiotic repair and knockout oligonucleotides is recommended for a typical annealing

reaction. For efficient ligation, the mutagenic oligonucleotide should be phosphorylated.

5. Mutant plasmid may be rapidly transferred from the *muts* host into a more suitable host for long-term maintenance and clonal segregation. The mutagenesis reaction products are cotransformed into the ES1301 *muts* strain along with R408 rfDNA. The cotransformed rfDNA causes the mutant phagemid to be replicated and packaged as an infectious particle which is secreted into the media. These particles are used to infect a suitable F$^+$ host such as JM109, and the tranfectants are selected by their antibiotic resistance encoded by the phagemid. The procedure requires only a single transformation step into ES1301 *muts* and reduces the total time required for the mutagenesis protocol by eliminating the plasmid miniprep and transformation into the final host strain. The number of colonies obtained after the cotransformation procedure is very dependent on the competency of the ES1301 *muts* cells; at least 10^6–10^7 cfu/µg DNA is required for efficient cotransformation.

a. Thaw competent ES1301 *muts* cells on ice. To 100 µL of cells add 15 µL of the mutagenesis reaction from Section 3.3. and 100 ng of R408 rfDNA, mix briefly.

b. Incubate cells on ice for 30 min.

c. Heat shock the cells at 42°C for 90 s to increase transformation efficiency.

d. Add 4 mL of LB medium without antibiotic and incubate at 37°C for 3 h with shaking to allow the cells to recover and produce infectious phagemid.

e. After the 3-hr incubation period:

   i. Transfer 3 mL of the described culture to two tubes and pellet cells by centrifugation at top speed in a microcentrifuge for 5 min. Remove the supernatants, combine, and add to 100 µL of an overnight culture of JM109 cells.

   ii. To the remaining 1 mL of unpelleted transformed ES1301 *muts* cells, add 4 mL of LB medium containing the appropriate selective antibiotic and incubate at 37°C overnight with shaking. This culture will serve as a backup, to be used if the cotransformation procedure yields too few transformants (*see* Section 3.5.).

f. Incubate the 3 mL JM109 culture from step 5a for 30 min at 37°C with shaking and plate 100 µL on each of four to five plates containing the appropriate selective media. A typical cotransformation should yield approx 50 colonies per plate. To obtain more colonies, plate the entire 3-mL culture. Pellet the cells by centrifuging 1 min in a microcentrifuge. Resuspend the cells in 500 µL of LB and plate 100 µL on each of five plates.

Acknowledgments

I thank Scott Lesley for his assistance in developing the Altered Sites II vectors and protocols and Ken Lewis and Dave Thompson for their work on the original Altered Sites protocols. I also thank Jerry Hildebrand for his assistance in preparing the figures.

References

1. Smith, M. (1985) *In vitro* mutagenesis. *Ann. Rev. Genet.* **19**, 423–462.
2. Hutchinson, C. A., Phillips, S., Edgell, M. H., Gillam, S., Jahnke, P., and Smith, M. (1978) Mutagenesis at a specific position in a DNA sequence. *J. Biol. Chem.* **253**, 6551–6559.
3. Wu, R. and Grossman, L. (1987) Site-specific mutagenesis and protein engineering, Section IV, Chapters 17–20. *Methods Enzymol.* **154**, 329–403.
4. Kunkel, T. A. (1985) Rapid and efficient site-specific mutagenesis without phenotype selection. *Proc. Natl. Acad. Sci. USA* **82**, 488–492.
5. Lewis, K. and Thompson, D. V. (1990) Efficient site directed in vitro mutagenesis using ampicillin selection. *Nucleic Acids Res.* **18**, 3439–3443.
6. Kramer, B., Kramer, W., and Fritz, H. J. (1990) Different base/base mismatched are corrected with different efficiencies by the methyl-directed DNA mismatch-repair system of E. Coli. *Cell* **38**, 879–887.
7. Siegel, E. C., Wain, S. L., Meltzer, S. F., Binion, M. L., and Steinberg, J. L. (1982) Mutator mutations in *Escherichia coli* induced by the insertion of phage mu and the transposable resistance elements Tn5 and Tn10. *Mutat. Res.* **93**, 25–33.
8. Zell, R. and Fritz, H. J. (1987) DNA mismatch-repair in *Escherichia coli* counteracting the hydrolytic deamination of 5-methyl-cytosine residues. *EMBO J.* **6**, 1809–1815.
9. Dotto, G. P., Enea, V., and Zinder, N. D. (1981) Functional analysis of bacteriophage fl intergenic region. *Virology* **114**, 463–473.
10. Dotto, G. P. and Zinder, N. D. (1983) The morphogenetic signal of bacteriophage fl. *Virology* **130**, 252–256.
11. Dotto, G. P., Horiuchi, K., and Zinder, N. D. (1984) The functional origin of bacteriophage fl DNA replication. Its signals and domains. *J. Mol. Biol.* **172**, 507–521.
12. *Altered Sites II in vitro Mutagenesis Systems Manual, #TM001* (1994) Promega Corp., Madison, WI.
13. Piechocki, M. P. and Hines, R. N. (1994) Oligonucleotide design and optimized protocol for site-directed mutagenesis. *BioTechniques* **16**, 702–707.
14. Sambrook, J., Fritsch, E. F., and Maniatis, T. (1989) *Molecular Cloning, A Laboratory Manual.* Cold Spring Harbor Laboratory Press, Cold Spring Harbor, NY.
15. Hanahan, D. (1985) Techniques for transformation of *E. coli*, in *DNA Cloning*, vol 1 (Glover, G. M., ed.), IRL Press, Oxford, UK.

CHAPTER 2

In Vitro Site-Directed Mutagenesis Using the Unique Restriction Site Elimination (USE) Method

Li Zhu

1. Introduction

In vitro site-directed mutagenesis has been widely used in vector modification, and in gene and protein structure/function studies *(1,2)*. This procedure typically employs one or more oligonucleotides to introduce defined mutations into a DNA target of known sequence *(2–9)*. A variation of this procedure, termed the USE (Unique Restriction Site Elimination) mutagenesis method *(1)*, offers two important—and unique—advantages: specific base changes can be introduced into virtually any double-stranded plasmid; and plasmids carrying the desired mutation can be highly enriched by selecting against the parental (wild-type) plasmid. The USE strategy employs two oligonucleotide primers: one primer (the mutagenic primer) produces the desired mutation, whereas the second primer (the selection primer) mutates a restriction site unique to the plasmid for the purpose of selection.

Unlike most other methods of in vitro mutagenesis *(4,7)*, the USE method does not require single-stranded vectors or specialized double-stranded plasmids. Cloned genes may be mutated in whatever vector they reside, thus eliminating days or even weeks of subcloning steps. The only requirement for the USE method is that the vector contain a unique restriction enzyme recognition site and an antibiotic-resistance gene that can be used in transformation as a selectable marker—conditions easily met

From: *Methods in Molecular Biology, Vol. 57: In Vitro Mutagenesis Protocols*
Edited by: M. K. Trower Humana Press Inc., Totowa, NJ

by most plasmids. Generally, any unique restriction site present in the plasmid can be used as the selection site in the mutagenesis experiment.

To carry out site-directed mutagenesis with the USE method, the mutagenic and selection primers are simultaneously annealed to one strand of the denatured target (parental) plasmid (Fig. 1). The annealing conditions favor the formation of hybrids between the primers and the DNA template, although some parental plasmids will simply reanneal. After new DNA strands are synthesized and ligated to the primer-annealed plasmids, the mixture of parental and hybrid plasmids is digested with a restriction enzyme whose recognition site is altered by annealing of the selection primer. This preliminary digestion with the selection enzyme linearizes parental plasmids, rendering them at least 100 times less efficient than closed circular forms in transformation of bacterial cells *(10,11)*. However, hybrid plasmids containing a mismatch in the enzyme recognition site are resistant to digestion and will remain in circular form. Because of the very high probability that both the selection primer and the mutagenic primer will simultaneously anneal to the same template, a plasmid that has an altered unique restriction site will have a high probability (>90%) of containing the targeted mutation *(12)*. Thus, this preliminary digestion step enriches for hybrid (mutant) plasmids while selecting against parental duplex plasmids.

The hybrid (mutant) plasmids are transformed into an *Escherichia coli* strain *(mutS)* defective in mismatch repair (first transformation), which generates both mutant and parental duplex plasmids. Transformants are pooled, and plasmid DNA is prepared from the resulting mixed plasmid population. The isolated DNA is then subjected to a second selective restriction enzyme digestion to eliminate the parental-type plasmids. Mutant plasmids lacking the restriction enzyme recognition site are resistant to digestion. A final transformation using the thoroughly digested DNA will result in highly efficient recovery of the desired mutated plasmids.

The combined use of two oligonucleotide primers in the USE method results in mutation efficiencies of 70–90%. The actual mutation efficiency achievable in any given experiment depends on a number of factors, including:

1. The ability of the restriction enzyme chosen for the selection steps to efficiently digest parental (unmutated) plasmids (*see* Note 1);
2. The complete denaturation of the target plasmid before annealing the primers;

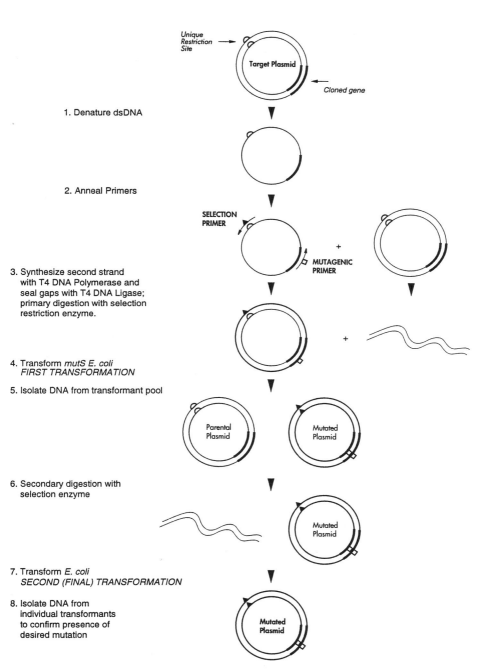

1. Denature dsDNA

2. Anneal Primers

3. Synthesize second strand
   with T4 DNA Polymerase and
   seal gaps with T4 DNA Ligase;
   primary digestion with selection
   restriction enzyme.

4. Transform *mutS E. coli*
   FIRST TRANSFORMATION

5. Isolate DNA from transformant pool

6. Secondary digestion with
   selection enzyme

7. Transform *E. coli*
   SECOND (FINAL) TRANSFORMATION

8. Isolate DNA from
   individual transformants
   to confirm presence of
   desired mutation

Fig. 1. Site-directed mutagenesis using the USE method. Note that the mutagenic primer contains the desired mutation and the selection primer contains a mutation to either eliminate a unique restriction site or to change it to a different unique site.

3. Simultaneous and saturated annealing of selection and mutagenic primers to the denatured target plasmid (*see* Note 2); and

4. The stable incorporation of the base changes brought about by the annealing of the primers (*see* Note 3).

Mutations that can be introduced using the USE system are: single or multiple specific base changes *(1,12–14)*; deletion of one or a few nucleotides *(1,12)*; precise, large deletions *(13)* (*see* Note 4); and addition (insertion) of a short stretch of DNA *(15)*.

Another useful feature of this method is that multiple successive rounds of mutagenesis may be performed on the gene of interest without recloning if the selection step is designed so that it changes the original unique restriction site into another unique restriction site—with no net loss of unique sites.

A list of ready-made selection primers available from Clontech (Palo Alto, CA) is shown in Table 1. Trans Oligos are designed to be suitable for use with many commonly used vectors and will maintain the reading frame as well as the amino acid sequence encoded by the target gene. Switch Oligos (also shown in Table 1) may be used to convert the mutated site back to the original restriction site when multiple rounds of mutagenesis are required. All Trans Oligos and Switch Oligos are phosphorylated at the 5' end during their synthesis, and therefore are ready for immediate use in the mutagenesis procedure.

2. Materials

All materials are stored at –20°C unless stated otherwise.

2.1. Reagents for USE Mutagenesis

1. 10X Annealing buffer: 200 mM Tris-HCl, pH 7.5, 100 mM MgCl$_2$, 500 mM NaCl (store at 4°C).
2. 10X Synthesis buffer: 100 mM Tris-HCl, pH 7.5, 5 mM each of dATP, dCTP, dGTP, and dTTP, 10 mM ATP, 20 mM DTT.
3. *E. coli* strains (store at –70°C in 50% glycerol):
   a. BMH 71-18 *mutS*, a mismatch repair-deficient strain: *thi, supE, Δ(lac-proAB)*, (*mutS*::Tn10)(F' *proAB, lacI*^{q} ZΔM15) *(16)* (*see* Note 5).
   b. Wild-type *mutS$^+$* strains, such as DH5α.
4. T4 DNA polymerase (2–4 U/μL).
5. T4 DNA ligase (4–6 U/μL).

Example of materials that can be used for a control mutagenesis (*see* Note 6 for discussion of the control materials provided in the Transformer Site-Directed Mutagenesis System from Clontech):

Name of primer	Catalog no.	Primer sequence	Applicable vectors
Trans Oligo *AatII/EcoRV*	(#6487-1)	GTGCCACCTG**GATATC**TAAGAAACC	1, 2, 4–7, 10, 11
Switch Oligo *EcoRV/AatII*	(#6378-1)	GTGCCACCTGA**CGT**CTAAGAAACC	1
Trans Oligo *AflIII/BglII*	(#6494-1)	CAGGAAAGAA**GATC**TGAGCAAAAG	1–3, 8, 11
Switch Oligo *BglIII/AflIII*	(#6372-1)	CAGGAAAGAA**ACATG**TGAGCAAAAG	1
Trans Oligo *AlwNI/SpeI*	(#6488-1)	GCAGCC**ACTAGT**AACAGGATT	1–3, 5, 6, 8–11
Switch Oligo *SpeI/AlwNI*	(#6373-1)	GCAGCCACT**GG**TAACAGGATT	1
Trans Oligo *EcoO109I/StuI*	(#6490-1)	GTATCACGAGGA**CCTTT**CGTCTC	1, 6, 11
Switch Oligo *StuI/EcoO109I*	(#6379-1)	GTATCACGAGG**CCC**TTTCGTCTC	1
Trans Oligo *EcoRI/EcoRV*	(#6496-1)	CGGCCAGTGA**TATC**GAGCTCGG	1, 6
Switch Oligo *EcoRV/EcoRI*	(#6374-1)	CGGCCAGTGAATTCGAGCTCGG	1
Trans Oligo *HindIII/MluI*	(#6497-1)	CAGGCATGCA**CGCG**TGGCGTAATC	1, 6
Switch Oligo *MluI/HindIII*	(#6376-1)	CAGGCATGCAAGC**TT**GGCGTAATC	1
Trans Oligo *NdeI/NcoI*	(#6493-1)	GAGTGCACCATG**GGC**GGTGTGAAAT	1, 4, 6
Switch Oligo *NcoI/NdeI*	(#6377-1)	GAGTGCACCAT**AT**GCGGTGTGAAAT	1
Trans Oligo *ScaI/StuI*	(#6495-1)	GTGACTGGTGA**GGCC**TCAACCAAGTC	1–11
Switch Oligo *StuI/ScaI*	(#6380-1)	GTGACTGGTGA**GTACT**CAACCAAGTC	1
Trans Oligo *SspI/EcoRV*	(#6498-1)	CTTCCTTTTC**GATATC**ATTGAAGCATTT	1, 2, 4–6
Switch Oligo *EcoRV/SspI*	(#6381-1)	CTTCCTTTTC**AATATT**ATTGAAGCATTT	1
Trans Oligo *XmnI/EcoRV*	(#6499-1)	GCTCATCATTG**GATATC**GTTCTTCGGG	1, 3, 4, 6, 8, 9
Switch Oligo *EcoRV/XmnI*	(#6375-1)	GCTCATCATTGGAAAACGTTCTTCGGG	1

[a]The Trans Oligo or Switch Oligo name denotes that a unique parental restriction site is replaced by a new unique restriction site. The underlined portions of the sequences represent the second restriction enzyme sites (after site conversion). Basepairs shown in bold are changed or deleted during mutagenesis, and ^ represents a basepair that has been deleted to create the new site. The vectors listed are examples of vectors that contain the indicated Trans Oligo sequences only once and thus are suitable for the USE method. Each Switch Oligo will anneal after mutagenesis to the same region that its corresponding Trans Oligo anneals. Some of the Trans Oligos may be used with additional vectors; for example, Trans Oligo *NdeI/NotI* is unique in 116 vectors found in GenBank. Note that all Trans Oligo and Switch Oligo sequences are unique in pUC19. However, Switch Oligo sequences may not be unique in other vectors after they have been mutated with the corresponding Trans Oligo. Before using a Trans Oligo or Switch Oligo with another vector not on the list, be sure to verify that the chosen restriction site is present in the target plasmid only once. Also verify that the base pair sequences flanking both sides of the restriction site (i.e., the primer arms) match with the plasmid sequence. Vector 1: pUC19; 2: pBR322; 3: pBluescript SKII+; 4: pGem3Z; 5: pET11c; 6: pNEB193; 7: pGemex-1; 8: pSPORT1; 9: pIBI25; 10: pGAD424; 11:pGBT9. All Trans Oligos and Switch Oligos are 5'-phosphorylated.

6. Control plasmid: pUC19M, 0.1 μg/μL (*see* Note 7).
7. Control mutagenic primer: 5'-Pi GAGGGTTTTCCCAGTCACGACG 3', 0.05 μg/μL (*see* Note 8).
8. Control selection primer: 5' Pi GAGTGCACCATGGGCGGTGTGAAAT 3', 0.05 μg/μL (*see* Note 9).
9. *Nde*I restriction enzyme (20 U/μL, for the control experiment).

Additional materials required for the experimental mutagenesis (*see* Notes 10–16 for tips on primer design).

10. 0.1 μg/μL Target plasmid (*see* Notes 17 and 18).
11. 0.05 μg/μL Mutagenic primer.
12. 0.05 μg/μL Selection primer.
13. 5–20 U/μL Selection restriction enzyme (*see* Note 19).

2.2. Primer Phosphorylation, Preparation of Competent E. coli Cells, and Transformations

1. T4 polynucleotide kinase (10 U/μL).
2. 10X T4 Kinase buffer: 500 mM Tris-HCl, pH 7.5, 100 mM MgCl$_2$, 50 mM DTT, 10 mM ATP.
3. Ampicillin: 100 mg/mL (1000X) stock solution in water. Filter sterilize and store at 4°C for no more than 1 mo.
4. Competent cells: Either electrocompetent cells or chemically competent cells (prepared ahead of time) may be used in the transformations. Electrocompetent BMH 71-18 *mutS* cells (#C2020-1) or DH5α cells (#2022-1), and chemically competent BMH 71-18 *mutS* cells (#C2010-1) may be purchased from Clontech.
5. IPTG (isopropyl β-D-thiogalactopyranoside): 20-mM stock solution in sterile, distilled water. Store at 4°C. Use 10 μL/10-cm plate.
6. LB agar plates containing 50–100 μg/mL ampicillin (LB + amp agar): LB + amp agar plates are used when performing the control mutagenesis with pUC19M and the control primers. LB agar plates containing a different antibiotic may be required for other target plasmids.
7. LB medium: 10 g/L bacto-tryptone, 5 g/L bacto-yeast extract, 10 g/L NaCl. Adjust pH to 7.0 with 5N NaOH. Autoclave to sterilize. For detailed information on the preparation of media for bacteriological work, please refer to the laboratory manual by Sambrook et al. *(2)*.
8. TE buffer: 10 mM Tris-HCl, pH 7.5, 1 mM EDTA.
9. Tetracycline: 5 mg/mL (100X) stock solution in ethanol. Wrap tube with aluminum foil and store at –20°C.
10. X-Gal (5-bromo, 4-chloro, 3-indolyl β-D-galactoside): 20 mg/mL stock solution in dimethylformamide (DMF). Store at –20°C. Use 40 μL/10-cm plate.

3. Methods

3.1. Primer Phosphorylation

Both the mutagenic and selection primers must be phosphorylated at their 5' end before being used in a USE mutagenesis experiment. Highly efficient 5' phosphorylation is commonly achieved by an enzymatic reaction using T4 polynucleotide kinase. (*See* Note 20 for an alternative phosphorylation procedure.) The control primers provided in the Transformer Kit have been phosphorylated and purified.

1. To a 0.5-mL microcentrifuge tube, add 2.0 μL of 10X kinase buffer, 1.0 μL of T4 polynucleotide kinase (10 U/μL), and 1 μg of primer (20–30 nucleotides long). Adjust the volume to 20 μL with water. Mix and centrifuge briefly.
2. Incubate at 37°C for 60 min.
3. Stop the reaction by heating at 65°C for 10 min.
4. Use 2.0 μL of the phosphorylated primer solution in each mutagenesis reaction.
5. Unused phosphorylated primers can be stored at –20°C for several weeks.

3.2. Denaturation and Annealing of Plasmid DNA

The following conditions are recommended for the annealing of phosphorylated primers to most plasmids *(1,12,13)*. Slow cooling is not necessary and, in many cases, may be detrimental. The alternative annealing protocol given in Note 21 is recommended for plasmids larger than 10 kb.

1. Prewarm a water bath to boiling (100°C) (*see* Note 22).
2. Set up the primer/plasmid annealing reaction in a 0.5-mL microcentrifuge tube as follows: 2.0 μL of 10X annealing buffer, 2.0 μL of plasmid DNA (0.05 μg/μL), 2.0 μL of selection primer (0.05 μg/μL), and 2.0 μL of mutagenic primer (0.05 μg/μL) (*see* Note 23).
3. Adjust with water to a total volume of 20 μL. Mix well. Briefly centrifuge the tube.
4. Incubate at 100°C for 3 min.
5. Chill immediately in an ice water bath (0°C) for 5 min. Briefly centrifuge to collect the sample.

3.3. Synthesis of the Mutant DNA Strand

1. Add to the annealed primer/plasmid mixture: 3.0 μL of 10X synthesis buffer, 1.0 μL of T4 DNA polymerase (2–4 U/μL), 1.0 μL of T4 DNA ligase (4–6 U/μL), and 5.0 μL of water.
2. Mix well and centrifuge briefly. Incubate at 37°C for 2 h.

3. Stop the reaction by heating at 70°C for 10 min to inactivate the enzymes.
4. Let the tube cool to room temperature for a few minutes.

3.4. Primary Selection
by Restriction Enzyme Digestion

After the mutant DNA strand synthesis and ligation, a majority (>95%) of the plasmids present in the total plasmid pool will be parental-type plasmids. The purpose of the first restriction enzyme digestion is to selectively linearize the parental DNA and thereby greatly enrich for mutant plasmids within the total DNA pool before the first transformation. This primary selection step facilitates the second (final) restriction digestion by reducing the percentage of plasmids that are susceptible to digestion.

1. For the control mutagenesis, simply add 1 µL of *Nde*I to the synthesis/ligation mixture and incubate at 37°C for 1–2 h.
2. For the experimental mutagenesis, use the buffer conditions that resulted in the most efficient digestion of the target plasmid, as determined by the relative reduction in the number of transformants in the preliminary test (*see* Note 19). If digestion was satisfactory (i.e., >99.9% of target plasmids were cut) using the annealing buffer, then simply add 20 U of the chosen restriction enzyme to the synthesis/ligation mixture and incubate at 37°C for 1–2 h. If the digestion was significantly better using the enzyme manufacturer's recommended buffer, then change or adjust the buffer accordingly (*see* Note 24).
3. After the primary restriction digestion, heat the tube containing the DNA at 70°C for 5 min to inactivate possible endo- or exonuclease contaminants that could damage the mutated DNA.

3.5. First Transformation

The purpose of the first transformation is to amplify the mutated strand (as well as the parental strand) in the BMH 71-18 repair-deficient *(mutS)* strain of *E. coli*. Either electroporation or chemical transformation may be used in this as well as all subsequent transformations. A detailed protocol for preparation of both types of competent cells can be found in refs. *17* and *18*. For best mutagenesis results, your transformation procedure should yield at least 1×10^7 transformants per microgram of DNA using chemical transformation, or at least 1×10^8 transformants per microgram of DNA using electrotransformation. The amount of plasmid/primer DNA solution and competent cell suspension used per tube depends on whether you are using chemical transformation or electrotransformation.

3.5.1. Chemical Transformation
1. Preheat a heating block or water bath to 42°C.
2. Add 5–10 µL of the primary restriction-digested plasmid/primer DNA solution to a 15-mL Falcon tube containing 100 µL of competent BMH 71-18 *muts* cells and incubate on ice for 20 min.
3. Transfer to 42°C for 1 min. Proceed to step 2.

3.5.2 Electroporation
1. Dilute the primary restriction-digested plasmid/primer DNA solution five-fold with water.
2. Add 2 µL of the diluted DNA to a separate tube containing 40 µL of electrocompetent BMH 71-18 *muts* cells on ice.
3. Perform the electroporation according to the manufacturer's instructions. (For example, if you are using the Bio-Rad [Hercules, CA] *E. coli* Pulser Electroporator, use a 0.1-cm cuvet and set the instrument at 1.8 kV, with constant capacitance at 10 µF and internal resistance at 600 W.)

3.5.3 Recovery
This applies to both chemical transformation and electroporation:
1. Immediately add 1 mL of LB medium (with no antibiotic) to each tube.
2. Incubate at 37°C for 60 min with shaking at 220 rpm.

3.5.4. Amplification
1. Add 4 mL of LB medium containing the appropriate selection antibiotic. (In the case of the control experiment with pUC19M, use LB medium containing 50 µg/mL ampicillin.)
2. Incubate the culture at 37°C overnight with shaking at 220 rpm.

3.6. Isolation of the Plasmid Pool and Second Restriction Enzyme Digestion

After overnight growth of transformed BMH 71-18 *muts* cells, both parental and mutated plasmid strands are segregated and amplified. Now the plasmid pool can be purified from the cells and subjected to a second restriction digestion to further enrich for the desired mutants by selecting against the parental (nonmutated) plasmids. A quick boiling-lysis method for plasmid preparation *(19)* is recommended, since it consistently results in clean "miniprep" DNA. However, other standard miniprep procedures such as the alkaline lysis method *(2)* may be used.

1. Dissolve the DNA pellets in 100 µL of TE buffer (each). The normal yield of plasmid DNA using the quick boiling-lysis method is approx 2–5 µg.

2. (Optional) Purify DNA on a spin column (e.g., Chroma SPIN + TE-400 Column, Clonetech, cat. no. K1323-1).
3. Set up the following restriction enzyme digestion: 5.0 µL of purified mixed plasmid DNA (approx 100 ng), 2.0 µL of 10X restriction enzyme buffer, and 1 µL of restriction enzyme (10–20 U). For the control experiment, use *Nde*I and 10X annealing buffer (which is functionally equivalent to 10X *Nde*I buffer). Adjust the final volume to 20 µL with sterile water.
4. Mix well. Incubate at 37°C for 1 h.
5. Add an additional 10 U of the appropriate restriction enzyme, and continue incubation at 37°C for another 1 h.

3.7. Final Transformation

The purpose of the final transformation is to amplify and stably clone the mutated plasmid in a mismatch repair-competent (MutS⁺) RecA⁻ strain of *E. coli* to avoid accumulation of random mutations in the plasmids. For this reason, the mismatch repair-deficient *E. coli* strain used for the first transformation (BMH 71-18 *mutS*) should not be used in the second transformation. For blue/white colony color conversion of transformants on X-gal/IPTG plates, an *E. coli* strain that is capable of *lacZα* complementation should be used; examples are DH5α, MV1190, or JM109. (Other *E. coli* strains can also be used if no color conversion is required.)

1. Use 5.0 µL of the digested plasmid (approx 25 ng) for transformation of chemically competent cells, or 1.0 µL of fivefold diluted (with water) plasmid (approx 1 ng) for transformation of electrocompetent cells. Follow the same procedure as for the first transformation.
2. Recovery:
   a. Immediately add 1.0 mL of LB medium (with no antibiotic) to each tube.
   b. Incubate at 37°C for 60 min with shaking at 220 rpm.
3. Prepare 10-, 100-, and 1000-fold dilutions of the cell/DNA mixture (100 µL each).
4. For transformation experiments in which you expect to see a blue/white colony color conversion, add 40 µL of a 20 mg/mL X-gal solution and 10 µL of a 20-m*M* IPTG solution to each tube containing cells (including controls).
5. Mix well and spread each suspension evenly onto LB agar plates containing the appropriate antibiotic for selection of transformants (50 µg/mL ampicillin for the control experiment).
6. Incubate the plates at 37°C overnight.

For pUC19M control transformations, the mutation efficiency is estimated by the number of blue (mutated) colonies divided by the total number of blue and white (unmutated) colonies on X-gal/IPTG plates. An efficiency rate of 70–90% is expected if the mutagenesis is performed successfully. For mutagenesis experiments that do not involve a visible phenotype, such as colony color, nutrition requirement, resistance to another antibiotic, or hybridization to a particular DNA probe, it may be necessary to isolate plasmid DNA to characterize the mutation. Depending on the type of mutation generated (such as a large deletion), the putative mutant plasmids may be screened by digestion with appropriate restriction enzymes. In any case, the mutations should be verified by directly sequencing the mutagenized region(s).

4. Notes

1. The success of this mutagenesis procedure is directly correlated with the success of the restriction enzyme digestions used for mutant enrichment. Thus, it is important to obtain complete digestion of the parental plasmid before each transformation. The chances of obtaining complete digestion will be maximized if the plasmid DNA is purified before the digestion steps as explained in Note 18 and the Methods section, and if you make sure that the target plasmid at low concentrations can be efficiently digested with the selection enzyme before beginning the mutagenesis experiment (Note 19). The extent of digestion of the plasmid DNA after the first and second digestion steps can be checked by electrophoresing two 5.0-µL samples on a 0.8% agarose minigel. Digested (linearized) plasmid DNA will run as a discrete band; undigested (circular) DNA will run as two bands, corresponding to the relaxed circular form and the supercoiled form, with relative mobilities less than and greater than the linearized form, respectively. Since the parental plasmid makes up a greater part (>95%) of the total plasmid pool at the first selection step, the bands corresponding to the uncut (mutant) plasmids may not be visible or, if visible, will be quite faint compared to the cut (parental) plasmid band. However, after the second selection digestion, the resistant bands will become significantly more intense.

2. If only one of the two mutations is incorporated into the newly synthesized strands, then the background of unmutated molecules following the second *E. coli* transformation will be high. Tips to ensure high coupling of the two types of mutations are given in Notes 13 and 23.

3. T4 DNA polymerase is used to extend the primers and to synthesize the mutant strand. Unlike the Klenow fragment of DNA polymerase I (an enzyme commonly used in in vitro mutagenesis), T4 DNA polymerase does not have strand displacement activity *(20,21)*. Thus, with T4 DNA polymerase, the primers (along with the desired base changes) will be incorporated into the newly synthesized strand. This property of T4 DNA

polymerase makes it possible to perform multiple site-directed mutageneses simultaneously using more than one mutagenic primer in the reaction mixture *(22)*. T4 DNA ligase is used to ligate the newly synthesized DNA strand to the 5' (phosphorylated) end of the oligonucleotide primer, a step that is necessary to obtain covalently closed circular DNA with high transforming ability. A specialized *E. coli* strain, BMH 71-18 *mutS*, defective in mismatch repair *(16)*, is used in the first transformation to prevent undesirable repair of the mutant DNA strand. The first transformation step also serves to amplify the entire mutagenesis process.

4. The USE method has been applied to generate precise deletions as large as several hundred basepairs. However, the efficiency is generally much lower than that of site-directed mutations *(13)*. The deletion mutagenesis efficiency will be improved if a unique restriction site within the targeted deletion region can be used for the mutant enrichment (our unpublished observations). This technique, which allows for a more direct selection for mutant plasmids, is the basis of the Quantum Leap Nested Deletion method described in Chapter 11.

5. *E. coli* strain BMH 71-18 *mutS* carries a Tn10 insertion in *mutS*; this Tn10 insertion causes a repair-deficiency phenotype as well as tetracyline resistance. For the repair-deficiency phenotype and Tn10 insertion to be maintained, this strain must be grown on medium containing 50 µg/mL tetracycline.

6. It is recommended to run a control mutagenesis in advance of—or concurrently with—the experimental mutagenesis. The control experiment should be designed to result in a specific, well-characterized mutation that can be detected easily, for example, by a change in colony phenotype. The control plasmid (pUC19M) and primers included in the Transformer Site-Directed Mutagenesis Kit (Clontech #K1600-1), result in a blue/white colony color conversion.

7. pUC19M has a stop codon in its *lacZ* gene and thereby makes white colonies on X-gal/IPTG plates when transformed into an appropriate host strain. pUC19M was derived from the wild-type pUC19 by a USE site-directed mutagenesis. pUC19M contains a mutation at nucleotide position 366, which interrupts the coding sequence of the *lacZ* gene on pUC19 by converting the UGG tryptophan codon to the amber stop codon UAG. (The amber mutation in the pUC19M *lacZ* gene is not sufficiently suppressed by the suppressor tRNA gene [*supE*] present in BMH 71-18 *mutS* strain.) Since this plasmid does not make functional β-galactosidase, it will form white colonies on LB agar plates containing X-gal and IPTG, when transformed into a *lacZ⁻* bacterial host (such as BMH 71-18 *mutS* or DH5α). The control plasmid, pUC19M, carries the gene for ampicillin resistance, which is used as the bacterial selectable marker. *E. coli* cells trans-

formed by pUC19M are selected by plating on medium containing 50 μg/mL ampicillin.

8. The control mutagenic primer reverts the stop codon in the *lacZ* gene of pUC19M back into a functional tryptophan codon. The reverted plasmid will produce blue colonies on X-gal/IPTG plates, thus allowing visual color discrimination of the base change when transformed into an appropriate *E. coli* host strain. Since there is no selective pressure on the mutagenic primer, it gives an objective indication of the mutagenesis process. The efficiency of mutagenesis can be determined by the number of blue (mutant) vs white (parental) colonies on X-gal/IPTG plates. If the mutagenesis has been successful, 70–90% of the ampicillin-resistant transformants will form blue colonies. For mutation experiments in which colony color conversion is not applicable, restriction analysis or sequencing is necessary to verify and characterize the mutations.

9. The control selection primer alters a unique *Nde*I recognition site on pUC19M, thus allowing for selection against parental (unmutated) plasmids by digestion with *Nde*I. Available premade selection primers are listed in Table 1.

10. The mutagenic and selection primers must anneal to the same strand of the plasmid. The distance between the selection primer and the mutagenic primer is not critical. These primers have been placed within 50 bp of each other or as far apart as 5 kb *(1,12)*. If possible, design the selection and mutagenic primers so that they will be relatively evenly spaced after annealing to the template; this will allow the DNA polymerase to extend both primers an equivalent distance. In rare cases, where the unique restriction site and the targeted mutagenic site are very close to each other, one single primer can be designed to introduce both mutations simultaneously.

11. The function of the selection primer is to eliminate the original unique restriction enzyme site. The selection primer can be designed by incorporating one or more basepair changes within the targeted unique restriction site. Since restriction enzymes recognize an exact DNA sequence, any base changes within the recognition sequence will abolish the restriction digestion.

12. If possible, use a restriction site located in an intergenic region as the selection site. If the selection restriction site must be located within a gene, avoid using a selection primer that will introduce changes that could interfere with the expression of that gene (e.g., by causing a reading-frame shift or a premature termination codon).

13. Length of primers: In most cases, 10 nucleotides of uninterrupted matched sequences on both ends of the primer (flanking the mismatch site) should give sufficient annealing stability, provided that the GC content of the primer is greater than 50%. If the GC content is less than 50%, the lengths

of the primer arms should be extended accordingly *(2)*. The mismatch bases should be placed in the center of the primer sequence. For optimum primer annealing, the oligonucleotides should start and end with a G or C. To ensure high coupling of the mutations introduced by the selection and mutagenic primers, the annealing strength of the mutagenic primer (to the target plasmid) should be greater than or equal to the annealing strength of the selection primer.

14. Number of base mismatches in the primer: There can be more than one base mismatch in the selection and mutagenic primers. However, the efficiency of targeted mutations is higher when there are fewer mismatches in the primers. Nevertheless, we have found that mutagenesis works well with primers having three consecutive bases deleted (such that one codon is excised and the reading frame is preserved), or three base mismatches *(12)*.

15. Annealing of more than one mutagenic primer to the target plasmid: Multiple mutagenic primers can be annealed to the same plasmid along with a single selection primer to simultaneously achieve mutagenesis at several sites *(22)*. Again, the main criterion in designing multiple mutagenic primers is that they do not overlap when annealed to the template. We have achieved a 39% success rate for introducing four targeted mutations simultaneously into the same plasmid using four mutagenic primers, in addition to the selection primer *(13)*.

16. Primers for generation of precise large deletions: If a large deletion is desired, the mutagenic primer should have at least 15 bp of matching sequences flanking both sides of the segment to be deleted. Using the Transformer Mutagenesis Kit, we have introduced precise deletions of 511 and 979 bp in pBR322 *(13)*. The upper limit on the size of deletions has not been determined, but it is presumed to be quite large, provided that no genes required for replication or selection of the plasmid are incapacitated.

17. Plasmids with tetracycline as the only selection marker are not suitable for mutagenesis, since the bacterial strain BMH 71-18 *mutS* has a Tn10 transposon that confers tetracycline resistance.

18. Because proteins and other impurities in the plasmid pool can significantly affect the degree of digestion obtained, it is important to use purified target plasmid DNA in the mutagenesis procedure. To achieve the maximum efficiency of cutting in the first digestion, the target plasmid should be purified by CsCl banding or a method that yields plasmid of comparable purity.

19. Restriction enzyme digestion is the sole selection mechanism operating in the USE procedure. Therefore, before using a particular restriction enzyme in a mutagenesis experiment, check to make sure that the target plasmid at low concentrations can be efficiently digested with the selection enzyme. I have found that the enzyme unit definition of 1 µg/h under defined buffer

and temperature conditions does not necessarily correspond to the enzyme's ability to cut very low concentrations of DNA.

a. Set up two digestions, each using 0.1 μg of the target plasmid with 5–20 U of the chosen restriction enzyme in a 30-μL (final vol) reaction. In one of the digestions, use the annealing buffer described in Section 2.1.; in the other digestion, use the buffer recommended by the enzyme manufacturer. The mutagenesis procedure is simpler if you can perform the first digestion in the annealing buffer used in the step preceding the digestion; the annealing buffer is functionally similar to *Nde*I buffer. If the glycerol concentration is greater than 5% (v/v) after adding the restriction enzyme, the reaction volume should be increased proportionally to avoid undesirable star activity. The same amount of DNA should be maintained.

b. Incubate for 1 h at 37°C.

c. Transform an appropriate *E. coli* strain separately with the two plasmid digests and with an equivalent amount of undigested plasmid. Plate out cells on appropriate selection medium and incubate overnight.

d. Compare the number of colonies obtained in each transformation. Ideally, you should see a 1000-fold reduction in transformation efficiency using the plasmid samples that have been restriction digested, compared to using undigested plasmid. If digestion of the target plasmid does not reduce the number of transformants to ≤1% of the control transformation, the final mutation efficiency may be less than expected. If this is the case, consider choosing a different restriction enzyme.

20. Alternatively, a 5' phosphate group can be added (with 100% efficiency) to an oligonucleotide during automated DNA synthesis using an appropriate CE-phosphoramidite reagent, such as 5'-phosphate-ON (Clontech cat. no. 5210-1). These phosphorylated synthetic oligonucleotides are stable for more than 6 mo at –20°C.

21. An alternative denaturing and annealing protocol that completely denatures the double-stranded DNA template is especially recommended when mutating large (i.e., >10 kb) plasmids. However, when a small amount (<1 μg) of plasmid DNA is used, care must be taken to avoid losing the DNA pellet during the ethanol wash (step 6). In general, it is safer to use larger quantities (1–2 μg) of DNA with this annealing procedure.

a. Mix at least 100 ng of plasmid (1–2 μL) in 16 μL of water with 4 μL of 2*M* NaOH in a microcentrifuge tube.

b. Incubate at room temperature for 10 min.

c. Neutralize with 4 μL of 3*M* NaOAc (pH 4.8).

d. Add 70 μL of ethanol and cool to –70°C.

e. Centrifuge for 10 min to pellet the precipitated DNA.

f. Carefully wash pellet with 70% ethanol. Collect pellet by centrifugation. Allow pellet to air dry.
g. Resuspend DNA in water to a concentration of >10 ng/µL. The resuspended DNA may be stored at 4°C for a few days.
h. For annealing, mix the desired (usually equal) amounts of the plasmid
   and primers (100 ng each for the control plasmid and primers). Adjust
   the volume to 18 µL with water and add 2 µL of annealing buffer.
i. Incubate at 37°C for 10 min and then place on to ice for another 10 min.
j. Proceed with synthesis and ligation.
22. Complete denaturation of the template DNA must occur. To achieve this,
    it is necessary to boil the DNA at 100°C. Lower temperatures do not suffice.
23. The recommended concentration of the plasmid is 0.05–0.1 µg/µL. To
    ensure high coupling of the mutations introduced by the selection and
    mutagenic primers, both primers should be present in a 200-fold molar
    excess to the single-stranded template DNA.
24. The concentration of NaCl in the synthesis/ligation mixture is 37.5 mM in
    a total vol of 30 µL. If the NaCl concentration must be increased for opti-
    mal digestion, the 10X annealing buffer (which contains 500 mM NaCl)
    can be used to make the adjustment. If the NaCl concentration must be
    reduced (or other undesirable components eliminated), the DNA mixture
    can be ethanol precipitated or passed through a spin column (e.g.,
    Clontech's Chroma Spin-30 Column, cat. no. K1301-1). The desalted DNA
    can then be resuspended in the new buffer.

Acknowledgments

I thank Wing P. Deng and Jac A. Nickoloff of Harvard University
School of Public Health for many helpful discussions over the past few
years. I also thank Hubert Chen, Ann Holtz, Megan Brown, and Paul Diehl
for technical assistance, and Kristen Mayo for editing the manuscript.

References

1. Deng, W. P. and Nickoloff, J. A. (1992) Site-directed mutagenesis of virtually any
   plasmid by eliminating a unique site. *Anal. Biochem.* **200,** 81–88.
2. Sambrook, J., Fritsch, E. F., and Maniatis, T. (1989) *Molecular Cloning: A Laboratory Manual,* 2nd ed, Cold Spring Harbor Laboratory Press, Cold Spring Harbor, NY.
3. Carter, P. (1987) Improved oligonucleotide-directed mutagenesis using M13 vectors. *Methods Enzymol.* **154,** 382–403.
4. Kunkel, T. A., Roberts, J. D., and Zakour, R. A. (1987) Rapid and efficient site-
   specific mutagenesis without phenotypic selection. *Methods Enzymol.* **154,** 367–382.
5. Kunkel, T. A. (1985) The use of phosphorothioate-modified DNA in restriction
   enzyme reactions to prepare nicked DNA. *Proc. Natl. Acad. Sci. USA* **82,** 488–492.

6. Lewis, M. K. and Thompson, D. V. (1990) Efficient site-directed in vitro mutagenesis using ampicillin selection. *Nucleic Acids Res.* **18,** 3439–3443.
7. Taylor, J. W., Ott, J., and Eckstein, F. (1985) The rapid generation of oligonucleotide-directed mutations at high frequency using phosphorothioate-modified DNA. *Nucleic Acids Res.* **13,** 8764–8785.
8. Taylor, J. W., Schmidt, W., Cosstick, R., Okruszek, A., and Eckstein, F. (1985) The rapid generation of oligonucleotide-directed mutations at high frequency using phosphorothioate-modified DNA. *Nucleic Acids Res.* **13,** 8779–8785.
9. Vandeyr, M., Weiner, M., Hutton, C., and Batt, C. (1988) A simple and rapid method for the selection of oligodeoxyribonucleotide-directed mutations. *Gene* **65,** 129–133.
10. Cohen, S. N., Chang, A. C. Y., and Hsu, L. (1972) Nonchromosomal antibiotic resistance in bacteria: genetic transformation of *Escherichia coli* by R-factor DNA. *Proc. Natl. Acad. Sci. USA.* **69,** 2110–2114.
11. Conley, E. C. and Saunders, J. R. (1984) Recombination-dependent recircularization of linearized pBR322 plasmid DNA following transformation of *Escherichia coli. Mol. Gen. Genet.* **194,** 211–218.
12. Zhu, L. (1992) Highly efficient site-directed mutagenesis of dsDNA plasmids. *CLONTECHniques* **VII(1),** 1–5.
13. Zhu, L. and Chen, H. (1992) In vitro generation of multiple-site mutations and precise large deletions. *CLONTECHniques* **VII(2),** 9–11.
14. Van Aelst, L., Barr, M., Marcus, S., Polverino, A., and Wigler, M. (1993) Complex formation between RAS and RAF and other protein kinases. *Proc. Natl. Acad. Sci. USA* **90,** 6213–6217.
15. Haught, C., Wilkinson, D. L., Zgafas, K., and Harrison, R. G. (1994) A method to insert a DNA fragment into a double-stranded plasmid. *BioTechniques* **16,** 46–48.
16. Zell, R. and Fritz, H. (1987) DNA mismatch repair in *Escherichia coli* counteracting the hydrolytic deamination of 5-methyl-cytosine residues. *EMBO J.* **6,** 1809–1815.
17. Chung, C. T., Niemela, S. L., and Miller, R. H. (1989) One-step preparation of competent *Escherichia coli*: transformation and storage of bacterial cells in the same solution. *Proc. Natl. Acad. Sci. USA* **86,** 2172–2175.
18. *Protocol for Transformer™ Site-Directed Mutagenesis Kit* (1994) Clontech #K1600-1, Palo Alto, CA.
19. Holmes, D. S. and Quigley, M. (1981) A rapid boiling method for the preparation of bacterial plasmids. *Anal. Biochem.* **114,** 193–197.
20. Masumune, Y. and Richardson, C. A. (1971) Strand displacement during deoxyribonucleic acid synthesis at single-strand breaks. *J. Biol. Chem.* **246,** 2692–2701.
21. Nossal, N. G. (1974) DNA synthesis on a double-stranded DNA template by the T4 bacteriophage DNA polymerase and the T4 gene 32 DNA unwinding protein. *J. Biol. Chem.* **249,** 5668–5676.
22. Perlak, F. J. (1990) Single-step, large-scale, site-directed in vitro mutagenesis using multiple oligonucleotides. *Nucleic Acids Res.* **18(24),** 7457–7458.

CHAPTER 3

Site-Directed Mutagenesis Using Double-Stranded Plasmid DNA Templates

Jeffrey Braman, Carol Papworth, and Alan Greener

1. Introduction

In vitro site-directed mutagenesis is an invaluable technique for studying protein structure–function relationships and gene expression and for modifying vectors. Several methods for performing this technique have appeared in the literature *(1–5)*. They generally require multiple enzymatic steps, specialized vectors, and convenient restriction sites or subcloning of the sequence of DNA to be mutated into a bacteriophage vector like M13 to produce and recover single-stranded DNA. These manipulations present major limitations to the routine use of these methods because they are time consuming and tedious.

A site-directed mutagenesis procedure was developed by Deng and Nickoloff *(6;* Fig. 1) that eliminated the need for subcloning and generating single-stranded DNA templates by employing double-stranded plasmid DNA. The procedure involves simultaneously annealing two oligonucleotide primers to the same strand of heat-denatured double-stranded plasmid DNA that contains a unique, nonessential restriction site. One primer (the mutagenic primer) introduces a chosen mutation into the plasmid and a second primer (selection primer) alters the sequence of the unique, nonessential restriction site in the plasmid. Extension of these primers by T4 DNA polymerase followed by ligation

From: *Methods in Molecular Biology, Vol. 57: In Vitro Mutagenesis Protocols*
Edited by: M. K. Trower Humana Press Inc., Totowa, NJ

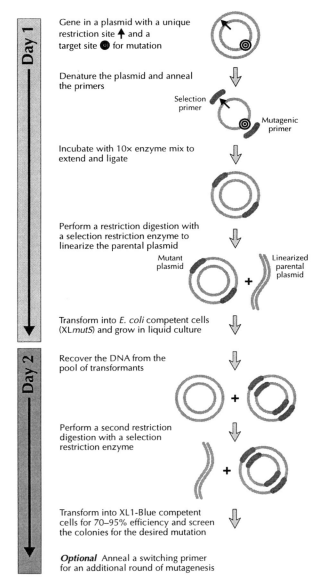

Day 1

Gene in a plasmid with a unique restriction site ⬆ and a target site ◉ for mutation

Denature the plasmid and anneal the primers

Selection primer

Mutagenic primer

Incubate with 10× enzyme mix to extend and ligate

Perform a restriction digestion with a selection restriction enzyme to linearize the parental plasmid

Mutant plasmid

Linearized parental plasmid

Transform into *E. coli* competent cells (XL*mutS*) and grow in liquid culture

Day 2

Recover the DNA from the pool of transformants

Perform a second restriction digestion with a selection restriction enzyme

Transform into XL1-Blue competent cells for 70–95% efficiency and screen the colonies for the desired mutation

Optional Anneal a switching primer for an additional round of mutagenesis

Fig. 1. Overview of the double-stranded, site mutagenesis protocol.

of the resulting molecules with T4 DNA ligase results in a population of plasmid molecules, some of which contain the desired mutation but no longer contain the unique restriction site. The plasmid is treated with a restriction enzyme that will digest the DNA that did not incorporate the selection oligonucleotide primer at the unique, nonessential restriction site. The unmutated parental plasmids are digested by the restriction enzyme while leaving the mutated plasmids undigested. The resulting restriction-enzyme-treated plasmid DNA is transformed into a mismatch repair-defective strain of *Escherichia coli* (BMH71-18*mutS*) that cannot distinguish the original unmutated strand of DNA from the newly created strand containing the desired mutation. The *mutS*-deficient strain randomly selects one of these strands as "correct" and changes the other strand to be complementary to the chosen strand. Since selection of the correct strand is random, half of the plasmids contain the desired mutation. Circular mutated plasmids are transformed by many orders of magnitude more efficiently than linear unmutated plasmid DNA. The transformed bacteria are cultivated overnight in liquid media, and plasmid DNA is recovered and treated once again with the restriction enzyme that digests plasmids containing the original unique, nonessential restriction site. Plasmid molecules that incorporate the selection primer, and presumably the chosen mutagenic primer, are not digested. Transformation of the resulting DNA into any desired *E. coli* strain results in colonies containing mutated plasmids. If a second round of mutagenesis is desired, a second mutagenic oligonucleotide primer can be incorporated with a "switching" primer that is used to convert the new unique, nonessential restriction site back to the original or another restriction site.

Several modifications to the Deng and Nickoloff protocol have been made to improve the reliability of the procedure and to increase the mutation efficiency *(7)*. These modifications and a detailed protocol are the subject of this article. The most significant change that has been made is the construction of a new mismatch repair-deficient *E. coli* host strain that is EndA⁻ and is referred to as XL*mutS*. The *endA* mutation eliminates an endonuclease that degrades miniprep plasmid DNA, prepared by either the boiling or alkaline lysis procedures. Removal of this endonuclease greatly improves the quantity and quality of plasmid DNA recovered from the mismatch repair-deficient *E. coli* host at this critical point in the mutagenesis procedure with a resultant improvement in the efficiency and reproducibility of mutated plasmid generation. Additional changes that have been made include the use of T7 DNA polymerase instead of T4 DNA polymerase *(8)* and optimization of the selection and mutagenic oligonucleotide primer-to-plasmid template ratio.

2. Materials

1. pWhitescript (pWS) control plasmid DNA was produced at Stratagene, (La Jolla, CA). The plasmid contains a stop codon (TAA) at the position where a glutamine codon (CAA) would normally appear in the α-complementing portion of the β-galactosidase gene of pBluescript II SK(–) corresponding to amino acid 9 of the protein. XL1-Blue *E. coli* cells transformed with this plasmid appear white on LB agar plates containing ampicillin and supplemented with IPTG and X-gal because active β-galactosidase has not been synthesized. Annealing of a "blue" mutagenic oligonucleotide primer to denatured pWS followed by polymerization and ligation results in a point mutation that converts the stop codon of pWS (TAA) back to the glutamine-encoding codon (CAA). Transformed XL1-Blue cells containing the mutated pWS plasmid appear blue on LB agar plates containing ampicillin supplemented with IPTG and X-gal because active β-galactosidase has been synthesized.
2. pUC18 control plasmid (0.1 ng/μL) was also obtained from Stratagene.
3. The "blue" mutagenic oligonucleotide primer was produced at Stratagene to test the efficiency of the procedure. The mutagenic oligonucleotide primer changes the stop codon (TAA) in the β-galactosidase gene of pBluescript II SK(–) to a glutamine-encoding codon (CAA) at amino acid 9 of the protein. This results in the conversion of white to blue bacterial colonies when pWS is converted to pBluescript and active β-galactosidase is synthesized; "blue" primer: GTG AGG GTT AAT TGC GCG CTT GGC GTA ATC ATG G.
4. High-transformation-efficiency *E. coli* strains were produced at Stratagene and their genotypes are as follows:
    a. XL*mutS* strain: *Δ(mcrA)183 Δ(mcrCB-hsdSMR-mrr)173 endA1 supE44 thi-1 gyrA96 relA1 lac mutS::Tn10* (Tet^r) (*F′ proAB lacI^{q}ZΔM15* Tn5 [Kan^r]).
    b. XL1-Blue strain: *recA1 endA1 gyrA96 thi-1 hsdR17 supE44 relA1 lac* (*F′ proAB lacI^{q}ZΔM15* Tn10 [Tet^r]).
5. 10X Mutagenesis buffer: 100 m*M* Tris-acetate, pH 7.5, 100 m*M* magnesium-acetate, 500 m*M* potassium acetate.
6. Enzyme dilution buffer: 20 m*M* Tris-HCl, pH 7.5, 10 m*M* KCl, 10 m*M* β-mercaptoethanol, 1 m*M* dithiothreitol (DTT), 0.1 m*M* EDTA, 50% (v/v) glycerol.
7. Deoxynucleotide (dNTP) mix: 2.86 m*M* dATP, 2.86 m*M* dCTP, 2.86 m*M* dGTP, 2.86 m*M* TTP, 4.34 m*M* rATP, 1.43X mutagenesis buffer.
8. 10X Enzyme mix: 0.25 U/μL of native T7 DNA polymerase, 1.0 U/μL of T4 DNA ligase, 0.6 μg/μL of single-stranded binding protein, in enzyme dilution buffer.

9. 1.4*M* β-mercaptoethanol.
10. SOB medium (per L): 20 g of tryptone, 5 g of yeast extract, 0.5 g of NaCl. Autoclave. Add 10 mL of 1*M* MgCl$_2$ and 10 mL of 1*M* MgSO$_4$/L of SOB prior to use. Filter sterilize.
11. SOC Medium (per 100 mL): Add 1 mL of 2*M* filter-sterilized glucose solution or 2 mL of 20% (w/v) glucose to 100 mL of SOB medium prior to use.
12. 2X YT Broth (per L): 10 g of NaCl, 10 g of yeast extract, 16 g of tryptone. Adjust to pH 7.5 with NaOH.
13. LB Agar (per L): 10 g of NaCl, 10 g of tryptone, 5 g of yeast extract, 20 g of agar. Adjust to pH 7.0 with 5*N* NaOH. Add deionized H$_2$O to a final volume of 1 L. Autoclave. Pour into Petri dishes (25 mL/100-mm plate). Store plates at 4°C.
14. LB-Ampicillin Agar (per L): One liter of LB agar. Autoclave. Cool to 55°C. Add 1 mL of 50 mg/mL filter-sterilized ampicillin. Pour into Petri dishes (25 mL/100-mm plate).
15. LB-Ampicillin-methicillin agar (use for reduced satellite colony formation [per L]): One liter of LB agar. Autoclave. Cool to 55°C. Add 0.4 mL of 50 mg/mL filter-sterilized ampicillin. Add 1.6 mL of 50 mg/mL filter-sterilized methicillin. Pour into Petri dishes (25 mL/100-mm plate).
16. Falcon 2059 polypropylene tubes (15 mL).
17. 5-bromo-4-chloro-3-indoyl-β-D-galactopyranoside (X-gal).
18. Isopropyl-β-D-thio-galactopyranoside (IPTG).

3. Methods
3.1. Mutagenic and Selection Oligonucleotide Primer Design

Mutagenic primers introduce specific experimental mutations, and mutagenic oligonucleotide primers for use in this protocol must be designed individually according to the desired mutation required. The following considerations should be made for designing mutagenic and selection oligonucleotide primers:

1. Both the mutagenic and the selection oligonucleotide primers must anneal and alter the same strand of the plasmid that is to be altered.
2. Mutagenic and selection oligonucleotide primers should be between 25 and 45 bases in length.
3. The mismatched portions of mutagenic oligonucleotide primers should be in the middle of the primer with approx 10–15 bases of correct sequence on either side.
4. Mutagenic and selection oligonucleotide primers should have a minimum GC content of 40% and should terminate in one or more C or G bases.

5. Mutagenic and selection oligonucleotide primers must be 5' phosphory-lated and should be purified by either FPLC or polyacrylamide gel electrophoresis prior to use.
6. Selection against sites having GATC, such as *Bgl*II, *Bam*HI, or *Pvu*I, has been found to be inefficient and primers using these sites are not recommended.
7. The distance between the selection site and the mutation target site oligonucleotide primers should be as far apart as possible for best results.

3.2. Selection and Switch Oligonucleotide Primer Sequences

Examples are given of selection and switch oligonucleotide primers and their sequences. The selection oligonucleotide primers change a unique, nonessential restriction site to the switch primer site and the switch oligonucleotide primer changes its restriction site back to the unique, nonessential restriction site.

1. *ALw*NI Selection oligonucleotide primer and *Nru*I switch primer: The *ALw*NI restriction site is located at basepair number 1569 in the *Col*EI origin of replication in the pBluescript II SK(−) phagemid. *ALw*NI to *Nru*I: CGC CAC TGG CAG CAG TCG CGA GTA ACA GGA TTA GCA GAG and *Nru*I to *ALw*NI: CGC CAC TGG CAG CAG CCA CTG GTA ACA GGA TTA GCA G.
2. *Kpn*I selection oligonucleotide primer and *Srf*I switch primer: The *Kpn*I restriction site is located at base pair number 657 in the polylinker of the pBluescript II SK(−) phagemid. *Kpn*I to *Srf*I: CTA TAG GGC GAA TTG GGT GCC CGG GCC CCC CTC GAG GTC G and *Srf*I to *Kpn*I: CTA TAG GGC GAA TTG GGT ACC GGG CCC CTC GAG GTC G
3. *Sca*I Selection oligonucleotide primer and *Mlu*I switch primer: The *Sca*I restriction site is located at basepair number 2526 in the ampicillin-resistance gene of the pBluescript II SK(−) phagemid. *Sca*I to *Mlu*I: CTG TGA CTG GTG ACG CGT CAA CCA AGT C and *Mlu*I to *Sca*I: GCT TTT CTG TGA CTG GTG AGT ACT CAA CCA AGT C.

3.3. Protocol for Mutagenesis

3.3.1. Step I: Annealing the Primers to the DNA

Simultaneously anneal the selection and mutagenic oligonucleotide primers to the double-stranded target plasmid DNA by preparing the following control and experimental reactions in 1.5-mL microcentrifuge tubes. For the purpose of demonstration, a control reaction is described that includes the use of the pWS plasmid DNA (*see* Section 2.) to be mutated and the *Kpn*I selection oligonucleotide primer (*see* Section 3.2.).

1. Control reaction: 1 µL (490 ng or 0.25 pmol) of pWS plasmid DNA (*see* Note 1), 5 µL (330 ng or 25 pmol) of *Kpn*I selection primer (*see* Note 2), 5 µL (281 ng or 25 pmol) of "blue" mutagenic primer (*see* Note 2), 2 µL of 10X mutagenesis buffer, 7 µL of double-distilled water (ddH₂O) to a final volume of 20 µL.
2. Experimental reaction: 0.25 pmol of the plasmid of interest (*see* Note 1), 25 pmol of the selection primer (*see* Note 2), 25 pmol of the mutagenic primer (*see* Note 2), 2 µL of 10X mutagenesis buffer, ddH₂O to a final volume of 20 µL.
3. Place the microcentrifuge tubes in a boiling water bath for 5 min and then immediately place the tubes on ice for 5 min. Centrifuge briefly in a table-top centifuge to collect the condensate.
4. Incubate the microcentrifuge tubes at room temperature (23–25°C) for 30 min.

3.3.2. Step II:
Extending the Primers and Ligating the New Strands

For both the control and experimental reactions, extend the primers with T7 DNA polymerase and ligate the new strands with T4 DNA ligase as indicated:

1. Prepare a fresh 1:10 dilution of the 10X enzyme mix by diluting 1 µL of the 10X enzyme mix in 9 µL of enzyme dilution buffer (*see* Note 3).
2. To each microcentrifuge tube, add 7 µL of the deoxynucleotide mix. The deoxynucleotide mix must be added to the reaction first or the 3'- to 5'-exonuclease activity of native T7 DNA polymerase will degrade the primers. Stir the 1:10 enzyme dilution with a pipet tip and add 3 µL of this fresh 1:10 enzyme dilution to the reaction. Stir the reaction mixture again with a pipet tip and centrifuge briefly.
3. Incubate the microcentrifuge tubes at 37°C for 1 h.
4. Inactivate the T7 DNA polymerase and T4 DNA ligase by incubating the microcentrifuge tubes at 70–80°C for 10–15 min to prevent religation of the digested strands during the subsequent digestion in Section 3.3.3. Cool the reactions to room temperature.

3.3.3. Step III:
Digesting with a Restriction Enzyme

After the reactions cool, digest both the control and experimental reactions with a restriction enzyme to eliminate those plasmids that did not anneal with the selection oligonucleotide primer.

1. Control reaction: Add the following components to the control reaction: 20 U of *Kpn*I restriction enzyme, ddH₂O to a total reaction vol of 60 µL. (Because *Kpn*I is active in 0.5 mutagenesis buffer, no buffer is added and

the control reaction is diluted to twice its volume, thus diluting the buffer concentration from 1–0.5X. For the buffer requirements of other restriction enzymes, please consult a restriction enzyme buffer chart available from the respective manufacturer of the restriction enzyme.)

2. Incubate the control reaction at 37°C for 1 h (*see* Note 4).
3. Experimental reaction: Digest the DNA at the selection restriction site by adding 20 U of the restriction enzyme. In order to prevent incomplete digestion owing to the glycerol concentration, the amount of restriction enzyme must not exceed 10% of the total digestion reaction volume, which includes the 3-μL volume of the fresh 1:10 enzyme dilution from step 2 in Section 3.3.2., and the required volume containing 20 U of the restriction enzyme. For example, if 2.5 μL is the required volume of restriction enzyme needed to provide 20 U, then the total enzyme volume is 5.5 μL (i.e., 3 + 2.5 μL). Because the total volume of enzyme (i.e., 5.5 μL) must not exceed 10% of the total digestion reaction volume, the final reaction volume must be 55 μL or more. The buffer must also be adjusted to the appropriate salt concentration for the restriction enzyme corresponding to the selection primer in use. Be sure to take into account the fact that the original 30 μL of the reaction is already 1X in mutagenesis buffer. For an example, see the control reaction description in step 1.
4. Incubate the experimental reaction at 37°C for 1 h.

3.3.4. Step IV:
Transforming into XLmutS Competent Cells

For both the control and experimental reactions, follow the transformation procedure outlined as follows (*see* Notes 5–10).

1. Thaw the XL*mutS* competent cells on ice.
2. Gently mix the cells by hand. Aliquot 90 μL of the XL*mutS* competent cells into two prechilled 15-μL Falcon 2059 polypropylene tubes.
3. Add 1.5 μL of the β-mercaptoethanol to the 90-μL aliquots of XL*mutS* competent cells to yield a final concentration of 25 m*M*.
4. Swirl the contents of the Falcon 2059 polypropylene tubes gently. Incubate the cells on ice for 10 min, swirling gently every 2 min.
5. Add 1/10 of the volume of the control and experimental reactions that have been digested with a restriction enzyme (*see* Section 3.3.3.) to each Falcon 2059 polypropylene tube and swirl gently. Use 6 μL for the control reaction.
6. Incubate the Falcon 2059 polypropylene tubes on ice for 30 min (*see* Note 11).
7. Heat pulse the Falcon 2059 polypropylene tubes in a 42°C water bath for 45 s. The length of time of the heat pulse is critical for obtaining the highest efficiencies.

8. Incubate the transformation mixture on ice for 2 min.
9. Add 0.9 mL of preheated SOC medium and incubate the Falcon 2059 polypropylene tubes at 37°C for 1 h with shaking at 225–250 rpm.
10. Plate 100 μL of the control reaction transformation on LB-ampicillin (100 μg/mL) agar plates, containing X-gal and IPTG, to verify the *lac* phenotype. For color selection, spread 20 μL of 0.2*M* IPTG and 20 μL of 10% (w/v) X-gal on LB ampicillin agar plates 30 min before plating the transformants (*see* Note 12).
11. Plate 1, 5, 25, and 200 μL of the transformation mixture, using a sterile spreader, onto the agar plates containing the appropriate antibiotic (*see* Note 13). If the transformants are ampicillin resistant, the transformation mixture may also be plated on LB-ampicillin (20 μg/mL)-methicillin (80 μg/mL) agar plates, if satellite colonies are observed.
12. Incubate the agar plates overnight at 37°C (*see* Note 14).

3.3.5. Step V:
Enriching for Mutant Plasmids

1. Enrich for mutated plasmids by adding the remaining transformation mixture that was not plated into 3 mL of 2X YT broth, supplemented with an appropriate antibiotic for the experimental plasmid.
2. Grow the culture overnight at 37°C with shaking.
3. For both the control and experimental reactions, perform a miniprep plasmid DNA isolation from 1.5 mL of the overnight culture in step 2 using a standard protocol *(9)*.
4. Perform restriction enzyme digestion of the miniprep plasmid DNA for both the control and experimental reactions as follows: Digest 10 μL (approx 500 ng) of the resulting miniprep plasmid DNA with the same selection restriction enzyme and appropriate buffer as described in Section 3.3.3. The reaction volume should be 10X the volume of added enzyme. Use at least 20 U of the restriction enzyme (*see* the following control reaction for an example).
5. Control reaction: 10 μL (approx 500 ng) of miniprep DNA, 1 μL of 10X mutagenesis buffer (0.5X final concentration), 20 U of *Kpn*I restriction enzyme, ddH$_2$O to a final volume of 20 μL. Incubate the digestion reaction for 1–2 h at 37°C.

3.3.6. Step VI:
Final Transformation into XL1-Blue Competent Cells

For both the control and experimental reactions, transform the digested DNA into the XL1-Blue competent cells or into a cell line of choice as outlined in the following.

1. Control reaction: Transform 40 µL of XL1-Blue competent cells with 1/10 of the volume (2 µL) of the digested DNA described in step 4 of Section 3.3.5.
2. Experimental reaction: Transform 1/10 of the volume of the digested DNA (but do not exceed 4 µL) into 40 µL of XL1-Blue competent cells or any desired competent cell line by following the transformation protocol given here and by referring to Notes 5–10:
   a. Thaw the competent cells on ice.
   b. Gently mix the competent cells by hand. Aliquot 40 µL of the competent cells into a prechilled 15-mL Falcon 2059 polypropylene tube.
   c. Add 0.68 µL of the β-mercaptoethanol to the 40 µL of competent cells to yield a final concentration of 25 mM.
   d. Swirl the contents of the Falcon 2059 polypropylene tube gently. Incubate the cells on ice for 10 min, swirling gently every 2 min.
   e. Add 1/10 of the volume of the experimental reaction (but do not exceed 4 µL) to the Falcon 2059 polypropylene tube and swirl gently. As an additional control, add 1 µL of the pUC18 control plasmid to a 40-µL aliquot of the XL1-Blue competent cells and swirl gently.
   f. Incubate the Falcon 2059 polypropylene tube on ice for 30 min (*see* Note 11).
   g. Heat pulse the Falcon 2059 polypropylene tubes in a 42°C water bath for 45 s. The length of time of the heat pulse is critical for obtaining the highest efficiencies.
   h. Incubate the transformation mixture on ice for 2 min.
   i. Add 0.45 mL of preheated SOC medium and incubate the Falcon 2059 polypropylene tubes at 37°C for 1 h with shaking at 225–250 rpm.
   j. The control reaction transformation should be plated on LB-ampicillin agar plates, containing X-gal and IPTG, to verify the *lac* phenotype. For color selection, spread 20 µL of 0.2M IPTG and 20 µL of 10% (w/v) X-gal on LB-ampicillin (100 µg/mL) agar plates 30 min before plating the transformants (*see* Note 12). If plating 5 µL, expect to see 150–300 colonies.
   k. Plate 1, 5, 25, and 200 µL of the experimental reaction transformation mixture, using a sterile spreader, onto the agar plates containing the appropriate antibiotic. If the transformants are intended to be ampicillin resistant, the transformation mixture may also be plated on LB-ampicillin (20 µg/mL)–methicillin (80 µg/mL) agar plates, containing IPTG and X-gal, if satellite colonies are observed (*see* Note 15).
   l. Incubate the plates overnight at 37°C (*see* Note 16).
   m. Observations that have been made during the course of developing this protocol and solutions to various problems associated with these observations are listed in Notes 17–20.

4. Notes

1. To determine the mass of template required to give 0.25 pmol (1 pmol = 1 × 10^{-12} mol), use the formula: mass of template required = [(0.25 × 10^{-12} mol)(660 g/mol/bp)(number of basepairs in the plasmid)]. For example, if the plasmid is 2960 bp, then mass of template required = [(0.25 × 10^{-12} mol)(660 g/mol/bp)(2960 bp)] = (4.88 × 10^{-7} g) = 488 ng.

2. The amount of selection and mutagenic oligonucleotide primer used should be 100X the picomole amount of template. To determine the mass of primer required to give 25 pmol, use the formula: mass of oligonucleotide primer = [(25 × 10^{-12} mol)(330 g/mol/base)(number of bases in the primer)]. For example, if the primer is 40 bases long, then mass of primer = [(25 × 10^{-12} mol)(330 g/mol/base)(40 bases)] = (3.30 × 10^{-7} g = 330 ng). To determine the concentration of oligonucleotide primer solutions, assume that a primer solution measuring 1 OD_{260} U is at a concentration of 33 µg/mL.

3. It is crucial to use the fresh 1:10 enzyme dilution within 6–8 h of preparation.

4. In order to keep the reaction volume as low as possible to obtain maximum digestion and transformation efficiency, use the highest concentration of high-quality restriction enzyme available.

5. Storage conditions: The competent cells are very sensitive to even small variations in temperature and must be stored at the bottom of a –80°C freezer. Transferring tubes from one freezer to another may result in a loss of efficiency. The XL*mutS* and XL1-Blue competent cells from Stratagene should be placed at –80°C directly from the dry ice shipping container. Cells stored in this manner should retain their guaranteed efficiency for 6 mo.

6. Aliquoting cells: When aliquoting, keep the competent cells on ice at all times. It is essential that the Falcon 2059 polypropylene tubes are placed on ice before the competent cells are thawed and that the cells are aliquoted directly into the prechilled tubes. When transforming the competent cells, it is important to use at least 90 µL of XL1*mutS* competent cells for each transformation and 40 µL of XL1-Blue competent cells for each transformation. Using smaller volumes will result in lower efficiencies.

7. Use of Falcon 2059 polypropylene tubes: It is important that Falcon 2059 polypropylene tubes are used for the transformation protocol, since other tubes may be degraded by the β-mercaptoethanol. In addition, the incubation period during the heat-pulse step is critical and has been calculated for the thickness and shape of the Falcon 2059 polypropylene tubes.

8. Use of β-mercaptoethanol: β-mercaptoethanol has been shown to increase transformation efficiencies two- to threefold.

9. Quantity of DNA added: Highest transformation efficiencies are observed by adding 1 µL of 0.1 ng/mL of supercoiled DNA to 100 µL of competent cells. An increasing number of colonies will be obtained when plating up to 50 ng, although the overall efficiency may be lower.

10. Length of the heat pulse: There is a defined "window" of highest transformation efficiency resulting from the heat pulse in Section 3.3.4., step 7 and Section 3.3.6., step 2. Optimal efficiencies are observed when cells are heat pulsed for 45–50 s. Heat pulsing for at least 45 s is recommended to allow for slight variations in the length of incubation. Efficiencies decrease sharply when incubating for <45 s or for >50 s.

11. Preheat the SOC medium to 42°C at this step.

12. Do not mix IPTG and X-gal, since these chemicals will precipitate. X-gal should be prepared in dimethylformamide (DMF). Prepare IPTG in sterile dH₂O.

13. When spreading bacteria onto the plate, tilt and tap the spreader to remove the last drop of the cells. For the XL*mutS* competent cells, if plating is >100 µL, the cells can be spread directly onto the plates. If plating is <100 µL of the transformation mixture, increase the volume of the transformation mixture to be plated to a total volume of 200 µL using SOC medium.

14. Approximately 45–50% of the colonies from the control reaction transformation should display the blue phenotype, and the expected colony numbers for the experimental transformations should be between 200 and 600 colonies per transformation plate.

15. When spreading bacteria onto the plate, tilt and tap the spreader to remove the last drop of the cells. For the competent cells, if plating is >100 L, the cells can be spread directly onto the plates. If plating is <100 µL of the transformation mixture, increase the volume of the transformation mixture to be plated to a total volume of 200 µL using SOC medium.

16. Approximately 70–95% of the control reaction transformation colonies should display the blue phenotype.

17. *Observation*: There are no colonies produced after the first transformation. *Suggestion*: Verify that the correct antibiotic selection was used. The control plasmid uses ampicillin, but the experimental plasmid may require another antibiotic. Check the quantity of the target plasmid DNA, which should be 0.25 pmol.

18. *Observation*: There are >1000 colonies produced after the first transformation. *Suggestion*: The expected colony numbers for the experimental reaction transformations should be between 200 and 600 colonies per transformation plate. If the expected colony numbers exceed 1000 following the first transformation, then incomplete digestion with the restriction enzyme may have occurred. Repeat the digestion step as outlined in Section 3.3.3.

19. *Observation*: The total number of colonies produced after the second transformation is low.
    Suggestion: The plasmid DNA yield from the miniprep may be low. Check the yield by electrophoresing a 10-µL sample of the digested DNA on a 1% (w/v) agarose gel and comparing the ethidium bromidestaining intensity with a known standard. Check the transformation efficiency of the competent cells with the pUC18 control plasmid DNA.
20. *Observation*: There are a large number of transformant colonies, but the mutation efficiency is low.
    Suggestion: Linearization of the parental plasmid may not have been complete. Ensure that the correct restriction enzyme is used for the selection oligonucleotide primer and that the restriction buffer is optimal for this enzyme. The miniprep plasmid DNA may contain impurities that could interfere with the restriction enzyme digestion. An additional purification step may be required to remove any RNA or protein remaining in the preparation. The extent of the restriction enzyme digestion can be monitored by visualizing a small aliquot of the digested DNA on a 1% (w/v) agarose gel. If necessary, add more restriction enzyme and digest the mixed plasmid DNA longer. Alternatively, there could be a problem with the incorporation of the selection and/or mutagenic primer into the newly synthesized DNA strand. If neither the experimental nor control reaction resulted in a reasonable number of mutants, there may be a problem with the T7 DNA polymerase and/or the T4 DNA ligase. Prepare a fresh 1:10 dilution of the 10X enzyme mix (*see* Section 2.) and use 3 µL of the fresh dilution in the reactions. Heat the reaction adequately to destroy the T4 DNA ligase after the extension and ligation step (*see* Section 3.3.2.). If the control reaction gave a reasonable number of mutants whereas the experimental reaction did not, there may be a problem with the experimental primers. Check to make sure the mutant primer is designed to hybridize to the same strand as the selection primer. Ensure that both of the primers have been phosphorylated and that both primers are of high purity and accurate concentration (*see* Section 3.1.). Occasionally, the mutation efficiency will be lower if the mutagenic primer is introducing a large insert or a deletion. This may also be the case when the target plasmid is very large (>8 kb). Try isolating a pool of plasmid DNA from the cells of the second transformation and repeat the restriction enzyme digestion step (*see* Section 3.3.3.) and then the transformation step (*see* Section 3.3.4.) a third time. This will further enrich for the mutant plasmid.

References

1. Kunkel, T. A. (1985) Rapid and efficient site-specific mutagenesis without phenotypic selection. *Proc. Natl. Acad. Sci. USA* **82,** 488–492.
2. Sayers, J. R., Schmidt, W., Wendler, A., and Eckstein, F. (1988) Strand specific cleavage of phosphorothioate containing DNA by reaction with restriction endonucleases in the presence of ethidium bromide. *Nucleic Acids Res.* **16,** 803–814.
3. Vandeyar, M. A., Weiner, M. P., Hutton, C. J., and Batt, C. A. (1988) A simple and rapid method for the selection of oligonucleotide-directed mutants. *Gene* **65,** 129–133.
4. Stanssens, P., Opsomer, C., McKeown, Y. M., Kramer, W., Zabeau, M., and Fritz, H.-J. (1989) Efficient oligonucleotide-directed construction of mutations in expression vectors by the gapped duplex DNA method using alternating selectable markers. *Nucleic Acids Res.* **17,** 4441–4454.
5. Lewis, M. K. and Thompson, D. V. (1990) Efficient site directed *in vitro* mutagenesis using ampicillin selection. *Nucleic Acids Res.* **18,** 3439–3443.
6. Deng, W. P. and Nickoloff, J. A. (1992) Site-directed mutagenesis of virtually any plasmid by eliminating a unique site. *Anal. Biochem.* **200,** 81–88.
7. Papworth, C., Greener, A., and Braman, J. (1994) Highly efficient double-stranded, site-directed mutagenesis with the Chameleon™ kit. *Strategies* **7,** 38–40.
8. Bebenek, K. and Kunkel, T. A. (1989) The use of native T7 DNA polymerase for site-directed mutagenesis. *Nucleic Acids Res.* **17,** 5408.
9. Sambrook, J., Fritsch, E. F., and Maniatis, T. (eds.) (1989) *Molecular Cloning: A Laboratory Manual*, 2nd ed., Cold Spring Harbor Laboratory Press, Cold Spring Harbor, NY.

CHAPTER 4

Site-Directed Mutagenesis Using a Uracil-Containing Phagemid Template

Christian Hagemeier

1. Introduction

The ability to introduce specific changes into almost any given DNA sequence has revolutionized the analysis of cloned genes. This technique has enabled researchers to identify regions necessary for the regulation of gene expression. Also, it was and still is instrumental to learn about the importance of functional domains or even single amino acids of proteins. Of the many useful methods available for site-directed mutagenesis, in this chapter I describe a protocol that is based on the "Kunkel Method" *(1,2)*. This method allows the generation of point mutations, deletions, and insertions for a given DNA sequence with high efficiency. I have used this procedure successfully many times and most recently to map protein interaction sites within the activation domain of the transcription factor E2F *(3)*.

1.1. Overview and Background Information

The method relies on synthetic oligonucleotides as carriers of the specific alteration one wishes to introduce into the target DNA sequence. The oligonucleotide is annealed to its cognate region of single-stranded DNA and elongated by DNA polymerase. This generates a mutant second-strand containing the specific alteration introduced through the synthetic oligonucleotide. This part of the method is very much similar to virtually all other procedures based on site-directed in vitro mutagenesis.

From: *Methods in Molecular Biology, Vol. 57: In Vitro Mutagenesis Protocols*
Edited by: M. K. Trower Humana Press Inc., Totowa, NJ

However, it is the principle of how to select against the nonmutant strand that distinguishes this method from all other protocols.

The selection is based on the use of template DNA containing a small percentage of uracil residues instead of thymine. This is achieved by passaging the vector carrying the target DNA through an *Escherichia coli* strain lacking the enzyme dUTPase (*dut⁻*) (Fig. 1A,B). The *dut⁻* deletion results in bacteria with high concentrations of dUTP and as a consequence, dUTP competes with thymine for incorporation into DNA. The *E. coli dut⁻* strain cannot repair the faulty incorporation since it also lacks the enzyme uracil *N*-glycosylase that normally leads to a removal of uracil residues from DNA (*ung⁻*). As a result, the *dut⁻ ung⁻ E. coli* produce double-stranded vector DNA containing a proportion of uracil residues.

The vector is designed such that single-stranded template DNA can be rescued from the bacteria with a helper phage (*see the following*, Fig. 1C). The single-stranded template is then used in the aforementioned standard site-directed mutagenesis reaction (Fig. 1D,E). It results in double-stranded vector DNA in which the nonmutant template strand, but not the in vitro synthesized strand with the desired mutation, contains uracil residues (Fig. 1E). By simply transforming an aliquot of the in vitro reaction into an *E. coli ung⁺* strain, the uracil-containing template strand will be degraded (Fig. 1F). Therefore, most of the progeny should contain the desired mutation (Fig. 1G).

1.2. General Considerations

As outlined herein, the choice of the right bacterial strain is absolutely essential for this mutagenesis procedure to succeed. But also the type of vector used in the reaction should be carefully considered. Usually, single-stranded template is obtained by subcloning the DNA fragment of interest into single-stranded phage vectors (e.g., M13). However, in order to save the time-consuming subcloning steps involved it would be most desirable to perform the mutagenesis reaction in the same vector that will then be used in an assay for the loss/gain of function the mutation will produce. Therefore, prior to the mutagenesis procedure it is worth cloning the DNA of interest into a vector harboring the intergenic region of a filamentous phage (phagemid). Like in the M13-system, this region then allows packaging of single-stranded vector DNA under two conditions: the use of a bacterial strain harboring an F1 episome (F'), and the use of helper phage for packaging the single-stranded vector DNA.

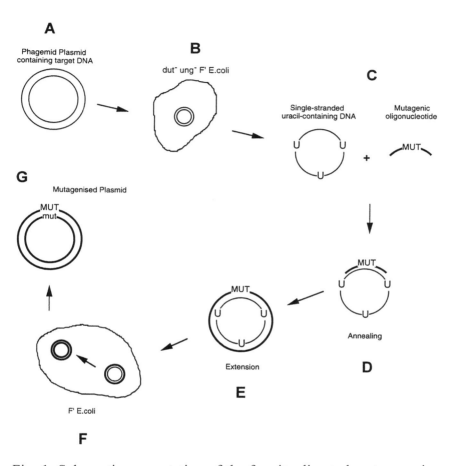

Fig. 1. Schematic presentation of the for site-directed mutagenesis pro-
edure using a uracil-containing phagemid template. *See* Section 1.1. for
etailed information.

Thus, with the right choice of bacterial strain (dut^- ung^- F') and vector
)NA (phagemid) the production of mutant clones can be achieved in a
ninimum of time. Since this mutagenesis reaction has a very high effi-
iency (usually greater than 50%) screening for mutants can be under-
aken directly by sequencing. Together, the high efficiency of this method
nd no need for subcloning steps make this mutagenesis procedure a valu-
ble and less expensive alternative to PCR-based methods. I always con-
ider this the method of choice when I need to introduce many independent

mutations into one gene. In that case I can rely on one scaled up preparation of uracil-containing single-stranded template DNA—the single most time-consuming step of this approach.

2. Materials

2.1. Preparation of Uracil-Containing Single-Stranded DNA

2.1.1. Preparation of Helper Phage Stock

1. *E. coli* : Any strain harboring an F' episome should be sufficient. However, I use JM101, which usually gives a reliably high titer phage preparation.
2. 2X YT medium: For 1 L medium, dissolve 16 g bactotryptone, 10 g yeast extract, and 10 g of NaCl in deionized H_2O. Aliquot into volumes of 100 mL, autoclave, and store at room temperature.
3. Bacteriophage: R408 (Stratagene, La Jolla, CA).
4. 0.45-μm filter and 10-mL syringe.

2.1.2. Transformation of Competent E. coli *(dut⁻ ung⁻ F')*

1. Competent bacteria of an *E. coli dut⁻ ung⁻* F' strain (e.g., RZ1032 or CJ236).
2. 2X YT medium: *see* Section 2.1.1.
3. 2X YT/Amp plates: Add 15 g of agar to 1 L of 2X YT medium prior to autoclaving. When cooled to approx 50°C add 100 μg/mL ampicillin. Pour the solution into sterile 90-mm Petri dishes such that the bottom of the plates is well covered.

2.1.3. Preparation of Single-Stranded DNA

1. 2X YT/Amp medium: Prepare medium as described in Section 2.1.1. Prior to use add 100 μg/mL ampicillin.
2. Bacteriophage R408 as described in Section 2.1.1.
3. PEG/ammonium acetate solution: $3.5M$ ammonium acetate, pH 7.5, 20% (w/v) polyetylene glycol (PEG) 8000. Store at room temperature.
4. TE buffer: 10 mM Tris-HCl, pH 8.0, 1 mM EDTA. Store at room temperature.
5. Phenol: Phenol equilibrated to pH 7.0–7.5. Aliquot into volumes of 100 mL and store in dark bottles at 4°C.
6. Chloroform/isoamyl alcohol: Mixture of 24 parts (v/v) of chloroform and 1 part (v/v) of isoamyl alcohol. Store in a dark bottle at 4°C.
7. $3M$ sodium acetate equilibrated to pH 5.2. Autoclave and store at 4°C.
8. Ice-cold ethanol (100%).

2.2. In Vitro Mutagenesis Procedure

2.2.1. Phosphorylation of the Synthetic Oligonucleotide

1. Synthetic mutagenic oligonucleotide: This oligonucleotide is complementary to the target DNA of the single-stranded vector and carries the desired mutation. Its concentration should be adjusted to 10 pmol/μL (*see* Note 1).
2. 10X Kinase buffer: 500 mM Tris-HCl, pH 7.4, 100 mM MgCl$_2$, 50 mM dithiothreitol (DTT). Store at −20°C.
3. ATP: 10 mM ATP in TE buffer. Store in small aliquots at −20°C.
4. T4 Polynucleotide kinase (10 U/μL).

2.2.2. Mutagenesis Reaction

1. Single-stranded target DNA (*see* Section 2.1.4.).
2. Phosphorylated mutagenic oligonucleotide (*see* Section 2.2.1.).
3. Annealing buffer: 500 mM NaCl, 100 mM Tris-HCl, pH 8.0, 100 mM MgCl$_2$, 50 mM DTT. Store at −20°C.
4. dNTP: mix 2.5 mM each of dATP, dTTP, dGTP, and dCTP. Store in small aliquots at −20°C (*see* Note 2).
5. ATP: 10 mM ATP in TE buffer. Store in small aliquots at −20°C.
6. 10X Ligase buffer: 660 mM Tris-HCl, pH 7.5, 50 mM MgCl$_2$, 50 mM DTT. Store at −20°C.
7. T4 DNA polymerase (1 U/μL).
8. T4 DNA ligase (1 U/μL).

2.3. Selection Against the Nonmutant Strand

1. Frozen competent bacteria of an *E.coli ung*[+] strain (e.g., JM101).
2. 2X YT medium: *See* Section 2.1.1.
3. 2X YT/Amp plates: *See* Section 2.1.2 .
4. Double-stranded vector DNA from the mutagenesis reaction.

3. Methods

3.1. Preparation of Uracil-Containing Single-Stranded DNA

3.1.1. Preparation of Helper Phage Stock

A single preparation of a helper phage stock usually will give an overall yield sufficient for hundreds of mutagenesis reactions. At the same time the phage stock is extremely stable and can be kept at 4°C for many months or years. Therefore, once this step has been accomplished further mutagenesis procedures will normally start with the transformation of phagemid DNA into competent *E. coli* (*see* Section 3.1.2.).

1. Grow an overnight culture of *E. coli* (F'; e.g., JM101) in 2X YT medium at 37°C.
2. On the next morning dilute 100 μL of the overnight culture into 10 mL of fresh 2X YT medium in a small sterile conical flask. Continue to grow the culture at 37°C until the OD_{600} reaches about 0.2 (mid-log-phase).
3. Infect the culture with 1 μL of R408 stock (Stratagene) and continue incubation for 6 h with vigorous shaking at 37°C (*see* Note 3).
4. Pellet the cells at 5000*g* for 10 min.
5. Pass the supernatant through a 0.45-μm filter into a sterile tube with screwcap using a 10-mL syringe.
6. Incubate the tube at 60°C for 10 min to kill residual bacteria (*see* Note 4).
7. Aliquot the phage preparation into 500-μL volumes in sterile reaction vials and store tubes at 4°C. The phage stock will be stable for months or years (*see* Note 5).

3.1.2. Transformation of Competent E. coli (dut⁻ ung⁻ F')

For the preparation of uracil-containing single-stranded phagemid DNA, the vector DNA has to be transformed into a *dut⁻ ung⁻* F' strain of *E. coli* (e.g., RZ1032 or CJ236).

1. Mix 50 μL of competent *E. coli* (*dut⁻ ung⁻* F') cells with approx 1–10 ng of phagemid vector containing the target DNA and incubate on ice for 30 min.
2. Transfer the tube to a 42°C water bath and heat shock for 1 min.
3. Add 150 μL of 2X YT and incubate for 30 min at 37°C with shaking.
4. Plate the contents of the tube onto one 2X YT/Amp plate and incubate overnight at 37°C. The yield should be approx 50–300 colonies.

3.1.3. Preparation of Single-Stranded Phagemid DNA

1. Pick two colonies from the plate and inoculate one small conical flask with 5 mL of 2X YT/Amp. Incubate at 37°C until OD_{600} is about 0.2 (mid-log-phase after 2.5–3 h).
2. Infect the culture with 10 μL of phage stock and continue the incubation with vigorous shaking for 5–6 h at 37°C (*see* Note 6).
3. Transfer the culture into 3 × 1.5 mL reaction vials and pellet the bacteria in a microfuge for 5 min. Meanwhile, add 250 μL of 20% PEG in 3.5*M* ammonium acetate to three more tubes.
4. Transfer 1 mL of supernatant from each tube into the PEG-containing reaction vials. Take care not to disturb the pellet! Mix the contents by briefly vortexing the tubes and precipitate the phage for 20 min at room temperature.
5. Pellet the phage in a microcentrifuge for 10 min at 4°C.

6. Carefully remove the supernatant and briefly respin the tubes to collect any remaining PEG solution. Make sure to aspirate all the supernatant using a drawn out Pasteur pipet attached to a vacuum line.
7. Resuspend each bacteriophage pellet in 100 μL of TE and pool contents of tubes in one reaction vial.
8. Extract once with 150 μL of phenol and once with an equal volume of chloroform:isoamyl alcohol.
9. Transfer the aqueous phase from the final extraction to a fresh tube. Take great care not to disturb the interphase! A clean preparation is more important than a maximum yield. Add 0.1 vol of 3 M sodium acetate and 2 vol of ice-cold ethanol. Mix well and allow DNA to precipitate for 30 min at −20°C.
10. Recover the DNA by centrifugation in a microfuge for 10 min at 4°C. Wash the pellet with 80% ethanol, respin the tube, and remove the supernatant with a drawn out Pasteur pipet attached to a vacuum line (*see* Note 7). Dry the pellet in a desiccator or speedvac for 3 min and dissolve the pellet in 50 μL TE.
11. Use an aliquot of 4 μL (should equal about 0.5 μg) for analyzing the single-stranded DNA preparation on a 1% agarose gel. Two bands of about equal intensity should be visible. The upper band refers to single-stranded plasmid DNA, the lower to single-stranded phage DNA.

3.2. In Vitro Mutagenesis Procedure

3.2.1. Phosphorylation of the Synthetic Oligonucleotide

To ligate the oligonucleotide to the 3' terminus of the newly synthesized strand in the mutagenesis reaction, it needs to be phosphorylated on its own 5' terminus.

1. Adjust concentration of the oligonucleotide to 10 pmol/μL.
2. Use 5 μL in the phosphorylation reaction and further add 1 mL of 10X kinase buffer, 1 μL of 10 m M ATP, and 2.5 μL of T4 polynucleotide kinase (10 U/μL).
3. Incubate the reaction for 30 min at 37°C.
4. Heat inactivate the enzyme at 65°C for 10 min. Spin the tube briefly to collect all droplets. The oligonucleotide can now be used directly in the mutagenesis reaction (*see* Note 8).

3.2.2. Mutagenesis Reaction

This reaction involves three steps. First, the phosphorylated oligonucleotide is annealed to the uracil-containing single-stranded DNA. Second, the oligonucleotide is extended along the template DNA from its 3' end. Third, the extended strand is ligated to the 5' end of the oligonucleotide.

1. Anneal 10 pmol of the phosphorylated oligonucleotide to 1 μg of single-stranded phagemid DNA by mixing 2 μL of the phosphorylation reaction (*see* Section 3.2.1.), 7 μL of the single-stranded DNA preparation (*see* Section 3.1.3.), and 1 μL of annealing buffer (*see* Note 9).
2. Incubate the reaction for 5 min at 65°C and then allow the reaction to slowly cool down to room temperature for about 30 min (*see* Note 10).
3. Add to the annealing reaction on ice: 4 μL of a 2.5 m*M* dNTP mix, 1 μL 10 m*M* ATP, 1 μL 10X ligase buffer, 2.5 U of T4 DNA polymerase, 2 U of T4 DNA ligase, and deionized H$_2$O to a total volume of 20 μL (*see* Note 11).
4. Incubate the reaction mix at room temperature for 10 min to allow efficient initiation of the polymerase reaction. Then incubate for a further 2 h at 37°C.

3.3. Selection Against the Nonmutant Strand

This step finally selects against the nonmutant strand. The plasmids are simply transformed into *ung$^+$ E. coli,* which will specifically degrade the uracil-containing (nonmutant) strand. The bacteria then synthesize a new strand along the template. The new double-stranded plasmid should contain the desired mutation in both strands.

1. Mix 50 μL of competent *ung$^+$ E. coli* (e.g., JM101) with 3 μL of the mutagenesis reaction and incubate on ice for 30 min.
2. Transfer the tube to a 42°C water bath and heat shock for 1 min.
3. Add 150 μL of 2X YT and incubate for 30 min at 37°C with shaking.
4. Plate the contents of the tube onto one 2X YT/Amp plate and incubate overnight at 37°C.

Owing to the high efficiency of the procedure on average one to two of three colonies should contain plasmid with the desired mutation. Therefore, pick three colonies per mutagenesis reaction, perform a standard DNA "miniprep," and sequence the DNA directly, without prior screening for mutants. If, for some reason, double-stranded sequencing does not give a satisfying result, single-stranded DNA easily can be rescued for sequencing according to the method described in Section 3.1.3.

4. Notes

1. This method allows the introduction of point mutations, insertions (loop in), and deletions (loop out) into the target DNA. In general the complementary region of the mutagenic oligonucleotide should be proportional to the number of mismatches. For instance, for point mutations involving up to five adjacent bases, the annealing of 12 bases either side of the mutated region is sufficient. An insertion of 12 bases should have 15 matches either

side and a larger deletion should have 20 bases on either side annealing to the template DNA. (I have successfully deleted 250 bp under these conditions.) Having cytosine and guanine bases at the termini of the mutagenic oligonucleotide ensures a tighter bond of the ends of the oligonucleotide to its template DNA. This is beneficial for the initiation of the polymerase reaction (at the 3' terminus) and the ligation of the synthesized strand to the 5' terminus of the oligonucleotide.

2. To avoid the risk of contaminating uracil, only high quality dNTPs should be used in the extension reaction.

3. Sufficient aeration of the culture is very important for bacteriophage growth. Therefore, even small volumes should be incubated in a conical flask and shaken at high speed (300 cycles/min).

4. Any bacteria passing this step would produce thymine-containing phage during the preparation of single-stranded DNA (*see* Section 3.1.1.).

5. Generally the supernatant will contain phage at a titer of about 5×10^{10} plaque forming units (pfu)/mL and phage titering is not essential. However, if preparations of single-stranded phagemid DNA give a low yield, phage titers should be checked.

6. The phage stock usually contains about 5×10^{10} pfu/mL or $5 \times 10^8/10$ µL. Ten milliliters of a bacterial culture with an OD_{600} of about 0.2 will contain approx 5×10^9 cells. Therefore, this configuration results in an MOI (multiplicity of infection) of 0.1. Consequently, after 5-6 h of further bacterial growth virtually all phage progeny will have evolved from the *dut⁻ ung⁻* strain of *E. coli* harboring uracil-containing DNA.

7. At this stage the pellet may not be visible. Try to use a flat bottom tube. In that case, after centrifugation the pellet will be in the top quarter of the bottom (with respect to its orientation in the microfuge) and all the supernatant can be removed easily with the tip of the Pasteur pipet being placed in the bottom quarter. If you use a flat bottom tube try to position the tube in the same orientation in the microfuge during the wash and respin steps. This avoids loosening of the pellet from the wall of the tube during centrifugation.

8. The successful incorporation of a phosphate group can be monitored by trace-labeling the oligonucleotide with $[\gamma^{32}P]ATP$ in the same reaction. The product can then be analyzed on a polyacrylamide gel.

9. The concentration of plasmid DNA is not too important. A ratio of 4:1 of phage and plasmid DNA will still work well in the mutagenesis reaction. One microgram of plasmid DNA is equivalent to about 0.5 pmol.

10. This can be achieved easily by using a beaker (with the tube placed in a floater) in a water bath. After 5 min at 65°C place the beaker on the bench and allow the reaction to cool to room temperature that will take about 30 min.

11. Traditionally, the Klenow fragment of *E. coli* DNA polymerase I has been used for the extension reaction. However, T4 (or T7) DNA polymerase offers the advantage that it can not displace the mutagenic oligonucleotide from the template DNA. Since the T4 DNA polymerase has a strong 3' exonucleotide activity the concentration of dNTPs should not be below 500 μM. A high dNTP concentration counteracts the exonuclease activity and leads to a more efficient extension reaction by the enzyme.

References

1. Kunkel, T. A. (1985) Rapid and efficient site-specific mutagenesis without phenotypic selection. *Proc. Natl. Acad. Sci. USA* **82**, 488–492.
2. Kunkel, T. A., Roberts, J. D., and Zakour, R. A. (1987) Rapid and efficient site-specific mutagenesis without phenotypic selection. *Methods Enzymol.* **154**, 367–382.
3. Hagemeier, C., Cook, A., and Kouzarides, T. (1993) The retinoblastoma protein binds E2F residues required for activation *in vivo* and TBP binding *in vitro*. *Nucleic Acids Res.* **21**, 4998–5004.

CHAPTER 5

Oligonucleotide-Directed Mutagenesis Using an Improved Phosphorothioate Approach

Susan J. Dale and Ian R. Felix

1. Introduction

Oligonucleotide-directed in vitro mutagenesis is an established tool for the investigation of protein structure and function, and increasingly for studying the role of DNA sequences in gene expression. The method described here is based on the phosphorothioate technique developed by Eckstein's group *(1,2)* that has been improved to make it quicker and more convenient *(3)*. Selection for the desired mutation takes place in vitro, allowing a high efficiency of mutagenesis to be achieved. Typically, an efficiency of greater than 85% mutants can be obtained with a range of types of mutation.

The principle of the method is illustrated in Fig. 1. The target for mutagenesis is produced as a single strand by cloning into either M13 *(4)* or phagemid *(5)* vectors. Specialized vectors are not needed. An oligonucleotide designed to introduce the desired mutation is annealed to the template. The annealed primer is extended using a DNA polymerase in the presence of T4 DNA ligase to produce a closed circular heteroduplex.

Unused single-stranded template DNA is removed by T5 exonuclease digestion, leaving heteroduplex DNA containing the mutation introduced by the oligonucleotide primer *(6)*. T5 exonuclease has single- and double-stranded exonuclease activities with a copurifying single-stranded endonuclease *(7)*. It can nick and digest the unwanted template DNA that would otherwise cause a nonmutant "background." Nicked, double-

From: *Methods in Molecular Biology, Vol. 57: In Vitro Mutagenesis Protocols*
Edited by: M. K. Trower Humana Press Inc., Totowa, NJ

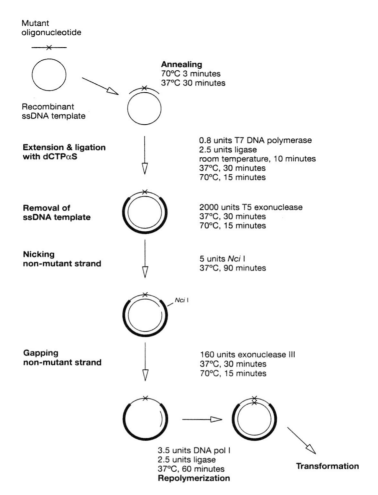

Fig. 1. Principle of mutagenesis using the improved phosphorothioate approach.

stranded DNA is also a substrate. However, the closed circular mutant heteroduplex is resistant to digestion and passes through the reaction undamaged.

The extension reaction incorporates dCTPαS into the mutant strand. This base analog has a sulfur atom substituted for oxygen at the alpha phosphate. Restriction enzyme *Nci*I is used to digest the heteroduplex DNA. It cannot cleave the phosphorothioate bonds in the mutant strand, so the product of this treatment is DNA with nicks in the nonmutant strand. This enables the selective destruction of the nonmutant strand, leading to a high efficiency of mutagenesis. Exonuclease III is used to digest the nicked nonmutant strand. Conditions have been optimized so that most of the nonmutant strand is digested, leaving a fragment of approx 800 bases *(2)* that acts as a primer for repolymerization. A double-stranded mutant homoduplex is generated using DNA polymerase I and T4 DNA ligase. Transformation of the products of the repolymerization reaction gives many clones of which a high proportion are mutants so that only a few need be selected for further analysis.

Protocols are given here for phosphorylation of mutant oligonucleotides, in vitro mutagenesis, preparation, and transformation of competent cells. Information on designing oligonucleotides to give high efficiency mutagenesis, and choice of polymerase to use to generate the mutant strand, is given in Notes 1–3.

2. Materials

1. Single-stranded template DNA prepared from M13 or phagemid vectors at 1 μg/μL *(8)*.
2. Mutant oligonucleotides of a sequence to direct the desired base change at 0.025 OD/mL/base. Oligonucleotides less than 30 bases long should be purified by desalting using an OPC column (Applied Biosystems, Foster City, CA). Longer oligonucleotides should be purified by electrophoresis through a 12–20% polyacrylamide gel *(8)*.
3. Reagents for mutagenesis are supplied as the Sculptor in vitro mutagenesis kit (Amersham, Arlington Heights, IL, RPN1526). This comprises:
   a. Native T7 DNA polymerase (0.8 U/μL);
   b. Klenow DNA polymerase (4 U/μL);
   c. T4 DNA ligase (2.5 U/μL);
   d. T5 exonuclease (1000 U/μL);
   e. *Nci*I restriction endonuclease (5 U/μL);
   f. Exonuclease III (160 U/μL);
   g. DNA polymerase I (3.5 U/μL);
   h. Buffer A: 1.4M MOPS, pH 8, and 1.4M NaCl;
   i. Buffer B: 70 mM Tris-HCl, pH 8, 10 mM MgCl$_2$, 45 mM NaCl;
   j. Buffer C: 700 mM Tris-HCl, pH 8, 350 μM EDTA, 200 mM DTT;
   k. Buffer D: 250 mM Tris-HCl, pH 8, 150 mM NaCl, 500 μM EDTA;
   l. dNTP mix A: 1.01 mM dATP, dCTPαS, dGTP, dTTP, 2.02 mM ATP, and 20 mM MgCl$_2$;
   m. dNTP mix B: 1.25 mM dATP, dCTP, dGTP, dTTP, 2.5 mM ATP, and 25 mM MgCl$_2$; and

n. *E. coli* TG1 host cells (Genotype: K12, Δ[lac-pro], supE, thi, hsdD5/ F'traD36, proA + B +, lacIq, lacZΔM15).
4. 2X TY medium: To make 1 L, add 16 g tryptone, 10 g yeast extract, and 5 g NaCl to water. Sterilize by autoclaving.
5. 10X M9 salts: To make 1 L add, 6 g anhydrous Na_2HPO_4, 3 g KH_2PO_4, 1 g NH_4Cl, 0.5 g NaCl in water.
6. Glucose/minimal media plates. Autoclave the following reagents separately, and cool before mixing aseptically; M9 salts with 15 g agar (1 L), $1M$ $MgSO_4$ (1 mL), $1M$ thiamine-HCl (1 mL), $0.1M$ $CaCl_2$ (1 mL), 20% glucose (10 mL).
7. H top agar: To make 1 L, add 10 g tryptone, 8 g NaCl, 8 g agar to water. Sterilize by autoclaving.
8. L plates: To make 1 L, add 10 g tryptone, 5 g yeast extract, 10 g NaCl, 15 g agar to water. Sterilize by autoclaving.
9. 10X Kinase buffer: $1M$ Tris-HCl, pH 8.0, 100 mM $MgCl_2$, 70 mM dithiothreitol, 10 mM ATP. Store at $-20°C$.
10. T4 polynucleotide kinase (Amersham, E70031, 10 U/μL).
11. 50 mM $CaCl_2$.
12. 10X TBE electrophoresis buffer: $0.89M$ Tris base, $0.89M$ boric acid, 0.02 mM EDTA.
13. 5 mg/mL Ethidium bromide solution. Wear gloves. Handle with care.
14. 5X Gel loading dye solution: 40% sucrose, 100 mM Tris-HCl, pH 8.0, 100 mM EDTA, 0.4 mg/mL Bromophenol blue.

3. Methods
3.1. Phosphorylation of Oligonucleotides

1. Measure the A_{260} of the purified oligonucleotide and calculate the concentration in OD/mL. Adjust an aliquot of the oligonucleotide solution to the concentration required for the phosphorylation reaction. This is 0.025 OD U/mL/base (equivalent to 1.6 pmol/μL); for example, a 20-mer should be at $20 \times 0.025 = 0.5$ OD/mL.
2. Add to a microcentrifuge tube, 30 μL oligonucleotide solution (0.025 OD/ mL/base), 3 μL 10X kinase buffer, 2 U T4 polynucleotide kinase. Mix by pipeting up and down. Incubate in a 37°C water bath for 15 min. Heat inactivate in a 70°C water bath for 10 min. The phosphorylated oligonucleotide can be used immediately or stored at $-20°C$.

3.2. The Mutagenesis Reaction

The complete mutagenesis reaction, including transformation of the mutants, can be carried out in 1 d if T7 polymerase is used in the initial polymerization. Alternatively, the reaction can be frozen after any stage (except annealing) and continued whenever convenient.

1. To anneal the mutant oligonucleotide and template, mix in a microcentrifuge tube, 2 μL single-stranded template (1 μg/μL), 1 μL phosphorylated oligonucleotide (1.6 pmol/μL), 1 μL buffer A, and 5 μL water. Incubate for 3 min in a 70°C water bath, followed by 30 min in a 37°C water bath. Spin the tube briefly in a microcentrifuge to collect condensation. Place on ice. The oligonucleotide:template ratio is 2:1, but alternative ratios can be used (*see* Note 2).

2. To extend and ligate the mutant strand, add to the annealing reaction 10 μL dNTP mix A, 2.5 U T4 DNA ligase, and 0.8 U T7 DNA polymerase. Mix by brief vortexing followed by spinning the tube briefly in a microcentrifuge. Incubate for 10 min at room temperature, followed by 1 h in a 37°C water bath. Heat inactivate the enzymes for 10 min in a 70°C water bath. A 1-μL sample may be removed, added to 9 μL water, and stored at –20°C for analysis by agarose gel electrophoresis. Some mutations can be created more efficiently using Klenow instead of T7 polymerase, and advice on when to use each enzyme is given in Note 3.

3. Single-stranded, nonmutant DNA is removed by adding 50 μL buffer B and 2000 U T5 exonuclease to the extension reaction. Mix and incubate for 30 min in a 37°C water bath, then heat inactivate for 15 min in a 70°C water bath. Heat inactivation must be no shorter than 15 min; this is necessary to prevent T5 exonuclease degrading nicked DNA during the next step. If a heat block is used instead of a water bath, the time should be extended to 20 min to allow for less efficient heat transfer. A 10-μL sample for electrophoresis may be removed and stored at –20°C.

4. To nick the nonmutant strand, add 5 μL buffer C and 5 U *Nci*I to the T5 exonuclease digestion. Mix and incubate for 90 min in a 37°C water bath. A 10 μL sample for electrophoresis may be removed and stored at –20°C. When a site for *Nci*I occurs within the mutant oligonucleotide sequence, an alternative nicking enzyme must be used (*see* Note 4).

5. For digestion of the nonmutant strand, add to the nicking reaction 20 μL buffer D and 160 U exonuclease III. Mix and incubate for 30 min in a 37°C water bath, then heat inactivate for 15 min in a 70°C water bath. A 10 μL sample for electrophoresis may be removed and stored at –20°C.

6. To repolymerize the gapped DNA, add 20 μL dNTP mix B, 3.5 U DNA polymerase, and 2.5 U T4 DNA ligase. Mix and incubate for 1 h in a 37°C water bath. A 15-μL sample for electrophoresis may be removed and stored at –20°C.

3.3. Preparation of Competent Cells

1. *E. coli* TG1 cells are recommended for use with this method, as they have been found to give a higher transformation efficiency with phosphoro-thioate DNA than other similar strains. Streak out some cells on to a glu-cose/minimal medium plate and incubate at 37°C for 24–36 h until single colonies are visible.
2. Pick a single colony from a glucose/minimal medium plate into 10 mL 2X TY medium. Incubate overnight at 37°C with shaking.
3. Inoculate 40 mL 2X TY medium in 250 mL flasks with 400 μL of overnight culture. If M13 vectors are to be transformed then inoculate a second flask to produce lawn cells. Incubate at 37°C with shaking until the A_{600} reaches about 0.3 (approx 2 h). (Store one flask on ice for use as lawn cells.)
4. Transfer 40 mL culture to a chilled 50 mL disposable centrifuge tube. Spin at 4°C for 5 min at 2500*g* in a prechilled rotor. Pour off all traces of the supernatant and place the pellet on ice. Add 20 mL chilled, sterile 50 m*M* $CaCl_2$. Gently resuspend the pellet. Leave on ice for 20 min. Spin the cells down as before. Resuspend the cell pellet in 4 mL 50 m*M* $CaCl_2$. Store the cells on ice, or at 4°C until required. The transformation efficiency increases after several hours storage, and begins to decrease after 24 h (*see* Note 5).

3.4. Transformation and Plating Out
3.4.1. Mutants in M13 Vectors

1. Dispense 300 μL competent cells into 15-mL polypropylene culture tubes for the transformations and place them on ice. (These tubes, available from Falcon, give better transformation efficiencies than microcentrifuge tubes or polystyrene tubes.)
2. Add 10 μL of each repolymerization reaction to 90 μL water and mix. Diluting the repolymerization reaction before transformation improves the yield of plaques. Add 100 μL of the diluted repolymerization to each tube containing competent cells and mix gently by flicking the tube. Leave on ice for 40 min. Meanwhile, prepare some molten H top agar and place it in a water bath at 45–50°C.
3. Heat shock the cells by incubating in a 42°C water bath for 45 s. Return them to ice for 5 min. Add 200-μL lawn cells to each tube. To one tube at a time, add 3–4 mL molten H top agar, mix by rolling, and immediately pour onto an L plate. Once the agar has set, invert the plates, and incubate at 37°C overnight.

3.4.2. Mutants in Phagemid Vectors

1. Carry out step 1 as for mutants in M13 vectors, aliquoting 100 µL competent cells per transformation. Molten H top agar and lawn cells are not needed. Follow the method as for M13 vectors until the samples have been subjected to heat shock.
2. After the heat shock, add 100 µL 2X TY medium to each tube. Incubate at 37°C with shaking for 30 min. Pour the contents of each tube onto an L plate containing a suitable antibiotic for selection of the phagemid vector used (*see* data sheet with vector). Allow to set before inverting and incubating overnight at 37°C.

3.5. Analysis of Mutagenesis
by Agarose Gel Electrophoresis

1. Defrost the samples taken throughout mutagenesis and add 2 µL gel loading dye to each. Also prepare markers of 200 ng single-stranded template DNA and RF DNA.
2. Prepare a 1% agarose gel using 1X TBE, and 20 µL 5 mg/mL ethidium bromide per 100 mL gel. Also prepare 1X TBE running buffer containing 300 µL 2-mercaptoethanol/L. The 2-mercaptoethanol reduces nicking of samples during electrophoresis.
3. Load the samples and separate by electrophoresis at about 100 V until the dye front is about 4–5 cm from the wells. The bands on the agarose gel can be assigned to the different forms of DNA produced during the mutagenesis procedure (Fig. 2). Owing to the various buffer conditions in each sample, the same form of DNA can have a slightly different mobility in each track.

4. Notes

1. Successful mutagenesis is dependent on the design of the mutagenic oligonucleotide, which is important for the degree of polymerization achieved in the initial extension reaction. The oligonucleotide should be long enough that mismatches do not occur within the last few bases at either end as these may destabilize annealing. Approximately 10 perfectly matched bases on either side of a point mutation are normally sufficient. This should be increased for multiple mismatches. The stability of binding of the 3' and 5' ends is important. The GC content of each end of the oligonucleotide on either side of the mutation site should be approximately equal and ideally be greater than 50%. This is to allow efficient priming and ligation of the mutant strand.

   Potential secondary structure around the mutation site should also be considered. Secondary structure, such as hairpin formation, within the tem-

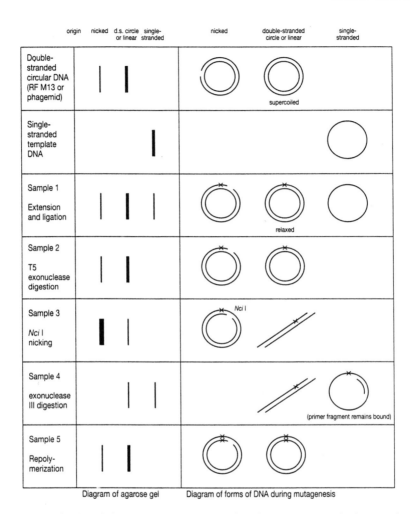

Fig. 2. Analysis of the mutagenesis reaction by agarose gel electrophoresis. The progress of the mutagenesis reaction can be monitored by agarose gel electrophoresis of samples taken after each step. The diagram shows the expected migration of the forms of DNA present in each sample relative to single- and double-stranded DNA markers.

plate may block the priming site. Within the oligonucleotide, it can prevent binding to the template or cause mispriming. Whenever possible, oligonucleotides should be positioned to avoid secondary structure. When this cannot be achieved, the length of the primer should be increased so that there are about 10 bases at each end complementary to regions outside the hairpin loop.

Analysis of the polymerization reaction by gel electrophoresis shows how successfully the mutant strand has been extended and ligated. The product of this reaction should be predominantly covalently closed circular DNA. Problems with this step may show as large amounts of single-stranded or nicked DNA, or as multiple bands due to incomplete polymerization. In this case, it may ultimately be necessary to redesign the oligonucleotide, but the strategies suggested in Notes 2 and 3 may be sufficient to resolve difficulties.

2. Increasing the oligonucleotide:template ratio in the annealing step can improve the degree of polymerization, particularly in cases of secondary structure (Note 1). Increasing the concentration of the oligonucleotide raises the amount of primer in the correct conformation to bind, and allows the oligonucleotide to compete successfully with template self-reannealing. Ratios of 5:1 or 10:1 are recommended, although increasing the oligonucleotide:template ratio also increases the probability of mispriming.

3. We have found that in cases of poor oligonucleotide binding, extension, and ligation are more successful when the reaction is performed at 16°C rather than 37°C. The lower incubation temperature appears to stabilize the bound oligonucleotide. T7 polymerase has very little activity at the reduced temperature, so Klenow polymerase is recommended for use when there is a possibility that secondary structure might interfere with extension and ligation. To use Klenow polymerase, 4 U should be substituted for T7 polymerase and the reaction should be incubated at 16°C overnight, followed by 15 min at 70°C.

4. When an *Nci*I site occurs within the mutant oligonucleotide it will not be protected from cleavage by incorporation of dCTPαS, so an alternative enzyme should be used. If a sample of the nicking reaction is analyzed by electrophoresis, the presence of a site in the oligonucleotide is seen as linear DNA instead of predominantly nicked DNA. Either *Ava*I (Amersham, E1007) or *Pvu*I (Amersham, E1075) can be used with minimal modifications to the standard protocol. *Pvu*I does not nick phosphorothioate-containing DNA as efficiently as either *Nci*I or *Ava*I. This results in an efficiency of mutagenesis of 40–66%. There is still a 90% probability of isolating a mutant if four transformants produced using *Pvu*I are analyzed. To use *Ava*I, 12 U should be substituted directly for *Nci*I. To use *Pvu*I, an alternative buffer B should be prepared (70 mM Tris-HCl, pH 8.0, 100 mM MgCl$_2$, 25 mM NaCl) and used in the T5 exonuclease reaction. For the nicking reaction use 24 U *Pvu*I and 5 μL standard buffer C.

5. Some apparent problems with mutagenesis can be traced to the preparation or transformation of competent cells. A low yield of transformants on all plates including the positive controls (single- or double-stranded template) suggests that the competent cell preparation has failed. It is important to keep the cells chilled at all times and handle them gently. A poor mutagenic efficiency coupled with transformants on the negative control plate (no DNA added) suggests that the competent cells are contaminated with nonmutants. Fresh cells should be prepared with fresh reagents, and disposable graduated pipets should be used for dispensing.

References

1. Taylor, J. W., Ott, J., and Eckstein, F. (1985) The rapid generation of oligonucleotide-directed mutations at high frequency using phosphorothioate-modified DNA. *Nucleic Acids Res.* **13**, 8764–8785.
2. Nakamaye, K. and Eckstein, F. (1986) Inhibition of restriction endonuclease *Nci*I cleavage by phosphorothioate groups and its application to oligonucleotide-directed mutagenesis. *Nucleic Acids Res.* **14**, 9679–9698.
3. Sayers, J. R., Krekel, C., and Eckstein, F. (1992) Rapid high efficiency site-directed mutagenesis via the phosphorothioate approach. *BioTechniques* **13**, 592–596.
4. Messing, J. (1983) New M13 vectors for cloning. *Methods Enzymol.* **101**, 20–78.
5. Viera, J. and Messing, J. (1987) Production of single-stranded plasmid DNA. *Methods Enzymol.* **153**, 3.
6. Sayers, J. R. and Eckstein, F. (1990) Properties of overexpressed phage T5 D15 exonuclease. *J. Biol. Chem.* **265**, 18,311–18,317.
7. Sayers, J. R. and Eckstein, F. (1991) A single-strand specific endonuclease activity copurifies with overexpressed T5 D15 exonuclease. *Nucleic Acids Res.* **19**, 4127–4132.
8. Sambrook, J., Fritsch, E. F., and Maniatis, T. (1989) *Molecular Cloning: A Laboratory Manual*, 2nd ed., Cold Spring Harbor Laboratory Press, Cold Spring Harbor, NY.

CHAPTER 6

Analysis of Point Mutations by Use of Amber Stop Codon Suppression

Scott A. Lesley

1. Introduction

It is often necessary to make multiple amino acid substitutions at a particular site to determine the function of the wild-type amino acid in protein structure and function studies. Each substitution requires a unique mutation at that site. An alternative to making a series of predetermined substitutions is to create a library of mutations at that site that encompasses all possible amino acid substitutions. The creation of such libraries is often simple. Screening the number of clones necessary to insure a complete representation of substitutions can be difficult and time consuming. Amino acid substitution by amber suppression provides an alternative to standard site-directed mutagenesis and library approaches *(1)*.

Secondary mutations were identified in *Escherichia coli* that suppressed the effects of amber (TAG) stop mutations in essential genes. These amber suppressors were found to map to tRNA genes and caused the insertion of a missense amino acid at the site of the amber stop codon and allowed translation to continue to produce a full-length functional protein. A number of these mutations were identified in different tRNAs which caused the insertion of different amino acids at the amber stop site. The anticodons of these tRNAs are a single base change away from recognizing an amber stop codon. tRNAs for insertion of other amino acids require multiple substitutions in the anticodon to allow them to recognize the amber stop. This precludes some of the tRNAs from being isolated as natural suppressors of amber stop codons. Many of these

From: *Methods in Molecular Biology, Vol. 57: In Vitro Mutagenesis Protocols*
Edited by: M. K. Trower Humana Press Inc., Totowa, NJ

tRNAs have been cloned and site-directed mutagenesis was used to change the anticodon for recognition of the amber stop codon *(2,3)*. The collection of natural and synthetic amber suppressors provides a set of strains, each of which causes the insertion of a different amino acid at the site of the amber stop mutation. The strains are used for protein structure/function studies by simply making a single amber stop mutation at the point of interest and transferring that amber mutant into each of the different suppressor strains *(see* Fig. 1). In this way a single point (amber) mutant can be used to determine the effect of up to 13 amino acid substitutions at a particular locus *(4–6)*.

This chapter describes the methods used for analysis by amber suppression. Amber stop mutations can be generated by any mutagenesis procedure. No description of the process of obtaining such mutants will be described here.

2. Materials

1. M9 minimal media plates: Dissolve 6 g of Na_2HPO_4, 3 g of KH_2PO_4, 0.5 g NaCl, and 1 g of NH_4Cl in 1 L of deionized H_2O. Add 15 g of agarose. Sterilize by autoclaving. Cool to 50°C and add 2 mL of $1M$ $MgSO_4$, 0.1 mL of $1M$ $CaCl_2$, 10 mL of 20% glucose, 10 mL of $0.1M$ thiamine-HCl, 10 mL of $0.1M$ methionine, and 10 mL of $0.1M$ proline. These solutions should be filter sterilized and added aseptically.
2. Resuspension buffer: 50 mM Tris-HCl, pH 7.5, 10 mM EDTA, 100 µg/mL RNaseA.
3. Lysis buffer: $0.2M$ NaOH, 1% SDS.
4. Neutralization buffer: $1.32M$ potassium acetate, pH 4.5.
5. Phenol:chloroform:isoamyl alcohol (25:24:1) mix.
6. Chloroform:isoamyl alcohol (24:1) mix.
7. Anhydrous and 70% ethanol.
8. TE: 10mM Tris-HCl, pH 7.5, 0.1 mM EDTA.
9. $0.1M$ $MgCl_2$.
10. $0.1M$ $CaCl_2$.
11. Sterile 80% glycerol.

3. Methods

3.1. Preparation of DNA for Transformation

The amber mutant for analysis should be generated in a construct that is compatible with all of the strains *(see* Notes 1 and 2). This mutant should be constructed such that the protein will be expressed in the *E. coli* host.

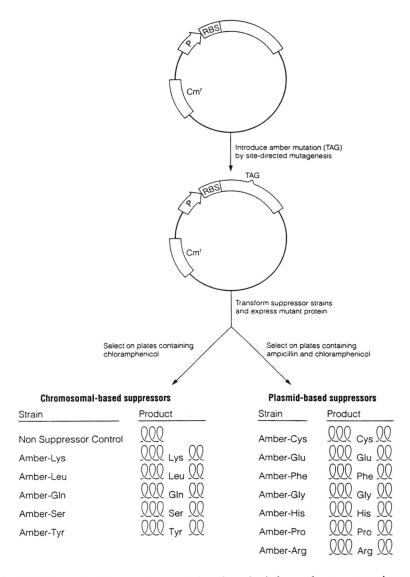

Fig. 1. Schematic diagram for mutational analysis by amber suppression using a vector with chloramphenicol resistance as an example. Strains are transformed with the expression vector containing the gene with the amber mutation. Those strains containing the suppressor tRNA on a plasmid are selected on media containing ampicillin as well as chloramphenicol. Expression of the amber mutant in the suppressor cell lines results in a missense incorporation at the site of the amber mutation. Cm^r (chloramphenicol resistance), P (promoter), rbs (ribosome binding site).

1. Prepare a culture for isolating the amber mutant plasmid by inoculating 50 mL of LB containing the appropriate antibiotic and incubating overnight at 37°C with shaking.
2. Pellet the cells from the overnight culture by centrifugation at 10,000g for 10 min.
3. Discard the supernatant and resuspend the cells in 10 mL of resuspension buffer.
4. Add 10 mL of lysis buffer to the cell resuspension and mix gently to lyse.
5. To the cleared lysate, add 10 mL of neutralization buffer and mix gently.
6. Pellet the cell debris by centrifugation at 10,000g for 15 min.
7. Remove the supernatant to a fresh polypropylene tube and add an equal volume of phenol:chloroform:isoamyl alcohol mix. Mix several times by inversion. Centrifuge at 10,000g for 10 min.
8. Remove the upper aqueous phase to a fresh polypropylene tube being careful to avoid any debris at the interface. Extract the aqueous phase with an equal vol of chloroform:isoamyl alcohol mix.
9. Centrifuge at 10,000g for 10 min to separate the phases. Remove the upper aqueous phase to a fresh tube and add 2 vol of anhydrous ethanol and mix by inversion. Let stand at room temperature for 30 min.
10. Pellet the DNA by centrifugation at 10,000g for 20 min. Discard the supernatant and rinse the pellet briefly with 70% ethanol. Allow the pellet to air dry.
11. Resuspend the pellet in 0.5 mL of TE.
12. DNA should be analyzed by agarose gel electrophoresis to determine purity and estimate the concentration.

3.2. Preparation of Competent Cells

Cells can be made competent by any of a number of established methods for inducing competency. The following method uses a traditional CaCl$_2$ protocol.

1. For each amber suppressor cell line, inoculate 5 mL of LB containing the appropriate antibiotic (*see* Table 1) from a stock. Incubate overnight at 37°C with shaking. Inoculate 50 mL of LB containing the appropriate antibiotic with 0.5 mL of overnight culture. Incubate at 37°C with shaking until an OD$_{600}$ nm of 0.5–0.8 is reached.
3. Place the culture on ice for 20 min.
4. Pellet the cells by centrifugation at 10,000g for 10 min in a sterile tube at 4°C. Discard the supernatant.
5. Resuspend the cells in 10 mL of 0.1M MgCl$_2$ at 4°C. Pellet the cells by centrifugation at 10,000g for 10 min in a sterile tube at 4°C. Discard the supernatant.

Table 1
Properties of Amber Suppressor Strains

Amino acid		Suppressor type	Locus	Antibiotic resistances
Alanine	A	Synthetic		amp
Cysteine	C	Synthetic		amp
Glutamic acid	E	Synthetic		amp
Phenylalanine	F	Synthetic		amp
Glycine	G	Synthetic		amp
Histidine	H	Synthetic		amp
Lysine	K	Natural	su5, *sup*G	tet
Leucine	L	Natural	su6, *sup*P	—
Proline	P	Synthetic		amp
Glutamine	Q	Natural	su2, *sup*E	—
Arginine	R	Synthetic		amp, tet
Serine	S	Natural	su1, *sup*D	—
Tyrosine	Y	Natural	su3, *sup*F	—

6. Resuspend the cells in 10 mL of $0.1M$ CaCl$_2$ at 4°C. Pellet the cells by centrifugation at $10,000g$ for 10 min in a sterile tube at 4°C. Discard the supernatant.
7. Resuspend the cells in 0.5 mL of $0.1M$ CaCl$_2$ at 4°C. Keep the cells on ice until ready to use.

3.3. Transformation of Suppressor Cell Lines

1. To 25 µL of competent cells prepared in Section 3.2., add approx 50–100 ng of the DNA prepared in Section 3.1. and incubate on ice for 30 min. The volume of the DNA should not exceed 2–5 µL for a 25-µL transformation.
2. Heat shock the cells for 2 min at 42°C and place on ice for 10 min.
3. Add 0.5 mL of LB to each transformation and incubate at 37°C with shaking for 1 h.
4. Plate 200 µL of each transformation onto LB plates containing the appropriate antibiotics. Incubate overnight at 37°C.

3.4. Analysis of Mutants

The method used for analysis of the various amino acid substitutions will depend on the protein to be assayed. This will require expression of the amber mutant in the suppressor strains and, unless a genetic screen is available, some type of enzyme assay (*see* Notes 3–7 for a discussion of important considerations for analysis). In preparation for this analysis, permanent stocks should be prepared from the transformants and their ability to suppress an amber stop confirmed.

1. Inoculate a tube containing 5 mL of LB plus the appropriate antibiotics for each transformant. Incubate with shaking overnight at 37°C.
2. Prepare a permanent stock from each culture by removing 0.8 mL of the overnight culture and adding it to 0.2 mL of sterile 80% glycerol and mixing by vortexing. Store the stock culture at −80°C.
3. Test the ability of the stock culture to suppress an amber stop by streaking from the stock culture onto a M9 (met pro thi glucose) plate described in Section 2.1. containing the appropriate antibiotics. Incubate at 37°C for 24–48 h to allow individual colony formation. Growth on M9 is an indication of suppressor function by suppression of the $argE^{am}$ mutation that allows growth in the absence of exogenous arginine.

4. Notes

1. Several of the suppressors are contained on plasmids. In order to use these suppressors, the gene containing the amber mutation must be able to cohabitate in the same cell. This can be done by infection of the suppressor cells with phage *(5)* or by the use of a compatible plasmid. The suppressors are on *col*E1-based plasmids that require the use of a plasmid containing a different origin of replication. Derivatives of pACYC184 that contain the p15a origin of replication are useful for cohabitation with the plasmid-based suppressors.
2. Expression of the protein in vivo requires the presence of the appropriate transcription and translation initiation signals. There are many examples of efficient bacterial expression systems that can be used. It is important to note that whatever system is used, all of the required components must be present in the cell. For example, T7 expression systems are inappropriate, since they require the presence of T7 RNA polymerase for expression. This polymerase typically is provided from the host strain and is not found in the suppressor strains. Expression systems that use *tac*, λP_L, or other promoters that utilize the host RNA polymerase are most suitable.
3. Expression levels of suppressed protein are dependent on the protein expression capability of the system used, the efficiency of the individual suppressor, and the stability of the suppressed protein in the cell. The expression systems recommended in Note 2 should provide sufficient protein for most applications. The efficiency of the suppression event is somewhat variable. Published suppression efficiencies typically range from 20–100% *(1)*. Any amber stop codon that is not suppressed results in a termination of translation and the formation of a truncated gene product. It

Table 2
Restrictions Sites That Can Be Introduced
in Conjunction with an Amber Stop Mutation

Restriction site	Recognition sequence	Potential amino acids		
		Position 1	Position 2	Position 3
*Bfa*I	5'CTAG 3'	G D V A S N I T C Y F R H L P	amber	
*Nhe*I	5' GCTAGC 3'	G S C R	amber	R Q H L P
*Spe*I	5' ACTAGT 3'	D N Y H	amber	W C Y L F S
*Xba*I	5' TCTAGA 3'	V I F L	amber	R S K N M L T
*Avr*II	5' CCTAGG 3'	A T S P	amber	G E D V A
*Bpu*1102 I	5' GCTTAGC 3'	A	amber	R Q H L P
*Bsu*36 I	5' CCTTAGG 3'	P	amber	G E D V A
*Sfc*I	5' CTRTAG 3'	L	amber	

is always prudent, therefore, to account for any residual activity of this truncated protein (*see* Note 6). The stability of a suppressed protein also effects its level in the cell, as does any mutation. Substitutions that cause misfolded products are likely to be degraded or insoluble. It is often desirable to determine the actual level of the suppressed gene product in order to get a more accurate determination of the substitution's effect on activity.

4. Amber mutations can be generated in the gene of interest by any number of procedures. It is often possible to incorporate a restriction site into the mutagenic oligo used that greatly facilitates the screening of such mutants. Table 2 lists a number of such sites and the amino acids that are tolerated in the adjacent positions. Owing to the degeneracy of the genetic code, 15 of the potential 20 amino acids in the proximal position to the amber can be incorporated with a *Bfa*I site.

5. The plasmid-based suppressors (especially the histidine and alanine suppressors) can be unstable when grown in the absence of selection for the suppressor function. The host strains contain an amber mutation in the arginine biosynthetic pathway. This mutation does not allow growth of these strains in the absence of added arginine except in the presence of the amber suppressor. It is prudent to maintain the cells on minimal media lacking arginine whenever possible to maintain the selection for the suppressor function.

6. A control strain lacking suppressor function should be used in all experiments to determine the activity of the truncated amber fragment. In most

Table 3
Amino Acid Substitutions for Phenylalanine at Position 25
in Chloramphenicol Acetyl Transferase by Amber Suppression

Amino acid substitution	In vivo phenotype[a]	Specific activity[b]
Cysteine	Cm[s]	dnb
Glutamic acid	Cm[s]	dnb
Phenylalanine	Cm[r]	150,000 U/mg
Glycine	Cm[s]	dnb
Histidine	Cm[r]	200,000 U/mg
Leucine	Cm[r]	20 U/mg
Proline	Cm[s]	dnb
Glutamine	Cm[s]	<5 U/mg
Serine	Cm[s]	<5 U/mg
Tyrosine	Cm[r]	500 U /mg
Stop	Cm[s]	nd

[a]Cm[r] = chloramphenicol resistant; Cm[s]= chloramphenicol sensitive.
[b]dnb = protein did not bind to affinity resin; nd = not determined.

cases, the truncated fragments have little or no activity. Since the suppression efficiency is not 100%, any residual activity of the truncated fragment should be accounted for. This control is also important to demonstrate the lack of any readthrough of the amber stop in the absence of the suppressor.

7. As with all types of mutagenesis, the affects of substitutions made by amber suppression are best characterized by specific activity rather than total activity in a cell lysate. In this way variations in the expression and stability of the mutant protein can be accounted for. Table 3 shows specific activity results for suppression of an amber mutation in the CAT gene. Suppressed protein was purified using a substrate analog affinity resin. Results in this case indicate that suppression with phe, his, tyr, or leu results in an enzyme that confers resistance to chloramphenicol but has dramatic differences in specific activity. The results also show that substitution with gln or ser results in an inactive protein without the loss of substrate binding. Substitution with other amino acids at this site results in a loss of substrate binding activity. These results demonstrate the amount of information that can be obtained from a single amber mutant.

Acknowledgments

Thanks to Mark Maffitt and Joe Ziegelbauer for their contributions to the results on the mutagenesis and analysis of the CAT enzyme.

References

1. Eggertsson, G. and Soll, D. (1988) Transfer ribonucleic acid-mediated suppression of termination codons in *Escherichia coli. Microbiol. Rev.* **52**, 354–374.
2. Kleina, L. G., Masson, J.-M., Normanly, J., Abelson, J., and Miller, J. H. (1990) Construction of *Escherichia coli* amber suppressor tRNA genes II. Synthesis of additional tRNA genes and improvement of suppressor efficiency. *J. Mol. Biol.* **213**, 705–717.
3. Normanly, J., Kleina, L. G., Masson, J.-M., Abelson, J., and Miller, J. H. (1990) Construction of *Escherichia coli* amber suppressor tRNA genes III. Determination of tRNA specificity. *J. Mol. Biol.* **213**, 719–726.
4. Miller, J. H. (1979) Genetic studies of the *lac* repressor XI. On aspects of *lac* repressor structure suggested by genetic experiments. *J. Mol. Biol.* **131**, 249–258.
5. Rennell, D., Bouvier, S. E., Hardy, L. W., and Poteete, A. R. (1991) Systematic mutation of bacteriophage T4 lysozyme. *J. Mol. Biol.* **222**, 67–87.
6. Markiewicz, P., Kleina, L. G., Cruz, C., Ehret, S., and Miller, J. H. (1994) Genetic studies of the *lac* Repressor XIV. Analysis of 4000 altered *Escherichia coli lac* repressor reveals essential and non-essential residues, as well as "spacers" which do not require a specific sequence. *J. Mol. Biol.* **240**, 421–433.

CHAPTER 7

A Simple Method
for Site-Directed Mutagenesis
with Double-Stranded Plasmid DNA

Derhsing Lai and Sidney Pestka

1. Introduction

Oligonucleotide-directed site-specific mutagenesis is a powerful tool to explore protein structure–function relationships. The single-stranded (M13) method *(1,2)*, the polymerase chain reaction (PCR) *(3–6)*, and the double-stranded plasmids method *(7–9)* are three basic procedures for these purposes. The single-stranded method developed by Zoller and Smith *(10)* has been modified to achieve a higher yield of mutants. Recently, the PCR method has become an easy and popular technique for site-directed mutagenesis. Both advantages and disadvantages of these methods have been discussed thoroughly *(11,12)*. Limitations of these methods include the availability of restriction sites for subcloning and the instability of large inserts in M13 vectors *(13)*, the low fidelity of *Taq* polymerase, the cost of multiple primers in the PCR protocols, and the low mutant yields with the double-stranded plasmid method.

Herein we describe a simple and efficient method for preparing site-specific mutations using double-stranded DNA requiring only a single synthetic primer for each mutant. Some subcloning steps are unnecessary and the mutant yield is theoretically 100% (*see* Note 1). A high mutation rate (58–97%) was achieved as measured by a phenotype assay restoring β-galactosidase activity (*see* Table 1). In theory, if two synthetic oligonucleotide primers are used, three separate mutations can be simultaneously created in a single reaction tube. In general, no special

From: *Methods in Molecular Biology, Vol. 57: In Vitro Mutagenesis Protocols*
Edited by: M. K. Trower Humana Press Inc., Totowa, NJ

Table 1
Mutation Rate

E. coli	DH5α	DH5α	JM109
Alkaline phosphatase	No	Yes	Yes
Blue/total	138/237[a]	16/18	126/130[a]
%	58	89	97

[a]Represents the combinations of three separate experiments.
The experiments with *E. coli* DH5α were performed as described
in Section 3., except as noted. An equal amount of fragment I (plasmid
pDL1 digested with *Xha*I, *Pst*I) and fragment II (*Xho*I, *Pst*I digested)
were incubated with a 500-fold excess of phosphorylated primer I.
Fragment I was dephosphorylated with alkaline phosphatase as noted
above. Site-specific mutagenesis was otherwise carried out as
described in the text. The ratio of blue to white colonies was used to
calculate the mutation efficiency. DNA from the blue colonies was
checked by restriction endonuclease *Cla*I digestion. The experiments
with *E. coli* JM109 were performed as the experiments with *E. coli*
DH5α with minor modifications: The *Xha*I, *Pst*I fragment (A–B fragment I, Fig. 1) was treated with alkaline phosphatase after the restriction enzyme digestion; *E. coli* JM109 competent cells and 2000-fold
excess of phosphorylated primer I were used. White colonies represented wild type and blue colonies, mutants.

Escherichia coli mutant strains, unusual nucleotides, or specific modification enzymes are required. The method may be used to generate base
changes, insertions, and deletions in a target DNA sequence.

A representative protocol for mutagenesis to generate site-directed
mutants directly with double-stranded plasmid DNA with high efficiency
is outlined herein. In this strategy (Fig. 1), restriction endonuclease A
must have complementary ends which are shared by the two double-
digested fragments I and II. There are no constraints for the other restriction endonucleases B and C except that they need to produce fragments I
and II. One or more B sites may be present in the gap produced by the A
and B double digestion (Fig. 1); and similarly one or more C sites may be
present in the gap produced by digestion with enzymes A and C (Fig. 1).
After reannealing and 3'-extension, duplexes I and II cannot religate since
they retain a 3'-overhang and a blunt end.

This mutation method has some advantages over others. Its efficiency
is as high as that of the single-stranded method. Moreover, the procedure
is more consistent and rapid compared to the single-stranded method
(1,2,10) because subcloning into either a single-stranded vector or a vec-

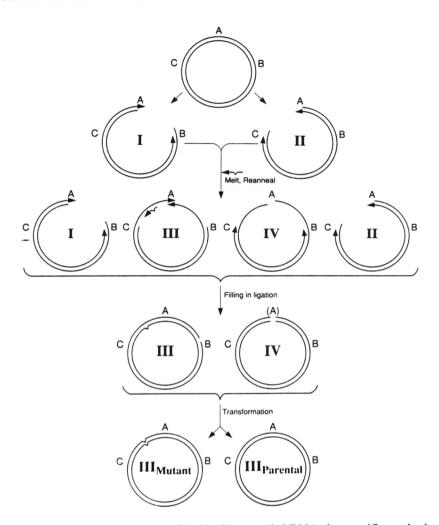

Fig. 1. Diagram of the strategy of the double-stranded DNA site-specific method with restriction endonuclease A producing a 3' overhang. The plasmids are digested with restriction endonucleases A and B and A and C to yield fragments I and II, respectively. In this example, the A restriction endonuclease site produces a 3'-protruding end. The B and C sites can be any sites flanking the target sequence. After denaturation and renaturation, the two homoduplexes (I, II) and two heteroduplexes (III, IV) are formed. The parental duplexes (I and II) and blunt-ended heteroduplex (IV) after filling in and ligation will yield no transformants. Only heteroduplex III can be extended and efficiently ligated. The A in parentheses means the site may no longer be intact after religation. The theoretical mutation percentage is 50%. In the example shown in the text and in Table 1, the restriction endonucleases are represented as follows: A, *Pst*I; B. *Xba*I; and C, *Xho*I. Arrowheads in the top half of the figure represent the 3' ends of the DNA strands. From ref. *14* with permission.

tor with an M13 origin can be omitted. In addition, the expense of primer synthesis is less than the cost of other PCR-based methods since only one primer is required. Recently, we have routinely used this method to create mutants of the extracellular domain of the murine interferon gamma receptor, mutant #4740 ($Lys^{111} \rightarrow$ Ala), mutant #4741 ($His^{196} \rightarrow$ Ala), and mutant #4136 ($Asp^{118} \rightarrow$ Ala) with mutation rates of 5, 3, and 10%, respectively.

2. Materials

1. Prepare double-stranded plasmid DNA using standard protocols. To demonstrate the utility of our method we constructed plasmid pDL 1. This is a pBluescript KS II phagemid vector modified by cutting the *Cla*I site within the polylinker, blunting the ends with the Klenow fragment of DNA polymerase I, and then religating. This eliminated the *Cla*I site and introduced a frameshift (two additional bases: CG) into the coding sequence for the *lac* α-peptide, resulting in a white colony phenotype on indicator plates.
2. Competent cells of *E. coli* DH5α and JM109 were prepared by the procedure of Nishimura et al. *(15)* (*see* Note 2).
3. Synthetic oligonucleotide primers (*see* Note 3). The mutagenic primer I (5'-CAAGCTTATCGATACCGTCG-3') was synthesized with a Millpore (Bedford, MA) DNA synthesizer model 8909. It was used to reconstruct the *Cla*I site in the *lacZ* gene of pDL1 by deletion of the two extra bases (CG) thereby restoring the wild-type *lac* α-peptide sequence, which in turn restores the blue colony phenotype. Primer I was incubated with T4 DNA kinase to phosphorylate the 5'-end (*see* Section 3.1., step 4).
4. Appropriate restriction endonucleases (Boehringer Mannheim, Indianapolis, IN).
5. Klenow fragment of DNA polymerase I (5 U/μL) (Boehringer Mannheim).
6. Alkaline phosphatase (Boehringer Mannheim).
7. T4 DNA ligase (2.5 U/μL) (Invitrogen, San Diego, CA).
8. 2.5 m*M* dNTP mix.
9. Geneclean kit (Bio 101, La Jolla, CA).
10. T4 Polynucleotide kinase (10 U/μL) (Gibco-BRL, Gaithersburg, MD).
11. Ampicillin (Sigma, St. Louis, MO).
12. Sequenase DNA polymerase (US Biochemicals, Cleveland, OH).
13. 200 mg/mL Isopropyl-β-D-thiogalactopyranoside (IPTG) (Calbiochem, La Jolla, CA).
14. 5-Bromo-4-chloro-3-indolyl-β-D-galactoside (X-gal): 20 mg/mL in dimethyl formamide.
15. TAE buffer: 0.04*M* Tris-acetate, 1 m*M* EDTA, pH 7.6.

16. Kinase buffer: 100 mM Tris-HCl, pH 7.6, 100 mM MgCl$_2$, 100 mM DTT, 50 mM EDTA, 100 mM spermidine-HCl.
17. 1 mM and 10 mM ATP solutions.
18. Ethanol: 70 and 95% solutions.
19. Hybridization solution: 172 mM NaCl, 12 mM Tris-HCl, pH 7.5, 14 mM MgCl$_2$, 1.7 mM 2-mercaptoethanol.

All other analytical grade chemicals were purchased from Fisher.

3. Method

The experimental procedure, a modification of that reported by Inouye and Inouye *(12)* is outlined in Fig. 1 or 2. The protocol is outlined here:

1. First, determine three restriction endonucleases sites (A, B, and C) to cover the mutagenesis target region (*see* Notes 3–5). In separate reaction tubes, digest the vector (5 µg) with 5 U each of enzymes A and B (pDL1 was double-digested with restriction endonucleases *Pst*I [A] and *Xha*I [B]) to produce fragment I, and A and C (for pDL1, *Pst*I [A] and *Xho*I [C] were used) to produce fragment II in a final reaction volume of 10 µL.
2. Without changing the buffer system, treat fragment I only (10 µL) with calf-intestinal alkaline phosphatase to remove 5'-phosphate termini by adding 1 U (1 U/µL) of this enzyme to the reaction mixture and then incubating for 15 min at 37°C. The addition of 1 µL of this modifying enzyme and the incubation period should be repeated.
3. Separate the digested fragments by gel electrophoresis in TAE buffer (1% agarose) at 94 V for 45 min and recover fragments I and II using a Geneclean kit.
4. Phosphorylate the mutagenic primer (150 pmol) (primer I for pDL1) with T4 polynucleotide kinase in kinase buffer and 1 mM ATP at 37°C for 1 h in a total volume of 50 µL. Precipitate the primer by addition of two volumes of ice-cold 95% ethanol at −20°C for 30 min and centrifugation at 14,000g at 4°C for 10 min to recover the DNA pellet. Wash the pellet with ice-cold 70% ethanol and recentrifuge at 14,000g for 5 min at 4°C. Repeat the wash and centrifugation step once more. Dry the pellet in a Speed-vac to remove any traces of ethanol and then resuspend it in a volume of 43 µL distilled water.
5. Mix equimolar amounts (0.3–0.4 µg) of DNA fragments I and II with either a 500- or 2000-fold molar excess of synthetic phosphorylated mutagenic primer in hybridization solution in a total volume of 35 µL. Control groups should be prepared containing no added primer. Cover reactions with 50 µL of light mineral oil to prevent evaporation and incubate in boiling water for 3 min to denature the DNA fragments.

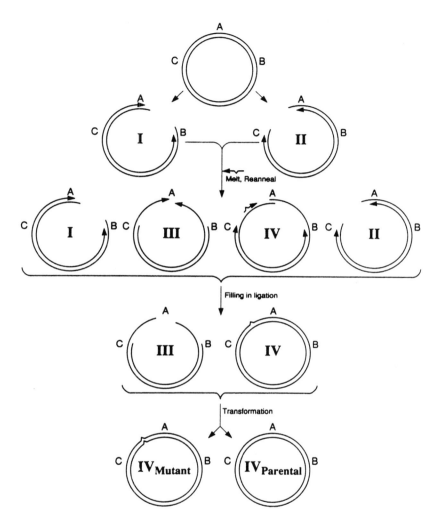

Fig. 2. Diagram of the strategy of the double-stranded DNA site-specific method with restriction endonuclease A producing a 5' overhang. If restriction endonuclease A is chosen to be one that produces a 5' overhang, then the mutation oligonucleotide must be complementary to the opposite strand as that shown in heteroduplex III of Fig. 1, and only heteroduplex IV produces a functional closed single-stranded circle after ligation. From ref. *14* with permission.

6. After denaturation, transfer mixtures to 30°C for 30 min then to 4°C for 30 min and then keep for at least 10 min on ice to allow the denatured DNA fragments to reanneal (*see* Note 6).

7. The formation of new heteroduplex DNAs (additional DNA band) is essential and should be confirmed by 1% agarose gel electrophoresis in TAE buffer before proceeding to the next step.

8. To extend the 3' ends and ligate the resulting heteroduplex plasmid (III, Fig. 1), incubate 11.6 μL of the reaction mixture with either 5 U of Sequenase or the Klenow fragment of DNA polymerase I (0.4 μL), 2 μL of T4 DNA ligase (2 U), 4 μL 2.5 mM dNTPs, and 2 μL 10 mM ATP in a final volume of 20 μL at 15°C overnight.

9. After the overnight incubation, transform competent bacteria with 5 μL of the mixture onto LB agar plates containing suitable antibiotics (e.g., 100 μg/mL ampicillin) at 37°C overnight (*see* Note 7).

10. This step is used only for the β-galactosidase phenotype assay. Prior to plating the bacteria, coat the surface of the plate with 44 μL X-gal solution and 4 μL IPTG solution *(16)*. Use the ratio of blue to white colonies to calculate the mutation efficiency. Because the transformation is performed with double-stranded DNA, each blue colony represents a 50% mixture of the wild-type and mutant plasmids.

11. To isolate the mutant plasmid, prepare a miniprep from each colony containing the mixture of wild-type and mutant plasmids using standard protocols *(16)*. Transform the plasmid DNA into competent *E. coli* cells as in step 10. Confirm that pure mutant plasmid DNA has been isolated by sequencing.

This method may be used with any plasmids containing three suitable restriction enzyme sites to generate base changes, deletions, and insertions in the target DNA. The method is a general one that is convenient and rapid. Insertion and deletion mutants can be easily identified without the need for sequencing by either PCR analysis or colony hybridizations. In fact, even single base changes can be identified rapidly by PCR by preparing an oligonucleotide with the mutant base at the 3'-end *(17,18)*. Since no specific plasmids or *E. coli* strains are required, the simplicity and high efficiency of this method should make it a useful general procedure for preparing site-specific mutations in double-stranded DNA.

In theory the same procedure can be modified by using two primers simultaneously to generate three mutants (two single mutants, one double mutant) in the same experiment (Fig. 3).

4. Notes

1. In practice, the mutant yield may be somewhat lower than the theoretical ratios although they approximated the theoretical values as shown in Table 1. This is assumed to be owing to such factors as incomplete in vitro DNA polymerization, primer displacement by the DNA polymerase used to fill

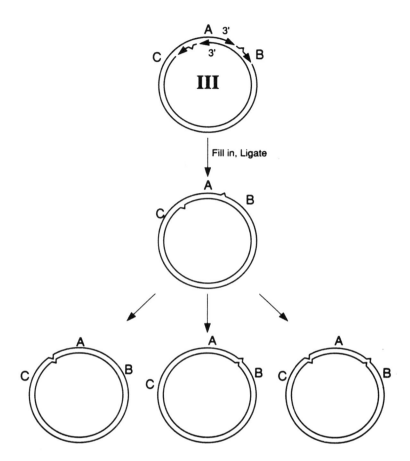

Fig. 3. Diagram of the strategy with two synthetic primers. This represents a variation of the procedure shown in Fig. 1 with the use of two oligonucleotide primers to produce two single and one double mutation simultaneously. Dephosphorylation of fragment I (Fig. 1) is not carried out. From ref. *14* with permission.

in the strands, and efficiency of primer phosphorylation. Also, the secondary structure of the single-stranded region may prevent the primer from hybridizing to the target sequence. The larger the single-stranded region, the higher the possibility of intrastrand secondary structure. The single-stranded gapped region should therefore be kept as short as possible. The PCR method may avoid this by use of high temperature annealing and polymerization. The only major source of background colonies results from strand extension without the primer hybridized to the target sequence. This can occur in all mutagenesis methods.

Double-Stranded Plasma DNA

83

2. We did not use a repair minus *E. coli* strain (e.g., BMH 71–18 *mutS*) *(19,20)* in these experiments because our actual mutation rates were almost equivalent to the theoretical rates. This strain suppresses in vitro mismatch repair and was used to construct two mutants of the soluble receptor for murine interferon gamma (data not shown). However, the mutation rate was not significantly different between the bacterial strains. Thus, special strains are not critical for this method.

3. Various computer programs including FOLDRNA and PRIME in the GCG package can be used to assist in primer design. If a unique restriction site is incorporated in the primer, positive clones can be easily identified by restriction enzyme digestion.

4. When restriction endonuclease A produces a 3' overhang (e.g., *Pst*I), Duplex IV produces a blunt-ended DNA that will not be religated significantly at the low concentrations of the ligase used. This was confirmed by demonstrating that blunt-ended heteroduplex DNA produced no colonies after this transformation method (data not shown). Duplex III, therefore, is the only one that can anneal and religate efficiently after 3'-extension. This design provides a theoretical mutation rate of 100%. Although it was not necessary to dephosphorylate fragment I, its dephosphorylation increased mutation efficiency significantly (Table 1).

5. It should be noted that if restriction endonuclease A is chosen with a 5' overhang, then duplex III cannot be extended and filled in (Fig. 2). The oligonucleotide must be complementary to the opposite strand as that shown in Fig. 1 (heteroduplex III) so that heteroduplex IV is the only one that religates the outer strand.

6. A thermal cycler may be used to create a continuous temperature gradient declining from 95–30°C over a period of 30 min.

7. In situations in which no indicator (e.g., the β-galactosidase phenotype assay) is available, prepare a total plasmid prep from the colonies plated out in Section 3., step 9. Clonal segregation may then be achieved by transformation of the plasmid DNA pool into a competent strain of *E. coli*. To ensure that this process is efficient, prolong the incubation period in the growth medium from the normal 1–2 to 2.5–3 h. After plating onto appropriate selection medium, either colony hybridization or PCR screening may be used to identify mutant clones.

Acknowledgments

We thank Eleanor Kells for her expert assistance in the preparation of this manuscript. This study was supported in part by United States Public Health Service Grants CA46465 and CA52363 from the National Institutes of Health awarded to S. Pestka.

References

1. Derbyshire, K. M., Salvo, J. J., and Grindley, N. D. F. (1986) A simple and efficient procedure for saturation mutagenesis using mixed oligodeoxynucleotides. *Gene* **46**, 145–152.
2. Li, B., Langer, J. A., Schwartz, B., and Pestka, S. (1989) Creation of phosphorylation sites in proteins: construction of a phosphorylatable human interferon α. *Proc. Natl. Acad. Sci. USA* **86**, 558–562.
3. Hignichi, R., Krummel, B., and Saiki, R. K. (1988) A general method of in vitro preparation and specific mutagenesis of DNA fragments: study of protein and DNA interactions. *Nucleic Acids Res.* **16**, 7351–7367.
4. Vallette, F., Mege, E., Reiss, A., and Adesnik, M. (1989) Construction of mutant and chimeric genes using the polymerase chain reaction. *Nucleic Acids Res.* **17**, 723–733.
5. Kadowaki, H., Kadowaki, T., Wondisford, F. E., and Taylor, S. I. (1989) Use of polymerase chain reaction catalyzed by Taq DNA polymerase for site-specific mutagenesis. *Gene* **76**, 161–166.
6. Ho, S., Hunt, H. D., Horton, R. M., Pullen, J. K., and Pease, L. R. (1989) Site-directed mutagenesis by overlap extension using the polymerase chain reaction. *Gene* **77**, 51–59.
7. Vlasuk, G. P. and Inouye, S. (1983) Site-specific mutagenesis vising synthetic oligodeoxyribonucleotides as mutagens, in *Experimental Manipulation of Gene Expression*, Appendix 2 (Inouye, M., ed.), Academic, New York, pp. 291–303.
8. Morinaga, Y., Franceschini, T., Inouye, S., and Inouye, M. (1984) Improvement of oligonucleotide-directed site-specific mutagenesis using double-stranded plasmid DNA. *Bio/Technology* **2**, 636–639.
9. DeChiara, T. M., Erlitz, F., and Tarnowski, S. J. (1986) Procedures for in vitro DNA mutagenesis of human leukocyte interferon sequences. *Methods Enzymol.* **119**, 403–415
10. Zoller, M. J. and Smith, M. (1982) Oligonucleotide-directed mutagenesis using M13-derived vectors: an efficient and general procedure for the production of point mutations in any fragment. *Nucleic Acids Res.* **10**, 6487–6500.
11. Jones, D. H. and Howard, B. H. (1990) A rapid method for site-specific mutagenesis and directional subcloning by using the polymerase chain reaction to generate recombinant circles. *BioTechniques* **8**, 178–183.
12. Inouye, S. and Inouye M. (1987) Oligonucleotide-directed site-specific mutagenesis using double-stranded plasmid DNA, in *Synthesis and Applications of DNA and RNA* (Narang, S. A., ed.), Academic, New York, pp. 181–206.
13. Cordell, B., Bell, G., Tisher, E., DeNoto, F. M., Ullrich, A., Pictet, R., Rutter, W. J., and Goodman, N. M. (1979) Isolation and characterization of a cloned rat insulin gene. *Cell* **18**, 533–543.
14. Lai, D., Zhu, X., and Pestka, S. K. (1993) A simple and efficient method for site-directed mutagenesis using double-stranded plasmid DNA. *Nucleic Acids Res.* **21**, 3977–3980.
15. Nishimura, A., Morita, M., Nishimura, Y., and Sugino, Y. (1990) A rapid and highly efficient method for preparation of competent *Escherichia coli* cells. *Nucleic Acids Res.* **18**, 6169.

16. Sambrook, J., Fritsch, E. F., and Maniatis, T. (1989) *Molecular Cloning: A Laboratory Manual*, 2nd ed., Cold Spring Harbor Laboratory Press, Cold Spring Harbor, NY.
17. Newton, C. R., Graham, A., Heptinstall, L. E., Powell, S. J., Summers, C., Kalsheker, N., Smith, J. C., and Markham, A. F. (1989) Analysis of any point mutation in DNA. The amplification refractory mutation system (ARMS). *Nucleic Acids Res.* **17,** 2503–2515.
18. Sommer, S. S., Cassady, J. D., Sobell, J. L., and Bottema, C. D. K. (1989) A novel method for detecting point mutations or polymorphisms and its application to population screening for carriers of phenylketonuria. *Mayo Clin. Proc.* **64,** 1361–1372.
19. Kramer, B., Kramer, W., and Fritz, H. J. (1984) Different base/base mismatches are corrected with different efficiencies by the methyl-directed DNA mismatch-repair system of *E. coli. Cell* **38,** 879–887.
20. Zell, R. and Fritz, H. J. (1987) DNA mismatch repair in *Escherichia coli* counteracting the hydrolytic deamination of 5-methyl-cytosine residues. *EMBO J.* **6,** 1809–1815.

CHAPTER 8

Double-Stranded DNA
Site-Directed Mutagenesis

Stéphane Viville

1. Introduction

It is now technically possible to create any desired mutation in a given DNA sequence. So-called site-directed mutagenesis allows the introduction of designed mutations into specific locations. This approach is invaluable for studying gene regulation as well as for functional assessment of proteins and their interactions. Several protocols have been successfully employed to generate such mutants. Here I describe a "linker-scanning" method that I have used to systematically mutate the murine major histocompatibility complex (MHC) class II Eα gene promoter (Fig. 1, ref. *1*).

1.1. General Considerations

All site-directed mutagenesis is based on the use of synthetic oligonucleotides that contain the desired mutations. Although single-stranded DNA vectors (generally based on M13) *(2)* and the polymerase chain reaction (PCR) *(3,4)* have been most widely employed, the linker-scanning method offers several advantages. Because mutations are introduced directly into a double-stranded plasmid template, the amount of subcloning required is minimal and PCR errors are completely eliminated. In addition, double-stranded templates allow cloning of larger target fragments and are much more stable than single-stranded templates.

In principle, this protocol is similar to those involving single-stranded DNA templates. Basically, a frame of single-stranded DNA encompassing

From: *Methods in Molecular Biology, Vol. 57: In Vitro Mutagenesis Protocols*
Edited by: M. K. Trower Humana Press Inc., Totowa, NJ

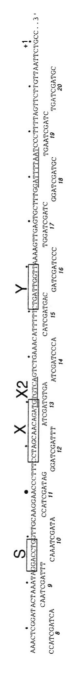

Fig. 1. Linker-scanning mutation of the Eα promoter: The sequence of each of the 10-bp linker-scanning mutations (numbered 1–20) is shown under the wild-type Eα promoter sequence. Class II regulatory motifs are underlined or boxed (reproduced from ref. 1).

only the region of interest is created within a double-stranded plasmid. The mutagenic oligonucleotide is used as a primer for the Klenow fragment of DNA polymerase I (Klenow) that synthesizes the second strand of the target region, and the free ends are joined by T4 DNA ligase. To generate the single-stranded target sequence, two distinct forms of the template plasmid are produced by digestion with appropriate restriction enzymes. For the first, the target sequence is completely excised from the plasmid; for the second, the plasmid is linearized outside the target sequence. The two forms are mixed, denatured, and allowed to reanneal. During this process four hybrids are produced: Two correspond to the original forms and two are heteroduplexes, each containing a stretch of single-stranded DNA encompassing the target sequence (Fig. 2). The mutagenic oligonucleotide will anneal to one of these heteroduplexes. Incubating a mixture of hybrid plasmids and mutagenic oligonucleotides with Klenow and T4 ligase will engender two types of viable plasmids: wild type and those carrying the desired mutation. Using the mutagenic oligonucleotide as a probe, it is fairly straightforward to screen colonies for the mutated plasmid. In practice, between 1 and 20% of the transformants carry the mutation. The protocol described in the following is based on the previously described "gapped heteroduplex" method *(5)* that I have simplified at several steps.

2. Materials

This protocol requires at least two or three restriction endonucleases, the Klenow fragment of DNA polymerase I, T4 ligase, polynucleotide kinase, and calf intestinal phosphatase (CIP). These enzymes are commonly used in a variety of molecular biology protocols and are commercially available. Complete descriptions of their activities are outlined in *Molecular Cloning: A Laboratory Manual (6)*. Storage, working conditions, and often appropriate buffers are supplied by the manufacturers. Solutions should be prepared using deionized water and molecular biology-grade reagents. Use high-quality phenol, chloroform, and ethanol.

2.1. Preparation of the Plasmid Fragment

1. Phenol: Phenol must be equilibrated to pH 7.0–7.5 with Tris-HCl prior to use. (Follow the protocol recommended by the supplier or in ref. *6*.) Equilibrated phenol can be stored (under water) at 4°C for 1 or 2 mo, but should be kept in aliquots at –20°C for long-term storage.

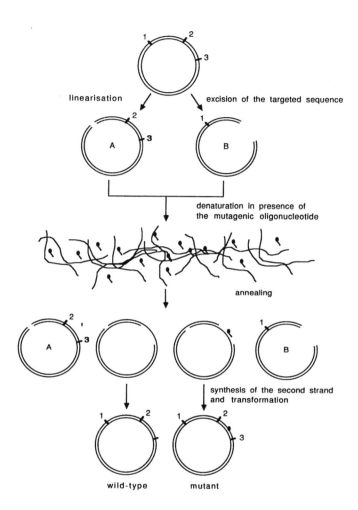

Fig. 2. Site-directed mutagenesis using a double-stranded DNA plasmid. This technique is based on the creation of a stretch of single-stranded DNA within double-stranded plasmids. To accomplish this, two forms of the plasmid are produced: **(A)** the plasmid is linearized outside of the target sequence, and **(B)** the target sequence is excised. When these two DNA fragments are denatured and allowed to reanneal in the presence of the mutagenic oligonucleotide, four distinct hybrids are formed. Two are heteroduplexes containing a stretch of single-stranded DNA. The mutagenic oligonucleotide hybridizes to one of these and serves as a primer for synthesis of the second strand. In theory, 33% of the transformed bacteria should contain the mutant plasmid.

Site-Directed Mutagenesis

2. 3*M* Na acetate (pH 5.6): Sterilize by autoclaving; store at room temperature.
3. TE buffer: 10 m*M* Tris-HCl, pH 7.4, 1 m*M* EDTA. Store at room temperature.
4. Gene-Clean kit: Available from Bio 101 (La Jolla, CA).

2.2. Phosphorylation of the Mutagenic Oligonucleotide

1. Mutagenic oligonucleotide: Appropriate design of mutagenic oligonucleotides is critical; each must contain an informative mutation along with sufficient homology to facilitate hybridization to the target plasmid *(see* Note 1). If you do not have access to an oligonucleotide synthesizer, oligonucleotides are commercially available from a variety of companies.
2. ATP: 10 m*M* adenosine triphosphate in TE buffer. Aliquot and store at −20°C.
3. 10X Nick translation NT buffer: 0.5*M* Tris-HCl, pH 7.5, 0.1*M* MgSO₄, 1 m*M* dithiothreitol, 500 µg/mL bovine serum albumin (Fraction V, Sigma, St. Louis, MO). Store in small aliquots at −20°C.

2.3. Site-Directed Mutagenesis

1. 1*M* NaCl: Sterilize by autoclaving; store at room temperature.
2. dNTP mix: 5 m*M* of each deoxynucleotide (dGTP, dATP, dCTP, and dTTP) in TE buffer. Store in small aliquots at −20°C.
3. Competent *Escherichia coli* cells: I have successfully used both MC1061 and DH5α strains *(see* Note 2).
4. 2X YT medium: To make 1 L dissolve 16 g of bactotryptone, 10 g yeast extract, and 10 g NaCl. Sterilize by autoclaving; store in a dark place.
5. 15% 2YT agar: To 1 L of 2X YT medium add 15 g of agar just prior sterilization; pour into sterile Petri dishes (30 mL/90-mm dish) after it has cooled to 50°C. For antibiotic plates, add the appropriate amount of antibiotic required immediately before pouring the medium *(see* Note 3).

3. Methods

3.1. Preparation of the Plasmid Fragments

3.1.1. Linearizing the Plasmid

As stated earlier, the plasmid containing the target must be linearized at a unique restriction site located outside of the target sequence. Subsequent treatment of the linearized plasmid with alkaline phosphatase, to eliminate the two 5' phosphates which are required for relegation of the plasmid, markedly decreases the efficiency of unwanted self-ligation.

1. Digest 10 µg of plasmid with the chosen enzyme; generally, incubation with 25 U of enzyme (2.5 U/µg) for 2 h under appropriate conditions (in a volume of 100 µL) is sufficient. A small aliquot (2–3 µL) should be run on an agarose gel to ensure that digestion is complete *(see* Note 4).

2. Increase the volume of the digestion reaction to 200 μL with water and add 0.5 U of CIP. Incubate for 30 min at 37°C. Inactivate the enzyme by heating the mixture for 15 min at 65°C.

3. Extract once with an equal volume of phenol:chloroform (1:1) and then with an equal volume of chloroform. Add 1/10 vol (20 μL) of 3*M* Na acetate (pH 5.6) and precipitate the DNA with 2.5 vol (500 μL) of 100% ethanol.

4. Pellet the DNA in a microfuge for 10 min and wash once with 500 μL of 70% ethanol. Dry and resuspend in 20 μL of TE.

5. To estimate the DNA concentration, run a 2-μL sample on an agarose gel with standard fragments of known concentration. The concentration should be approx 400–500 ng/μL. Hereafter, I will refer to this fragment as "A" (DNA fragment A, Fig. 2).

3.1.2. Excision of the Target Locus

The target region should be between 400 bp and 1 kb in length and can be excised by one enzyme for which two sites exist (one on each side of the sequence of interest) or by two enzymes (which cut at two unique restriction sites that flank the target locus; *see* Note 5). If one enzyme is used, CIP treatment will be required; if two are used, this will not be necessary unless they generate cohesive ends (which is rare).

1. Digest 10 μg of the plasmid as described in Section 3.1.1.

2. Separate the two fragments on an appropriate agarose gel and cut out a slice of agarose containing the plasmid with the targeted region excised.

3. Purify using the Gene-Clean kit (*see* Note 6).

4. Evaluate the concentration of the DNA solution by electrophoresis as in Section 3.1.1. It is preferable to run fragment A alongside.

This fragment is referred to as DNA fragment B (Fig. 2).

3.2. Phosphorylation of the Mutagenic Oligonucleotide

To serve as a substrate for T4 DNA ligase, the mutagenic oligonucleotide must be phosphorylated.

1. Add 7 μL of oligonucleotide (10 pmol/μL), 1 μL of 10 m*M* ATP, 1 μL of 10X NT buffer, 1 U of T4 polynucleotide kinase, and water to a final volume of 10 μL.

2. Incubate for 30 min at 37°C. To inactivate the enzyme, incubate for 10 min at 65°C (*see* Note 7).

No further purification is required.

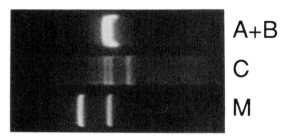

Fig. 3. Assessment of the denaturation/annealing step. If denaturation/
annealing of the two DNA fragments, A + B, results in the formation of heteroduplexes, an additional band, C, should be apparent when the annealed mixture is run on an agarose gel. Lane 1, fragments A and B prior to denaturation/
annealing; lane 2, fragments A and B after denaturation/annealing; lane 3 size
markers (M).

3.3. Site-Directed Mutagenesis

1. To create the heteroduplex plasmid and allow hybridization of the
   mutagenic oligonucleotide, assemble 200–400 ng of DNA fragment A,
   200–400 ng of DNA fragment B, 2.5 µL of 10X NT buffer, 2.5 µL of 1M
   NaCl, 3 µL of 5'-phosphorylated oligonucleotide (21 pmol), and water to a
   final volume of 24 µL. Remove 8 µL to use as a control later.
2. Denature-anneal the fragments by heating the mixture to 100°C for 3 min.
   Put at room temperature for 20 min and then cool on ice for 30 min. Centrifuge for 30 s in a microfuge.
3. Remove 8 µL and run on a 1% agarose gel with the control aliquot from step
   1. If heteroduplex plasmids have formed, an additional band (larger than
   the two initial fragments) will be apparent in the denatured/annealed DNA
   sample (*see* Fig. 3). If this band is not visible, do not proceed.
4. Mix 8 µL of annealed fragments, 2 µL of 10 mM ATP, 2 µL of 5 mM
   dNTP, 0.5 µL of Klenow enzyme (4 U/µL), 2 µL of T4 DNA ligase (0.6 U/
   µL), and water to a final volume of 15 µL. Incubate this mixture overnight
   (or longer than 8 h) at 15°C.
5. Mix 7 µL of the elongation-ligation mixture with 100 µL of competent
   E. coli (*see* Note 8) and incubate for 20 min in an ice/water mix.
6. Follow by heat shock for 3 min at 37°C. Dilute the cells with 700 µL of 2X
   YT and incubate for 45 min at 37°C with shaking.
7. Plate 200 µL of the bacteria onto each of four agar plates containing an
   appropriate selective antibiotic (*see* Note 9).

Screening of transformants (*see* Note 10) can be carried out in a number of ways, but one of the most reliable is that described by Hanahan and Meselson *(7)*. Essentially, the colonies are transferred to a membrane (nitrocellulose or nylon), the bacteria lysed, and the DNA denatured with NaOH. The DNA is fixed to the membrane and can then be hybridized with the mutagenic oligonucleotide. Detailed, reliable protocols can also be found in ref. *6*. Once the clones of interest have been identified, it is a good idea to confirm the mutation by sequencing (*see* Note 11). Double-stranded sequencing can be carried out on DNA from minipreps following the method described by Jones and Schofield. *(8)*.

4. Notes

1. In general, the length of homologous sequence should be proportional to the mismatches that create the mutation, and each should be between 5 and 15 bp. Long oligonucleotides (>35 bp) are expensive and occasionally difficult to synthesize. It is possible to design the oligonucleotides such that a restriction site is either created or eliminated in the mutant. This strategy simplifies the characterization of the mutants and can facilitate further manipulation of the DNA.
2. Many bacterial strains are available and can be used.
3. For ampicillin add 1 mL of a 50 mg/mL solution of ampicillin to 1 L of 2X YT agar.
4. Avoid loading samples directly from the refrigerator or freezer since in some cases the DNA may form secondary structures that are stable at low temperature. Heat samples 5 min at 65°C to eliminate this effect.
5. If the enzymes require different NaCl concentrations, digest first at the lower concentration, then increase the volume and adjust the NaCl concentration for the second enzyme.
6. Any method for purifying DNA from agarose gels can be used. One other method I recommend is electrophoresis onto DEAE-cellulose membrane as described in ref. *6*.
7. This reaction can be monitored by adding 1 μL of [γ-^{32}P]ATP (3000 Ci/mmol) to the reaction. If the reaction works properly, the [^{32}P]ATP will be incorporated; this can be assessed by TCA precipitation or by running a small sample on a polyacrylamide gel and exposing it to film.
8. Competent bacteria with transformation efficiencies >10^6 colonies/μg of DNA should be used. This can be easily achieved by the following protocol: Inoculate 10 mL of 2X YT with a single colony of fresh DH5α and grow at 37°C until an OD_{600} 0.4–0.6 is reached (it should take 3–5 h). Pellet the bacteria (5 min at 4000 rpm), discard the supernatant, and wash

with 10 mL of cold CaCl$_2$ (100 mM). Pellet again and resuspend the bacteria in 2 mL of cold CaCl$_2$ (100 mM). Store at 4°C for 2–48 h. One hundred microliters are used for each transformation following the standard protocol *(6)*.

9. All transformations should include at least two controls: one sample in which no DNA is added and one in which 1 ng of an intact plasmid is present.

10. There could be many reasons for the lack of colonies after the transformation (e.g., the bacteria are not competent; Klenow and/or T4 DNA ligase are deficient, etc.).

11. The two main problems that can occur with this site-directed mutagenesis method are: First, it is possible not to get the desired mutation. This is generally owing to either the poor quality of the DNA fragments or of the oligonucleotide used. Repurification of the DNA is recommended before repeating the experiment. The oligonucleotide can be purified by polyacrylamide gel electrophoresis. Second, it is possible to get the mutation at the wrong site. In this case, it is owing to the fact that the complementary sequences of the mutagenic oligonucleotide are not sufficiently long enough on either side of the target base(s) to be mutagenized. In such a case, new, longer mutagenic primers should be prepared.

References

1. Viville, S., Jongeneel, V., Koch, W., Mantovani, R., Benoist, C., and Mathis, D. (1991) The E promoter: a linker-scanning analysis. *J. Immunol.* **146,** 3211–3217.
2. Wallace, R. B., Schold, M., Johnson, M. J., Dembek, P., and Itakura, K. (1981) Oligonucleotide directed mutagenesis of the human -globin gene: a general method for producing specific point mutations in cloned DNA. *Nucleic Acids Res.* **9,** 3647–3656.
3. Nelson, R. M. and Long, G. L. (1989) A general method of site-specific mutagenesis using a modification of the *Thermus aquaticus* polymerase chain reaction. *Anal. Biochem.* **180,** 147–151.
4. Hemsley, A., Arnheim, N., Toney, M. D., Cortopassi, G., and Galas, D. J. (1989) A simple method for site directed mutagenesis using the polymerase chain reaction. *Nucleic Acids Res.* **16,** 6545–6551.
5. Inouye, S. and Inouye, M. (1987) Oligonucleotide-directed site-specific mutagenesis using double-stranded DNA, in *Synthesis and Application of DNA and RNA,* (Narang, S. A., ed.), Academic, Orlando, FL, pp. 181–206.
6. Maniatis, T., Fritsch, E., and Sambrook, J. (1989) *Molecular Cloning: A Laboratory Manual,* 2nd ed., Cold Spring Harbor Laboratory Press, Cold Spring Harbor, NY.
7. Hanahan, D. and Meselson, M. (1980) Plasmid screening at high colony density. Gene **10,** 63–67.
8. Jones, D. S. and Schofield, J. P. (1990) A rapid method for isolating high quality plasmid DNA suitable for DNA sequencing. *Nucleic Acids Res.* **18,** 7463,7464.

CHAPTER 9

Solid-Phase In Vitro Mutagenesis Using a Plasmid DNA Template

Roy Edward

1. Introduction

Oligonucleotide-mediated mutagenesis is a predictable and flexible means of introducing very specific changes into cloned DNA sequences to facilitate study of structure–function relationships or modification of restriction endonuclease restriction sites. Several novel polymerase chain reaction (PCR)-based methods of in vitro mutagenesis have been described *(1–6)*. Site-specific mutations are created by introducing mismatches into the oligonucleotides used to prime the in vitro amplification step. Among these PCR-based mutagenesis systems is splicing by overlap extension *(1–5)*, which involves a two-step PCR, followed by cloning of blunt-end products requiring restriction digestion of the PCR product as well as a ligation step. A modification *(7)* simplifies the removal of excess primers and wild-type template, utilizing biotinylated primers and streptavidin-coated magnetic beads to purify the PCR products. Alternatively, PCR amplification is used to create recombinant plasmid circles with discrete, cohesive single-stranded ends *(6)*. This method also requires purification steps to remove excess primers. These circles, formed without the use of restriction enzyme digestion or ligation, provide high yields of mutants. However, since the entire vector sequence must be PCR amplified, this method may be limited to relatively small vectors when using standard *Taq* polymerase because of both its frequency of misincorporation and difficulties with amplification of larger

From: *Methods in Molecular Biology, Vol. 57: In Vitro Mutagenesis Protocols*
Edited by: M. K. Trower Humana Press Inc., Totowa, NJ

fragments. The nonspecific mutations often introduced by *Taq* polymerase during PCR *(8)* necessitate sequencing the entire amplicon. Hultman et al. *(9)* described an elegant in vitro mutagenesis procedure based on solid-phase technology employing magnetic beads (Dynabeads M-280 Streptavidin) onto which both vector and insert fragment are immobilized separately via a biotin molecule incorporated into one of the strands. The basic concept is outlined in Fig. 1. In the case of the fragment to be mutated, a single-stranded template suitable for primer-directed polymerase extension is obtained by elution of the nonimmobilized strand with alkali. Ordinarily a general primer, complementary to the vector portion of the immobilized fragment, is hybridized simultaneously with the specific mutagenesis primer. An extension reaction using T4 DNA polymerase and T4 DNA ligase yields a mutated strand containing the desired mismatch that is eluted and hybridized with the single-stranded vector fragment. The result is a gap-duplex plasmid comprising small double-stranded regions of overlap and large stretches that are single-stranded. The mutated region is single-stranded specifically in order to avoid mismatch repair. *Escherichia coli* are transformed directly with the gap-duplex plasmid and clones are screened by conventional methods, preferably DNA sequencing, in order to identify mutated plasmids.

This simple protocol, requiring no special bacterial strains or vectors, has yielded more than 80% mutants *(9)*. Additionally, this protocol has the advantage that the same result may be accomplished with or without PCR. A solid-phase approach circumvents the potential problem of accumulated polymerase errors by allowing one to produce the vector by non-PCR means. The cloning is achieved without the use of either restriction enzymes or DNA ligase.

2. Materials

Solutions and reagents are stored at room temperature unless specified otherwise and are of molecular biology grade.

2.1. Biotinylation and Immobilization of Plasmid DNA

1. *E. coli* strain RRIΔM15 as plasmid host cell.
2. Appropriate plasmid containing multiple cloning site into which the target DNA sequence is cloned.
3. Appropriate restriction enzymes. Store at –20°C.

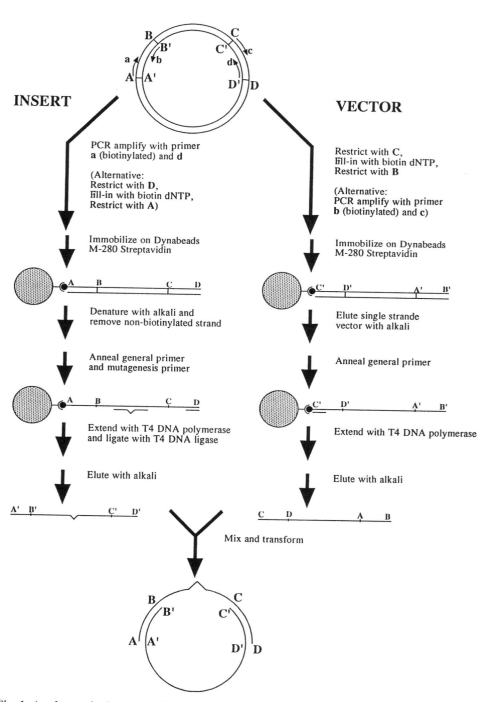

Fig. 1. A schematic drawing of the basic concept of solid-phase in vitro mutagenesis.

4. Klenow DNA polymerase. Store at –20°C.
5. Biotin dNTP 3' labeling mix: 2 m*M* biotin-16-dUTP, 2 m*M* each of dATP, dGTP, and dCTP. Store at –20°C.
6. 5X Klenow DNA polymerase buffer: 0.25*M* Tris-HCl, pH 7.2, 50 m*M* MgSO₄, 0.5 m*M* DTT. Store at –20°C.
7. Sephadex G-50 column (Pharmacia Biotech, Uppsala, Sweden).
8. Ethanol.
9. TE buffer: 10 m*M* Tris-HCl, pH 7.5, 1 m*M* EDTA, pH 8.0. Autoclave. Store at 4°C.
10. Dynabeads M-280 Streptavidin (Dynal AS, Oslo, Norway), 10 mg/mL. Store at 4°C.
11. Magnetic rack for 1.5-mL microcentrifuge tubes: Dynal MPC-E or Dynal MPC-E-1 (Dynal AS).
12. TEN buffer: TE as described containing 1*M* NaCl. Autoclave. Store at 4°C.
13. 0.5*M* EDTA, pH 8.0.

2.2. Elution of Single-Stranded Vector DNA

1. 0.15*M* NaOH. Freshly prepared. Store at +4°C.
2. 10X TE buffer: 100 m*M* Tris-HCl, pH 7.5, 10 m*M* EDTA, pH 8.0. Autoclave. Store at +4°C.
3. 1.25*M* Acetic acid.

2.3. Amplification and Immobilization of Template for In Vitro Mutagenesis

1. 1X PCR buffer: 25 m*M* TAPS-HCl, pH 9.3, 50 m*M* KCl, 0.1% Tween-20.
2. 1X PCR master mix: PCR buffer supplemented with 2 m*M* MgCl₂, 10 pmol/μL of each PCR primer (one 5' biotinylated) (primers **a** and **d** in Fig. 1), 200 μ*M* of the four dNTPs. Store at –20°C.
3. Mineral oil.
4. *Taq* DNA polymerase (5 U/μL). Store at –20°C.

2.4. Solid-Phase In Vitro Mutagenesis
2.4.1. Double Primer System

1. General extension primer. Store at –20°C.
2. 5' Phosphorylated mutagenesis primer. Store at –20°C.
3. Annealing buffer: 10 m*M* Tris-HCl, pH 7.5, 10 m*M* MgCl₂, 100 m*M* NaCl, 100 μg/mL bovine serum albumin (BSA). Store at –20°C.
4. T4 DNA polymerase. Store at –20°C.
5. T4 DNA ligase. Store at –20°C.
6. T4 DNA polymerase buffer: 20 m*M* Tris-HCl, pH 8.8, 2 m*M* DTT, 10 m*M* MgCl₂, 1.0 m*M* ATP, 100 μg/mL BSA, 0.5 m*M* each of the four dNTPs. Store at –20°C.

2.4.2. 5' Phosphorylation of the Mutagenic Primer
1. T4 Polynucleotide kinase. Store at –20°C.
2. 10X Polynucleotide kinase buffer: 500 mM Tris-HCl, pH 7.5, 100 mM MgCl$_2$, 50 mM DTT, 0.5 mg/mL nuclease-free BSA. Store at –20°C.
3. 10 mM ATP solution. Store at –20°C.

2.4.3. Single Primer System
Combined extension/mutagenesis primer.

2.5. Transformation of Gap-Duplex Plasmids
1. IPTG/X-Gal plates for blue/white selection.
2. Competent *E. coli* RRIΔM15.

3. Methods
3.1. Plasmid Purification
E. coli strain RRIΔM15 *(10)* can be used as a plasmid host. Plasmid purification is performed as described elsewhere *(11)*.

3.2. Biotinylation and Immobilization of Plasmid DNA
1. Digest 10 µg of plasmid DNA with a restriction endonuclease that generates a 5' overhang (Enzyme C in Fig. 1), e.g., *Hin*dIII. This site must be unique in the vector. Such sites may conveniently be found in the vector polylinker.
2. Fill in the 5' extension using Klenow DNA polymerase, biotin-16-dUTP, and appropriate dNTPs (*see* Notes 1–3). Mix the restricted plasmid DNA, 10 µL of 5X Klenow buffer, 1 µL of biotin dNTP 3' labeling mix, 5 U Klenow DNA polymerase, and make up to 50 µL with distilled water. Incubate at room temperature for 45 min. Inactivate by addition of EDTA solution to a final concentration of 15 mM and heat to 60°C for 15 min.
3. Remove unincorporated biotin-16-dUTP using a Sephadex G-50 desalting column pre-equilibrated with TEN buffer, followed by ethanol precipitation (*see* Note 4).
4. Redissolve the plasmid in TE buffer, and digest with a second restriction endonuclease that again cuts the vector uniquely and is located at a position that flanks both the first restriction site and the region of mutagenesis (Enzyme B in Fig. 1). This again may be conveniently situated in the flanking polylinker (*see* Note 5).
5. Wash 600 µg Dynabeads M-280 Streptavidin twice in 100 µL TEN buffer using the magnetic rack and resuspend in 60 µL of TEN buffer.
6. Mix the digested biotinylated double-stranded DNA with the Dynabeads. Incubate at room temperature for 15 min. Place the tube in the magnetic

rack for at least 30 s, and remove the supernatant using a pipet. Wash the Dynabeads and immobilized vector DNA twice with TEN buffer using the magnetic rack.

3.3. Elution of the Single-Stranded Vector DNA

Add exactly 20 µL 0.15M NaOH and incubate for 10 min at room temperature (*see* Note 6). Place the tube in the magnetic rack, and transfer the supernatant containing the single-stranded vector to a clean tube. Neutralize the single-stranded vector by adding exactly 2.2 µL 10X TE, pH 7.5, and 1.3 µL 1.25M acetic acid using the same pipetor (*see* Notes 7 and 8).

The immobilized single-stranded vector DNA may be washed in TE and stored for several weeks at 4°C and may be used later for generation of further single-stranded vector DNA by primer extension with T4 DNA polymerase (*see* Note 9).

3.4. Amplification and Immobilization of Template for In Vitro Mutagenesis

When designing the biotinylated and nonbiotinylated primers for the amplification of the template insert, it is of critical importance to achieve the correct orientation and complementary overlapping sequences that will form the gap-duplex molecule. (Figure 1 can be used as a guide in this design process.) It is recommended that the double-stranded overlap should be 50–100 bases in length. If sequences are chosen carefully, then these primers can be used to amplify inserts from a wide range of pUC/M13 derived vectors.

1. Pick a single colony of *E. coli* harboring the plasmid with an insert to be mutated from an agar plate with a sterilized Pasteur pipet. Suspend the colony in 10 µL PCR buffer and lyse the bacteria by boiling for 5 min.
2. To each PCR tube add the PCR Mastermix (98 µL) containing the primer pair flanking the region for mutagenesis (*see* primers **a** and **d** in Fig. 1). One of the primers must be biotinylated at its 5'-end. Add 2 µL of the bacteria lysate and 2 U of *Taq* polymerase and cover the reaction mixture with a layer of mineral oil. Run a 20-cycle PCR program with denaturation at 96°C for 0.5 min, annealing at 60°C for 1 min and extension at 72°C for 1 min.
3. Mix the PCR reaction mixture with 600 µg Dynabeads M-280 Streptavidin, previously washed with TE containing 1.0M NaCl. Incubate at room temperature for 15 min. Place the tube in the magnetic rack for at least 30 s, and remove the supernatant using a pipet.

4. Add 20 µL 0.15*M* NaOH and incubate for 10 min at room temperature to convert the immobilized double-stranded DNA to single-stranded form. Place the tube in the magnetic rack.
5. Remove the supernatant, and wash the immobilized single-stranded template DNA once in 50 µL 0.15*M* NaOH and three times in 50 µL TE. The washed, immobilized template is now ready for site-directed mutagenesis and may be stored for several weeks at 4°C.

3.5. Solid-Phase In Vitro Mutagenesis

A single-stranded template suitable for primer directed DNA polymerase reaction is obtained by elution of the nonimmobilized strand with alkali (*see* Section 3.4.). The in vitro mutagenesis can then either be performed using a double primer system or a single primer system (*see* Fig. 2). In the double primer system, a general primer that overlaps the vector polylinker sequence of the immobilized fragment is used together with the specific mutagenesis primer harboring a mismatch in the region to be changed (*see* Fig. 2A). An extension reaction using DNA polymerase and DNA ligase is subsequently performed to yield a mutated strand containing the desired mismatch. The synthesized strand is finally eluted, neutralized, and mixed with the single-stranded vector fragment, which yields a gap-duplex plasmid with overlapping double-stranded regions.

To be able to use the single primer system, the mutation site must be in close proximity to the vector polylinker allowing a combined mutation/extension primer to be used (*see* Fig. 2B). This strategy eliminates the need for the ligation step. This will result in a rather short region of overlap, however the gap-duplex plasmid can still be used successfully for transformation.

3.5.1. Solid-Phase In Vitro Mutagenesis Using the Double Primer System (Fig. 2A)

1. To the immobilized template DNA add 10 µL annealing buffer, 15 pmol of the general extension primer, and 15 pmol of the 5' phosphorylated mutagenesis primer (*see* Note 10). Heat the reaction mixture to 65°C and allow to cool to 0°C. Place the tube in the magnetic rack and remove the annealing buffer using a pipet.
2. Add the T4 DNA polymerase buffer, 3.5 U T4 DNA polymerase, and 1 U T4 DNA ligase to a total volume of 30 µL. Incubate on ice for 10 min and follow by a 2 h extension at 37°C. Place the tube in the magnetic rack and remove the supernatant.

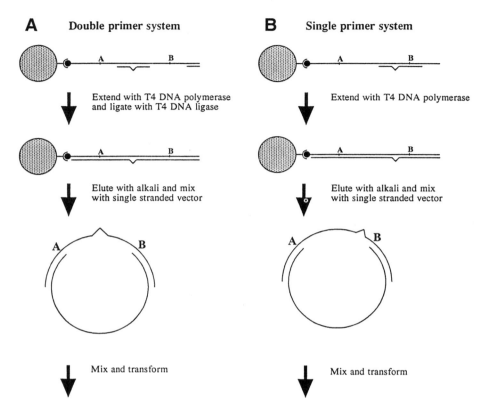

Fig. 2. A schematic drawing of the two systems for solid-phase in vitro mutagenesis using a double **(A)** or single **(B)** primer system.

3. Wash the Dynabeads once in 50 µL TE and elute off the mutated insert by incubation in exactly 20 µL $0.15M$ NaOH. Place the tube again in the magnetic rack and transfer the supernatant to a clean tube.
4. Neutralize the supernatant by adding exactly 2.2 µL 10X TE, pH 7.5, and 1.3 µL $1.25M$ acetic acid.

3.5.2. Solid-Phase In Vitro Mutagenesis Using the Single Primer System (Fig. 2B)

A combined mutagenesis/extension primer is used for annealing. The subsequent synthesis of a single-stranded insert is performed under the same conditions as in the double primer approach, but with the T4 DNA ligase excluded. Elution and neutralization steps are carried out as for the double primer approach.

3.6. Transformation of Gap-Duplex Plasmids

1. Mix 10 µL of the eluted and neutralized single-stranded vector DNA with 10 µL of the synthesized single-stranded DNA containing the mutated insert (*see* Note 11). Incubate at 70°C for 10 min and allow to cool to room temperature.
2. Transform competent *E. coli* cells directly with the reaction mixture and spread the cells on IPTG/Xgal plates (with appropriate antibiotics) for blue and white selection. Positive clones should be analyzed by DNA sequencing *(11)*.

4. Notes

1. There are two alternative ways to introduce the biotin into one of the DNA strands (*see* Fig. 1): by site-specific restriction, followed by a fill-in reaction using biotin-dNTPs and DNA polymerase, or by PCR amplification using a 5' biotinylated primer.
2. The restriction/fill-in route will yield a biotinylation at the 3' end of the DNA fragment, whereas the PCR amplification will yield a biotinylation at the 5' end of the DNA fragment. Thus, the choice of biotinylation must be carefully considered to ensure that complementary strands are obtained for both the vector and insert.
3. The single-stranded vector is preferably produced by the restriction/fill-in procedure. A non-PCR approach is recommended, since accumulation of polymerase errors are a major concern whenever PCR products are cloned *(8)*.
4. The fractions coming off the Sephadex G-50 column containing DNA can be readily detected by a spot test. For this, 2-µL aliquots of each collected fraction are mixed with an equal volume of a 2-µg/mL solution of ethidium bromide. These stained aliquots are then placed on the inside of an empty Petri dish. This Petri dish is then inverted on a standard UV transilluminator. Those drops that fluoresce represent fractions containing DNA *(12)*.
5. It may be informative to check biotinylation of vector/template DNA by gel electrophoresis. This is easily achieved by running small aliquots of the biotin-labeled DNA before and after binding to streptavidin-coated Dynabeads. Comparison of the band intensity will give an indication of the efficiency of the Klenow fill-in reaction and the binding capacity of the beads for your vector/template combination.
6. Always use freshly prepared NaOH. Old or poorly stored NaOH will be inefficient in the elution of the strand complementary to the Dynabeads-immobilized strand. It will also cause poor titration of the eluted complementary strand.

7. Careful and accurate pipeting is essential to ensure that the eluted strand is correctly neutralized. It will be beneficial to use the same pipetor to dispense the NaOH, TE, and acetic acid to eradicate the possibility of calibration variances between pipetors.

8. The initial eluted alkali-treated and -neutralized single-stranded vector can be used directly for combination with the mutated template generated in either Sections 3.5.1. or 3.5.2.

9. The Dynabeads with the immobilized single-stranded vector can be washed and resolved in TE and stored at 4°C for several weeks. This immobilized vector can be used as a template for synthesis of pure, single-stranded vector, giving enough material for many mutagenesis experiments *(9)*. To perform this, follow the procedure in Section 3.5.1., but exclude T4 DNA ligase and the mutagenic primer.

10. The insert fragment can be cloned directly into different vectors ready for transformation provided that complementary overlap regions exist between the vector and the insert.

11. In the double primer system, the mutagenesis primer must be phosphorylated to facilitate ligation using T4 DNA ligase. Primer phosphorylation may be performed using the reagents given in Section 2.4.2. Mix 1 µL of 10X T4 polynucleotide kinase buffer, 15 pmol of mutagenic primer, 1 µL of ATP, 5 U polynucleotide kinase, and 6.5 µL of distilled water. Incubate at 37°C for 60 min. Inactivate the kinase at 70°C for 5 min. The primer can now be added directly to the mutagenesis reaction in Section 3.5.1.1. Alternatively, it can be purified for storage.

Acknowledgments

I thank Erik Hornes (Dynal A/S, Oslo, Norway) for his assistance in this work.

References

1. Higuchi, R., Krummel, B., and Saiki, R. K. (1988) A general method of *in vitro* preparation and specific mutagenesis of DNA fragments: Study of protein and DNA interaction. *Nucleic Acids Res.* **16,** 7351–7367.

2. Ho, S. N., Hunt, H. D., Horton, R. M., Pullen, J. K., and Pease, L. R. (1989) Site directed mutagenesis by overlap extension using polymerase chain reaction. *Gene* **77,** 51–59.

3. Landt, O., Grunert, H. P., and Hahn, U. (1990) A general method for site-directed mutagenesis using the polymerase chain reaction. *Gene* **96,** 125–128.

4. Nelson, R. M. and Long, G. L. (1989) A general method for site-specific mutagenesis using the *Thermus aquaticus* polymerase chain reaction. *Anal. Biochem.* **180,** 147–151.

5. Sarkar, G. and Sommer, S. S. (1990) The "megaprimer" method of site-directed mutagenesis. *BioTechniques* **8,** 404–407.

6. Jones, D. H. and Howard, B. H. (1990) A rapid method for site-specific mutagenesis and directional subcloning by using the polymerase chain reaction to generate recombinant circles. *BioTechniques* **8,** 178–183.

7. Hall, L. and Emery, D. C. (1991) A rapid and efficient method for site-directed mutagenesis by PCR, using biotinylated universal primers and streptavidin-coated magnetic beads. *Pro. Eng.* **4(5),** 601.

8. Tindall, K. R. and Kunkel, T. A. (1988) Fidelity of DNA synthesis by the *Thermus aquaticus* DNA polymerase. *Biochemistry* **27,** 6008–6013.

9. Hultman, T., Murby, M., Ståhl, S., Hornes, E., and Uhlén, M. (1990) Solid phase *in vitro* mutagenesis using plasmid DNA template. *Nucleic Acids Res.* **18(17),** 5107–5112.

10. Rüther, U. (1982) *Nucleic Acids Res.* **10,** 5765–5772.

11. Hultman, T., Ståhl, S., Hornes, E., and Uhlen, M. (1989) Direct solid-phase sequencing of genomic and plasmid DNA using magnetic beads as solid support. *Nucleic Acids Res.* **17(13),** 4937–4946.

12. Gabrielsen, O. S. and Huet, J. (1993) Magnetic DNA affinity purification of yeast transcription factor. *Methods Enzymol.* **218,** 508–525.

CHAPTER 10

Targeted Mutagenesis Mediated by the Triple Helix Formation

Peter M. Glazer, Gan Wang, Pamela A. Havre, and Edward J. Gunther

1. Introduction

Oligonucleotides can bind in the major groove of duplex DNA and form triple helices in a sequence-specific manner *(1–4)*. Progress in elucidating the third strand binding code has raised the possibility of developing nucleic acids as sequence-specific reagents for research and possibly clinical applications. Oligonucleotide-mediated triplex formation has been shown to prevent transcription factor binding to promoter sites and to block mRNA synthesis in vitro and in vivo *(5–8)*. Instead of using triplex formation to transiently block gene expression, however, we reasoned that it would be advantageous to use triple helix formation to target mutations to specific sites in selected genes in order to produce permanent, heritable changes in gene function and expression *(9–11)*. In this approach, mutations are targeted to a selected site by linking the triplex-forming oligonucleotide to a mutagen so that the sequence specificity of the triplex formation can be imparted to the action of the mutagen (Fig. 1).

As a potential research tool for inducing mutations in a selected gene, triple helix targeted mutagenesis has several unique attributes. Although this technique may be useful for generating targeted mutations in duplex DNA in vitro, it may have greater value as an approach to generate gene-specific mutations in vivo. In our recent work, we have found that triplex-forming oligonucleotides can enter mammalian cells and introduce

From: *Methods in Molecular Biology, Vol. 57: In Vitro Mutagenesis Protocols*
Edited by: M. K. Trower Humana Press Inc., Totowa, NJ

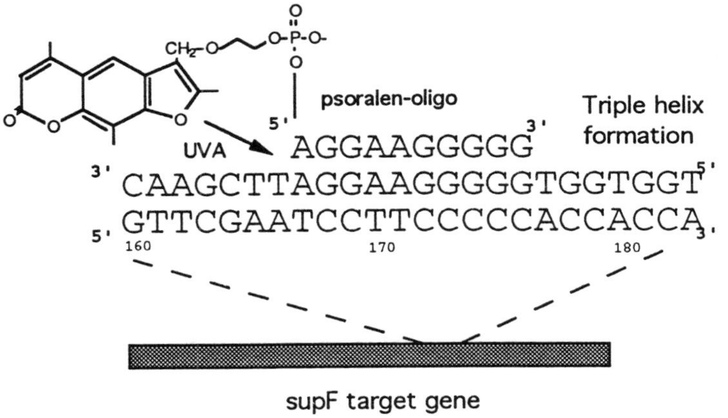

psoralen-oligo

Triple helix formation

5' AGGAAGGGGG 3'
3' CAAGCTTAGGAAGGGGGTGGTGGT 5'
5' GTTCGAATCCTTCCCCCACCACCA 3'
160   170   180

supF target gene

Fig. 1. Strategy for triple helix-targeted mutagenesis. The 10-base triple helix-forming oligonucleotide is shown positioned above its target site in the *supF* gene (bp 167–176). The oligonucleotide is conjugated to a mutagen, 4'-hydroxymethyl-4,5',8-trimethylpsoralen, which is targeted to intercalate between basepairs 166 and 167, as indicated by the arrow. Photoactivation of the psoralen generates adducts and thereby mutations at the targeted site.

targeted lesions and thereby mutations in a chosen gene *(12)*. The same strategy could be used to target mutations to selected genes within bacteria or yeast. Efforts are also underway in our laboratory to use this technique on *Drosophila* embryos. Ultimately, triplex-mediated targeting may offer an alternative to standard gene transfer techniques for the genetic manipulation of cells, especially for gene knockout experiments. This would bypass the need for several complicated experimental steps, including in vitro site-directed mutagenesis of the chosen gene, construction of a selection vector for homologous recombination and gene replacement, transfer of that construct into the recipient cells, and selection for successful gene replacement or disruption.

Triplex-mediated targeting depends on the sequence-specific formation of a triple helix at a selected site in double-stranded DNA. Our current understanding of DNA triple helices and the current collection of nucleotide analogs limits triple helix formation to regions of DNA with polypurine:polypyrimidine sequences. The general applicability of this technique will depend on the extension of the third strand binding code and on the development of nucleotide analogs so that triplex formation can occur at any sequence with the required specificity. Much work in this regard is underway *(6,13–15)*.

Operationally, triplex-directed mutagenesis involves using the third strand to position a mutagen at the desired location in the DNA. We have used psoralen, but other mutagens, such as alkylating agents, could be employed to produce a different spectrum of mutations. Following triplex formation and site-specific psoralen intercalation, the psoralen is photoactivated with long wavelength UV light (UVA). This generates a targeted psoralen adduct in the DNA. A mutation is produced when this targeted premutagenic lesion is processed by cellular repair and replication activities into a mutation. Hence, the DNA must be on a replicon that can replicate in either bacteria or, preferably, mammalian cells. For in vivo mutagenesis, the target gene will be either on a chromosome or in a viral genome. Our work has shown that mostly T:A to A:T transversions are produced at the targeted psoralen intercalation site. However, other basepair changes and small deletions encompassing the target site are occasionally observed. The yield and specificity of the mutagenesis will depend on the replicon used and on the host cell in which the targeted vector is replicated. We observed only 0.2% mutations on replication of a damaged lambda vector in *Escherichia coli (10)*, but we found 7.4% mutations when a simian virus 40 (SV40) replicon containing the targeted adduct was replicated in monkey COS cells *(11)*. The SV40 replicon must be a shuttle vector that also contains a bacterial plasmid origin of replication and an antibiotic resistance gene. This allows cloning of the mutated vectors in bacteria following isolation of the vector DNA from the COS cells, facilitating rapid analysis of the mutagenesis and manipulation of the resulting gene (Fig. 2).

Only targeted mutagenesis mediated by in vitro triple helix formation is described in this chapter. Although our recent work suggests that in vivo targeted mutagenesis is also possible *(12)*, our understanding of the parameters governing in vivo triplex formation and mutation targeting is incomplete. It is premature to consider it a reliable technique at this time.

2. Materials

Solutions are stored at room temperature unless stated otherwise.

1. Oligonucleotides: Psoralen-linked oligonucleotides can be obtained from Oligos Etc. (Wilsonville, OR) or can be synthesized by standard automated methods using materials from Glen Research (Sterling, VA). The psoralen

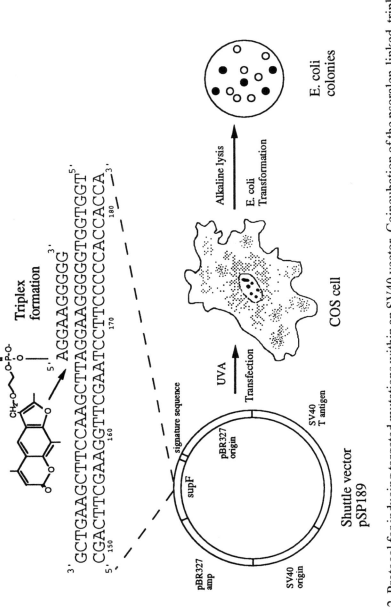

Fig. 2. Protocol for inducing targeted mutations within an SV40 vector. Coincubation of the psoralen-linked, triplex-forming oligonucleotide with the SV40 vector (containing the selected gene to be mutated) allows triplex formation to deliver the psoralen to the target site. Photoactivation of the psoralen generates targeted adducts, which are turned into mutations during repair and replication of the SV40 vector transfected into monkey COS cells. The vector DNA is

112

is incorporated into the oligonucleotide synthesis as a psoralen phosphor-amidite, resulting in an oligonucleotide linked at its 5' end via a two-carbon linker arm to 4'-hydroxymethyl-4,5',8-trimethylpsoralen, as illustrated in Fig. 1. Oligonucleotides are stored at –20°C, protected from light.

2. Vectors: An SV40-based shuttle vector, pSP189, containing the SV40 origin of replication and T-antigen gene and the pBR327 replication origin and β-lactamase gene, was used in our work (Fig. 2; obtained from Michael Seidman, Otsuka Pharmaceuticals, Rockville, MD; *[16]*). This vector also contained the *supF* gene, an amber suppressor tRNA gene, that was used as a model gene in our initial experiments. This gene is cloned into unique *Xho*I and *Eag*I sites in the vector, and can be replaced with the gene of interest. Unique *Eco*RI and *Bam*H1 sites are also present.

3. Cells: Monkey COS-7 cells are available from the American Type Culture Collection (#1651-CRL). Standard *E. coli* K12 cells used as hosts for plasmid transformation and growth are suitable for vector rescue.

4. Triplex-binding buffer: 10 m*M* Tris-HCl, pH 7.4, 1 m*M* spermidine, and 20 m*M* MgCl$_2$.

5. Light source for psoralen photoactivation: Psoralen photoactivation is accomplished using broad band UVA light centered at 365 nm. UVA lamps are available from Southern New England Ultraviolet Co. (Branford, CT). Dosimetry should be performed using a radiometer, such as the IL1400 from International Light (Newburyport, MA). A typical UVA irradiance is 5 mW/cm^2.

6. COS cell growth medium (DMEM/10% FCS): Dulbecco's Modified Eagle Media (DMEM) supplemented with 10% fetal calf serum (FCS) (available from Gibco-BRL, Gaithersburg, MD, or other standard supplier).

7. Cell resuspension solution: 50 m*M* Tris-HCl, 10 m*M* EDTA, pH 8.0, 100 μg/mL RNase A.

8. Cell lysis solution: 0.2*M* NaOH, 1% SDS.

9. Neutralization solution: 3*M* potassium acetate, pH 5.5.

10. Bacterial plates: Standard LB agar supplemented with ampicillin. Add 10 g bactotryptone, 5 g bactoyeast extract, and 10 g NaCl/L of water. Adjust pH to 7.5 with NaOH. Add 15 g bactoagar/L. Autoclave. Allow to cool to 55°C before adding ampicillin to a final concentration of 50 μg/mL.

11. Ampicillin stock: 10 mg/mL of the sodium salt of ampicillin in water. Sterilize by filtration and store at –20°C.

12. TE: 10 m*M* Tris-HCl, pH 8.0, 1 m*M* EDTA.

3. Methods

3.1. Target Site Choice

Choose a target site consisting of polypurine:polypyrimidine sequences, since triple helix-targeted mutagenesis is generally limited to such sites.

Triple helices do not efficiently form at sites of mixed sequence. Ideally, choose a site with an A:T basepair at the 3' end of the homopurine run as the target for psoralen photomodification. If another mutagen is used, this is not necessarily required (*see* Note 5). In this way, the psoralen at the 5' end of the third strand is positioned adjacent to the T:A basepair to be mutated (*see* Fig. 1 and Note 6).

3.2. Oligonucleotide Design and Synthesis

1. For G:C basepair rich target sites, synthesize third strand oligonucleotides containing A and G to form antiparallel triple helices *(9–11)*. In this motif *(1,2)*, G binds to G:C basepairs and either A or T can be used to bind to A:T basepairs (Fig. 3). The third strand binds in the major groove of the DNA to the purine strand of the duplex and is oriented antiparallel to the duplex purine strand, in terms of 5' to 3' polarity (*see* Fig. 1 for an example, Fig. 3 for basic guidelines, and refs. *1* and *2* and Notes 1–4 for further discussion).
2. For A:T basepair rich target sites, synthesize T and C containing oligo-nucleotides, which bind in an orientation parallel to the purine-rich strand of the duplex.
3. Incorporate psoralen at the 5' end in the synthesis using psoralen phosphoramidites.

3.3. Triplex Formation

1. Form a triple helix with the psoralen-conjugated oligonucleotide and the target gene (inserted into an SV40-based shuttle vector, *see* Section 2.2.) by coincubation of the SV40 vector DNA at 50 nM with the oligonucle-otide at 1 μM in triplex-binding buffer for 2 h at 37°C (*see* Notes 7 and 8).
2. In the case of a pyrimidine motif triple helix (T and C-containing third-strand oligonucleotide), adjust the pH of the binding buffer to 5.5–6.0 to enhance triplex formation (*see* Note 9).

3.4. Mutagenesis Protocol

1. Irradiate the triple helix complex with 1.8 J/cm^2 of UVA light to generate psoralen photoadducts at the targeted sites (*see* Note 10).
2. Transfect the complex into COS cells as in steps 3–7.
3. Grow the COS cells to 70% confluence. Detach the cells from the culture dish by treatment with trypsin, and resuspend them in DMEM/10% FCS.
4. Wash the cells in growth medium three times by centrifugation at 900g for 5 min (4°C) using a Sorvall RT6000D. Resuspend the cells at 1×10^7 cells/mL.
5. Add the plasmid DNAs at 3 μg DNA/10^6 cells and incubate the cell/DNA mixtures on ice for 10 min.

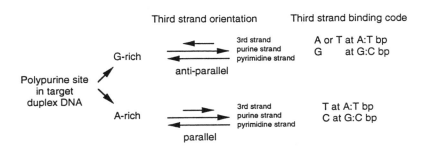

Fig. 3. Guidelines for the design of triple helix-forming oligonucleotides. Triple helices form most readily at polypurine:polypyrimidine sites in DNA. If these sites are G:C basepair rich, triplex formation in the antiparallel motif is favored, whereas A:T basepair rich sites are conducive to parallel triple helix formation, as indicated. The arrows indicate the 5'–3' direction of the strands.

6. Transfect cells by electroporation using a BioRad (Richmond, CA) gene pulser at a setting of 25 µF/250 W/250 V in the 0.4 cm cuvet. Following electroporation, keep the cells on ice for 10 min.
7. Dilute the cells with growth medium and transfer them to culture dishes for 48 h, at which time isolate the vector DNA (*see* Section 3.5.).

3.5. Rescue of Mutated Vectors for Analysis

Isolate the vector DNA from the COS cells using a modified alkaline lysis procedure.

1. Detach the cells by trypsinization, wash once, and resuspend in 100 µL of cell resuspension solution.
2. Add an equal volume of cell lysis solution, followed by 100 µL of neutralization solution.
3. Incubate for 15 min at room temperature and then centrifuge in a microcentrifuge for 10 min.
4. Extract the supernatant with an equal volume of phenol/chloroform (1:1) once, and precipitate the DNA with 2.5 vol of ethanol at –70°C for 10 min.
5. Collect the DNA by centrifugation for 10 min, wash with 70% ethanol once, and allow to air dry for 5 min at room temperature. Dissolve the DNA pellet in 10 µL of TE buffer.
6. Use 1 µL of the sample of vector DNA to transform the *E. coli* host by electroporation (BioRad, setting 25 µF/250 W/1800 V, using a 0.1-cm cuvet). Plate the transformed *E. coli* cells onto LB plates containing 50 µg/mL of ampicillin.

3.6. Identification of Mutants

Colonies containing mutations in the target gene can be identified by several methods, including colony hybridization with oligonucleotide probes matching the desired mutant sequence *(11)*. Another useful technique is allele-specific PCR or some variant of it *(17)*. We have used colony hybridization with good specificity *(11)*. A discussion of these techniques is beyond the scope of this chapter.

4. Notes

1. Some interruptions of the homopurine sequence in the duplex DNA may be acceptable, but the ability of a proposed third strand to bind to the target sequence should be tested in vitro, using a gel mobility shift assay *(10)*.
2. Triplex formation can also occur in the parallel motif in which the third strand consists of T binding to A:T basepairs and C binding to G:C basepairs *(3,4,6,7)*. The third strand is oriented parallel to the purine strand of the duplex. Target sites with a majority of A:T basepairs (as opposed to G:C basepairs) are preferred for parallel motif triplex formation. However, our understanding of this is evolving.
3. Triplex formation by A and G or T and G containing oligonucleotides has the advantage that it is not sensitive to pH. In contrast, triplex formation in the parallel motif by a polypyrimidine oligonucleotide (containing C and T) requires acidic pH because of the need for protonation of the cytosine.
4. We have found a 10-bp homopurine:homopyrimidine run to be sufficient for efficient and specific triplex formation in vitro. An 8-bp site was found to be insufficient.
5. If an alkylating agent is tethered to the triplex-forming oligonucleotide as the mutagen, then the target base may be G, to give G:C to A:T transversions. However, this is has not yet been demonstrated.
6. Currently, incorporation of psoralen in automated oligonucleotide synthesis is conveniently done only at the 5' end of the oligonucleotide.
7. Triplex formation will occur at lower temperatures, but the specificity will be reduced.
8. A greater excess of oligonucleotide may lead to a some nonspecific mutagenesis.
9. Triplex formation in the pyrimidine or parallel motif requires protonation of C in the third strand, which is favored at low pH *(5)*.
10. If the target site consists of either a 5' TpA 3' or 5' ApT 3' sequence, then psoralen interstrand crosslinks (between Ts in opposite strands of the duplex) as well as psoralen monoadducts will be formed. Only psoralen monoadducts will form at an isolated T *(9)*.

Acknowledgments

We thank F. P. Gasparro, R. Franklin, and S. J. Baserga for their help. P. M. Glazer is supported by the Charles E. Culpeper Foundation, the Leukemia Society of America, the American Cancer Society, and the NIH (ES05775).

References

1. Beal, P. A. and Dervan, P. B. (1991) Second structural motif for recognition of DNA by oligonucleotide-directed triple-helix formation. *Science* **251,** 1360–1363.
2. Beal, P. A. and Dervan, P. B. (1992) The influence of single base triplet changes on the stability of a Pur-Pur-Pyr triple helix determined by affinity cleaving. *Nucleic Acids Res.* **20,** 2773–2776.
3. Duval-Valentin, G., Thuong, N. T., and Helene, C. (1992) Specific inhibition of transcription by triple helix-forming oligonucleotides. *Proc. Natl. Acad. Sci. USA* **89,** 504–508.
4. Fossella, J. A., Kim, Y. J., Shih, H., Richards, E. G., and Fresco, J. R. (1993) Relative specificities in binding of Watson-Crick basepairs by third strand residues in a DNA pyrimidine triplex motif. *Nucleic Acids Res.* **21,** 4511–4515.
5. Cooney, M., Czernuszewicz, G., Postel, E. H., Flint, S. J., and Hogan, M. E. (1988) Site-specific oligonucleotide binding represses transcription of the human c-*myc* gene in vitro. *Science* **241,** 456–459.
6. Giovannangeli, C., Rougee, M., Garestier, T., Thuong, N. T., and Helene, C. (1992) Triple-helix formation by oligonucleotides containing the three bases thymine, cytosine, and guanine. *Proc. Natl. Acad. Sci. USA* **89,** 8631–8635.
7. Grigoriev, M., Praeuth, D., Guieysse, A. L., Robin, P., Thuong, N. T., Helene, C., and Harel-Bellan, A. (1993) Inhibition of gene expression by triple helix-directed DNA crosslinking at specific sites. *Proc. Natl. Acad. Sci. USA* **90,** 3501–3505.
8. Postel, E. H., Flint, S. J., Kessler, D. J., and Hogan, M. E. (1991) Evidence that a triplex-forming oligodeoxyribonucleotide binds to the c-*myc* promoter in HeLa cells, thereby reducing c-*myc* mRNA levels. *Proc. Natl. Acad. Sci. USA* **88,** 8227–8231.
9. Gasparro, F. P., Havre, P. A., Olack, G. A., Gunther, E. J., and Glazer, P. M. (1994) Site-specific targeting of psoralen photoadducts with a triple helix-forming oligonucleotide: characterization of psoralen monoadduct and crosslink formation. *Nucleic Acids Res.* **22,** 2845–2852.
10. Havre, P. A., Gunther, E. J., Gasparro, F. P., and Glazer, P. M. (1993) Targeted mutagenesis of DNA using triple helix forming oligonucleotides linked to psoralen. *Proc. Natl. Acad. Sci. USA* **90,** 7879–7883.
11. Havre, P. A. and Glazer, P. M. (1993) Targeted mutagenesis of SV40 DNA mediated by a triple-helix forming oligonucleotide. *J. Virol.* **67,** 7324–7331.
12. Wang, G., Levy, D. D., Seidman, M. M., and Glazer, P. M. (1994) Targeted mutagenesis in mammalian cells mediated by intracellular triple helix formation. *Mol. Cell. Biol.* **15,** 1759–1768.

13. Griffin, L. C., Kiessling, L. L., Beal, P. A., Gillespie, P., and Dervan, P. B. (1992) Recognition of all four basepairs of double-helical DNA by triple-helix formation: Design of nonnatural deoxyribonucleosides for pyrimidine-purine basepair binding. *J. Am. Chem. Soc.* **114,** 7976–7982.

14. Koh, J. S. and Dervan, P. B. (1992) Design of nonnatural deoxyribonucleoside for recognition of GC base pairs by oligonucleotide-directed triple helix formation. *J. Am. Chem. Soc.* **114,** 1470–1478.

15. Stilz, H. U. and Dervan, P. B. (1993) Specific recognition of CG basepairs by 2-deoxynebularine within the purine.purine.pyrimidine triple helix motif. *Biochemistry* **32,** 2177–2185.

16. Parris, C. N. and Seidman, M. M. (1992) A signature element distinguishes sibling and independent mutations in a shuttle vector plasmid. *Gene* **117,** 1–5.

17. Li, H., Cui, X., and Arnheim, N. (1990) Direct electrophoretic detection of the allelic state of single DNA molecules in human sperm by using the polymerase chain reaction. *Proc. Natl. Acad. Sci. USA* **87,** 4580–4584.

CHAPTER 11

A Universal Nested Deletion Method Using an Arbitrary Primer and Elimination of a Unique Restriction Site

Li Zhu and Ann E. Holtz

1. Introduction

The generation of nested deletions within cloned fragments of DNA has important applications in molecular biology. For DNA sequencing, nested deletions provide a series of overlapping templates that can be used to generate a composite sequence with a single sequencing primer; in gene and protein functional studies, nested deletions allow researchers to locate and define a variety of functional domains based on regions of deletions.

There are several existing techniques for making nested deletions, including *Bal*31 digestion *(1)*, exonuclease III digestion *(2)*, and M13 single-stranded template-based, primer-mediated methods *(3)*. Some of these methods rely on a very special arrangement of multiple restriction sites *(2)*; some require single-stranded DNA as the starting template *(3)*; and some do not generate unidirectional deletions, which complicates further analysis and sequencing of the resulting clones *(1)*. Additionally, none of these methods allow one to control directly the scale of incremental deletion sizes.

The nested deletion method described here is a simple and highly efficient means of introducing unidirectional, ordered deletions into virtually any double-stranded plasmid in vitro. This deletion method is based

From: *Methods in Molecular Biology, Vol. 57: In Vitro Mutagenesis Protocols*
Edited by: M. K. Trower Humana Press Inc., Totowa, NJ

119

on a modification of USE (<u>u</u>nique restriction <u>s</u>ite <u>e</u>limination) site-directed mutagenesis (*4*; Chapter 2 of this book) and, indeed, many components and procedures in these two methods are very similar. Although this nested deletion method is similar to an M13-based method introduced by Shen and Waye *(3)*, no specialized vectors or single-stranded templates are required. The only requirements are that the starting plasmid contain a unique restriction site adjacent to the gene of interest targeted for deletions, and a bacterial selection marker (e.g., antibiotic resistance); these conditions are easily met by most cloning vectors.

Briefly, this deletion method employs a single oligonucleotide deletion primer and uses restriction enzyme digestion at a unique site as an efficient means to enrich for plasmids with deletions of all sizes (Figs. 1 and 2). This single oligonucleotide primer serves two functions simultaneously: It generates the nested deletions, and it eliminates a unique restriction site. The oligonucleotide primer consists of two structural domains: On the 5' side is an anchoring domain whose sequence is complementary to the primer binding site on the template (and serves as the protection site); and on the 3' side is a short tail consisting of an arbitrary sequence of four or five nucleotides that does not anneal to the region immediately contiguous with the primer binding site. Thus, when the anchoring domain of the primer is annealed to a denatured target (i.e., parental) plasmid, the 3' tail anneals (semirandomly) to complementary sequences within the cloned gene sequence; the intervening segment of parental DNA that has no homology within the deletion primer will loop out. The length of looped out DNA in a particular primer/plasmid hybrid is determined by the number and location of sites to which the 3' tail may anneal.

After new DNA strands are synthesized and ligated, the mixture of parental and hybrid plasmids is subjected to digestion by a restriction

---

Fig. 1. *(opposite page)* Strategy for generating nested deletions using a deletion primer with an arbitrary 3' tail, and restriction enzyme digestion to enrich for mutants. Note: Although the deletion primer is typically designed to anneal to sequences within or flanking the MCS, it can be designed to anneal anywhere within the target sequence. The only requirement is that a unique restriction site must be located between the primer annealing site and the sequence targeted for deletion.

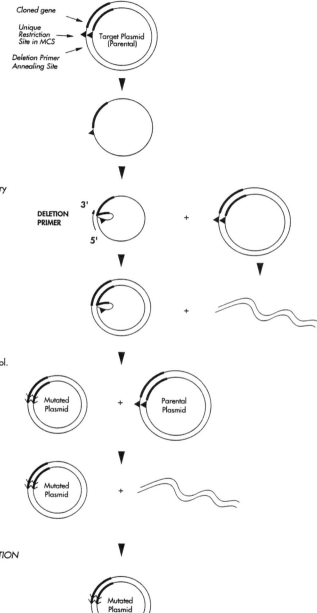

1. Denature dsDNA

2. Anneal Deletion Primer: 5' end of primer anneals specifically to sequences flanking MCS; 3' end anneals randomly to complementary sequences within the cloned gene.

3. Synthesize second strand with T4 DNA polymerase and seal gaps with T4 DNA ligase.

4. Perform primary selection using restriction enzyme digestion of reannealed parental plasmids.

5. Transform *mutS E. coli*.
   FIRST TRANSFORMATION

6. Isolate DNA from transformant pool.

7. Perform secondary selection using restriction enzyme digestion of parental plasmids. Mutated plasmids have deletions of varying lengths within the cloned gene.

8. Transform *E. coli*.
   SECOND (FINAL) TRANSFORMATION

9. Isolate plasmids from individual transformants and estimate deletion sizes

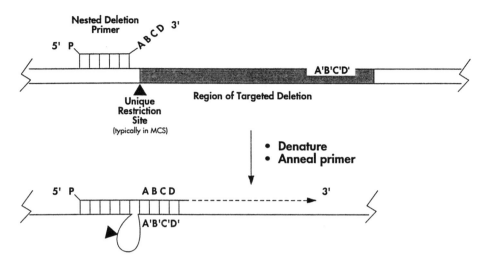

Fig. 2. Details of the deletion primer used in the nested deletion method. The arbitrary sequence on the short 3' tail of the nested deletion primer anneals semirandomly to complementary sequences within the region targeted for deletions. The intervening nonhomologous sequence is looped out and will be lost when the new DNA strand is synthesized.

enzyme whose unique recognition site lies within the looped-out segment on the hybrid. Typically, any one of the unique restriction sites present in the multiple cloning site (MCS) on either side of the inserted sequence can be used as the selection site. Hybrid plasmids containing the looped out segment are resistant to digestion. The parental DNA, however, is sensitive to digestion and will be linearized, rendering it at least 100 times less efficient in transformation of bacterial cells *(5)*. The mixture of mutated and unmutated plasmids is transformed into a repair-deficient *mutS⁻* strain of *Escherichia coli* (first transformation). Transformants are pooled, and plasmid DNA is prepared from the bacteria harboring the mixed plasmid population. The isolated DNA is then subjected to a second selective restriction enzyme digestion. This destroys many of the remaining parental target plasmids and enriches for mutated (i.e., deletion-containing) forms. The thoroughly digested DNA is then used in a second (final) transformation (this time in a repair-competent strain of *E. coli*), which results in highly efficient recovery of the desired mutated plasmids. Plasmid DNA is isolated from antibiotic-resistant transformants by a quick-lysis (or equivalent) method *(6)* and analyzed by gel electrophoresis for the sizes and order of deletions *(7)*.

The semi-random annealing of the deletion primers typically generates deletions falling within roughly discrete size categories. One significant advantage of our unique nested deletion system is that, by modifying the length and composition of the arbitrary tail of the deletion primer, the size of the incremental jumps in deletion sizes can be tailored to meet the needs of a specific application. The average distance separating groups of deletion endpoints is directly related to the length of the arbitrary sequence chosen for the 3' tail of the deletion primer, and the presence of degenerate or partially degenerate nucleotide positions within the tail sequence (*see* Note 1 and Table 1). Typical examples of deletion primers, designed for use with vectors containing T3 or T7 promoter sequences, are provided in Note 2 and Table 2.

The strategy employed in this nested deletion method results in consistently very high (>95%) deletion efficiencies. However, as is the case for site-directed mutagenesis using the USE method (Chapter 2), the actual mutation efficiency for this nested deletion method depends on several factors, including:

1. The specificity of the restriction enzyme chosen for the selection steps, and its ability to efficiently digest parental (unmutated) plasmids (*see* Notes 3 and 14);
2. The complete denaturation of the target plasmid before annealing the deletion primer;
3. The saturated annealing of the deletion primer to the denatured target plasmid; and
4. The stable incorporation of the deletion following the annealing step (*see* Note 4).

2. Materials

All materials are stored at –20°C unless stated otherwise.

2.1. Reagents for Generation of Nested Deletions

1. 10X Annealing buffer: 200 mM Tris-HCl, pH 7.5, 100 mM MgCl$_2$, 500 mM NaCl. Store at 4°C.
2. 10X Synthesis buffer: 100 mM Tris-HCl, pH 7.5, 5 mM each of dATP, dCTP, dGTP, and dTTP, 10 mM ATP, 20 mM DTT.

Table 1
Relationship Between the Length of the Arbitrary 3' Tail
and the Average Size of Deletions

Length of tail	Number of degenerate nucleotide positions	Average distance between groups of deletion endpoints
3-mer	0	$4 \times 4 \times 4 = 64$ bp
4-mer	0	$4 \times 4 \times 4 \times 4 = 256$ bp
5-mer	0	$4 \times 4 \times 4 \times 4 \times 4 = 1024$ bp
5-mer	1 (partial[a])	$4 \times 4 \times 4 \times 4 \times 2 = 512$ bp
6-mer	0	$4 \times 4 \times 4 \times 4 \times 4 \times 4 = 4096$ bp

[a]One position synthesized as a mixture of two nucleotides (e.g., G and C).

Table 2
Example of Typical Deletion Primers

Oligo[a]	Oligo sequence[b]
T3	5'p– CGCAATTAACCCTCACTAAAGGG^CGCC –3'
T7	5'p– GTAATACGACTCACTATAGGGCG^GTGG –3'

[a]The name denotes that the deletion primer contains a deletion relative to the sequence of the target plasmid. Thus, when the primer is annealed to the target plasmid, a portion of the parental plasmid corresponding to the deletion loops out in the hybrid. In this process, one or more unique parental restriction sites are deleted. The T3 and T7 oligos may be used with any vector that contains the T3 or T7 promoter sequence, respectively. However, before using these oligos with your vector, be sure to verify that the sequence of the complementary region matches with a sequence flanking the MCS, that the restriction site to be used in the selection procedure is present in the target plasmid only once, and that the selection site is located between the primer binding site and the targeted region.
[b]The ^ symbol marks the beginning of the arbitrary 3' tail.

3. *E. coli* strains (store at –70°C in 50% glycerol):
   a. BMH 71-18 *mutS*, a mismatch repair-deficient strain: *thi, supE*, Δ(*lac-proAB*), (*mutS*::Tn10)(F' *proAB, lacI*q ZΔM15) *(8)* (*see* Note 5).
   b. Wild-type *mutS*+ strains such as DH5α.
4. T4 DNA polymerase (2–4 U/μL).
5. T4 DNA ligase (4–6 U/μL).
6. TE buffer: 10 m*M* Tris-HCl, pH 7.5, 1 m*M* EDTA.
7. STET buffer: 0.1*M* NaCl, 10 m*M* Tris-HCl, pH 8.0, 1 m*M* EDTA, 5% Triton X-100.
8. BSA 100X stock solution: 10 mg/mL BSA, for use with some restriction enzymes, including *Eco*RV. Optional.

Example of materials that can be used for a control deletion mutagenesis (*see* Note 6):

9. Control plasmid: pBR322, 0.05 μg/μL (*see* Note 7).
10. Control deletion primer: 5'-Pi GCCGGTACTGGCGGGCCTCTTGCG-GGCG-3', 0.10 μg/μL (see Note 8).
11. *Eco*RV restriction enzyme (20 U/μL, for the control experiment) (*see* Note 9).

Additional materials required for the experimental deletion mutagenesis (*see* Notes 10 and 11 for tips on primer design):

12. Target plasmid, 0.05 μg/μL (*see* Notes 12 and 13).
13. Deletion primer, 0.1 μg/μL.
14. Selection restriction enzyme (5–20 U/μL) (*see* Note 14).

2.2. Primer Phosphorylation, Preparation of Competent E. coli Cells, and Transformations

1. T4 Polynucleotide kinase (10 U/μL).
2. 10X T4 Kinase buffer: 500 mM Tris-HCl, pH 7.5, 100 mM MgCl$_2$, 50 mM DTT, 10 mM ATP.
3. Ampicillin: 100 mg/mL (1000X) stock solution in water. Filter sterilize and store at 4°C for no more than 1 mo.
4. Competent cells: Either electrocompetent cells *(9)* or chemically competent cells (prepared ahead of time) *(10)* may be used in the transformations. Electrocompetent BMH 71-18 *mutS* cells (#C2020-1) or DH5α cells (#2022-1), and chemically competent BMH 71-18 *mutS* cells (#C2010-1) may be purchased from Clontech.
5. LB agar plates containing 50–100 μg/mL ampicillin (LB/+amp): LB/+amp plates are used when performing the control mutagenesis with pBR322 and the control primer. LB agar plates containing a different antibiotic may be required for other target plasmids.
6. LB agar plates containing 100 μg/mL ampicillin and 50 μg/mL tetracycline (LB/+amp/+tet): LB/+amp/+tet plates are used to determine the efficiency of deletion mutagenesis in the control experiment.
7. LB medium: 10 g/L bactotryptone, 5 g/L bactoyeast extract, 10 g/L NaCl. Adjust pH to 7.0 with 5N NaOH. Autoclave to sterilize. For detailed information on the preparation of media for bacteriological work, please refer to the laboratory manual by Sambrook et al. *(11)*.
8. TE buffer: 10 mM Tris-HCl, pH 7.5, 1 mM EDTA.
9. Tetracycline: 5 mg/mL (100X) stock solution in ethanol. Wrap tube with aluminum foil and store at –20°C.

3. Methods

3.1. Primer Phosphorylation

Deletion primers must be phosphorylated at the 5' end before being used in a deletion mutagenesis experiment. Highly efficient 5' phosphorylation is commonly achieved by an enzymatic reaction using T4 polynucleotide kinase (#8408-1). (*See* Note 15 for an alternative phosphorylation procedure.) The control deletion primer provided in the Quantum Leap Kit has been phosphorylated and purified.

1. To a 0.5-mL microcentrifuge tube, add 2.0 μL of 10X kinase buffer, 1.0 μL of T4 polynucleotide kinase, and 1 μg of primer (20–30 nucleotides long). Adjust the volume to 20 μL with water. Mix and centrifuge briefly.
2. Incubate at 37°C for 60 min.
3. Stop the reaction by heating at 65°C for 10 min.
4. Use 2.0 μL of the phosphorylated primer solution in each mutagenesis reaction.
5. Unused phosphorylated primers can be stored at –20°C for several weeks.

3.2. Denaturation and Annealing of Plasmid DNA

The following conditions are recommended for the annealing of phosphorylated primers to most plasmids *(4,12)*. Slow cooling is not necessary and, in many cases, may be detrimental. The alternative annealing protocol given in Note 16 may give better results for plasmids larger than 10 kb.

1. Prewarm a water bath to boiling (100°C) (*see* Note 17).
2. Set up the primer/plasmid annealing reaction in a 0.5-mL microcentrifuge tube as follows: 2.0 μL of 10X annealing buffer, 2.0 μL of plasmid DNA (0.05 μg/μL), and 2.0 μL of deletion primer (0.1 μg/μL) (*see* Note 18).
3. Adjust with water to a total volume of 20 μL. Mix well. Briefly centrifuge the tube.
4. Incubate at 100°C for 3 min.
5. Chill immediately in an ice water bath (0°C) for 5 min. Briefly centrifuge to collect the sample.

3.3. Synthesis of the Mutant DNA Strand

1. Add to the annealed primer/plasmid mixture: 3.0 μL of 10X synthesis buffer, 1.0 μL of T4 DNA polymerase, 1.0 μL of T4 DNA ligase, and 5.0 μL of water.
2. Mix well and centrifuge briefly. Incubate at 37°C for 2 h.

3. Stop the reaction by heating at 70°C for 10 min to inactivate the enzymes.
4. Let the tube cool to room temperature for a few minutes.

3.4. Primary Selection
by Restriction Enzyme Digestion

After the mutant DNA strand synthesis and ligation, a majority (>95%) of the plasmids present in the total plasmid pool will be parental-type plasmids. The purpose of the first restriction enzyme digestion is to selectively linearize the parental DNA and thereby greatly enrich for mutant plasmids within the total DNA pool before the first transformation. This primary selection step facilitates the second (final) restriction digestion by reducing the percentage of plasmids that are susceptible to digestion.

1. For the control mutagenesis, simply add 1 μL of *Eco*RV, and BSA to a final concentration of 100 μg/mL, to the synthesis/ligation mixture, and incubate at 37°C for 1–2 h.
2. For the experimental mutagenesis, use the buffer conditions that resulted in the most efficient digestion of the target plasmid, as determined by the relative reduction in the number of transformants in the preliminary test (*see* Note 14). If digestion was satisfactory (i.e., >99.9% of target plasmids were cut) using the annealing buffer, then simply add 20 U of the chosen restriction enzyme to the synthesis/ligation mixture and incubate at 37°C for 1–2 h. If the digestion was significantly better using the enzyme manufacturer's recommended buffer, then change or adjust the buffer accordingly (*see* Note 19).
3. After the primary restriction digestion, heat the tube containing the DNA at 70°C for 5 min to inactivate possible exonuclease or nonspecific endonuclease contaminants that could damage the mutated DNA.

3.5. First Transformation

The purpose of the first transformation is to amplify the mutated strand (as well as the parental strand) in the BMH 71-18 repair-deficient (*mutS*) strain of *E. coli*. Either electroporation or chemical transformation may be used in this as well as all subsequent transformations. Detailed protocols for preparation of competent cells can be found in refs. *9–11*. For best mutagenesis results, your transformation procedure should yield at least 1×10^7 transformants/μg of DNA using chemical transformation, or at least 1×10^8 transformants/μg of DNA using electrotransformation. The amount of plasmid/primer DNA solution and competent cell suspension used per tube depends on whether you are using electrotransformation or chemical transformation. After the recovery step, transformants are grown on agar medium rather than in liquid culture to avoid biasing the plasmid population toward those containing the largest deletions (*see* Note 20).

3.5.1. Chemical Transformation

1. Preheat a heating block or water bath to 42°C.
2. Add 5–10 μL of the primary restriction-digested plasmid/primer DNA solution to a 15-mL tube containing 100 μL of competent BMH 71-18 *mutS* cells and incubate on ice for 20 min.
3. Transfer to 42°C for 1 min. Proceed to step 2.

3.5.2. Electroporation

1. Dilute the primary restriction-digested plasmid/primer DNA solution five-fold with water.
2. Add 2 μL of the diluted DNA to a separate tube containing 40 μL of electrocompetent BMH 71-18 *mutS* cells on ice.
3. Perform the electroporation according to the manufacturer's instructions. (For example, if you are using the BioRad [Hercules, CA] *E. coli* Pulser Electroporator, use a 0.1-cm cuvet and set the instrument at 1.8 kV, with constant capacitance at 10 μF and internal resistance at 600 Ω.)

3.5.3. Recovery

This applies to both chemical transformation and electroporation.

1. Immediately add 1 mL of LB medium (without antibiotic) to each tube.
2. Incubate at 37°C for 60 min with shaking at 220 rpm.

3.5.4. Amplification

1. After the 60-min recovery period, centrifuge the tube at 2000*g* for 5 min to pellet the cells.
2. Remove most of the supernatant and resuspend the pellet in the remaining medium.
3. Spread the entire transformation mixture onto an LB agar plate containing the appropriate selection antibiotic. In the case of the control experiment with pBR322, use LB/+amp (*see* Note 20).
4. Incubate the culture at 37°C overnight.

3.6. Isolation of the Plasmid Pool and Second Restriction Enzyme Digestion

After overnight growth of transformed BMH 71-18 *mutS* cells, both parental and mutated plasmid strands are segregated and amplified. Now the plasmid pool can be purified from the cells and a second restriction digestion can be applied to further enrich for the desired mutants by selecting against the parental (nonmutated) plasmids. A quick boiling lysis method for plasmid preparation *(6)* is recommended, since it consistently results in clean "miniprep" DNA. However, other standard miniprep procedures, such as the alkaline lysis method *(9)*, may be used.

1. Add a small amount of LB medium to the LB-agar selection plate and carefully scrape the colonies together using a sterile glass rod.
2. Resuspend the colonies in ~100 µL of STET buffer and proceed with the plasmid miniprep.
3. Dissolve the DNA pellets in 100 µL of TE buffer (each). The normal yield of plasmid DNA using the quick boiling lysis method is approx 2–5 µg.
4. (Optional) Purify DNA on a spin column. (e.g., Chroma Spin + TE-400 column).
5. Set up the following restriction enzyme digestion: 5.0 µL of purified mixed plasmid DNA (approx 100 ng), 2.0 µL of 10X restriction enzyme buffer, and 1 µL of restriction enzyme (10–20 U). For the control experiment, use *Eco*RV and 10X annealing buffer with 100 µg/mL BSA (which is functionally equivalent to 10X *Eco*RV buffer). Adjust the final volume to 20 µL with sterile water.
4. Mix well. Incubate at 37°C for 1 h.
5. Add an additional 10 U of the appropriate restriction enzyme, and continue incubation at 37°C for another 1 h.

3.7. Final Transformation

The purpose of the final transformation is to amplify and stably clone the mutated plasmid. To avoid accumulation of random mutations in the plasmids, the mismatch repair-deficient *E. coli* strain (BMH 71-18 *mutS*) used for the first transformation should not be used in the second transformation.

1. Use 5.0 µL of the digested plasmid (approx 25 ng) for transformation of chemically competent cells, or 1.0 µL of fivefold diluted (with water) plasmid (approx 1 ng) for transformation of electrocompetent cells. Follow the same procedure as for the first transformation (*see* Section 3.5.).
2. Recovery:
   a. Immediately add 1.0 mL of LB medium (with no antibiotic) to each tube.
   b. Incubate at 37°C for 60 min with shaking at 220 rpm.
3. Prepare 10-, 100-, and 1000-fold dilutions of the cell/DNA mixture (100 µL each).

4. Mix well and spread each suspension evenly onto LB agar plates containing the appropriate antibiotic for selection of transformants (LB/+amp50 for the control experiment).
5. Incubate the plates at 37°C overnight.

3.8. Characterization of Mutant Plasmids

1. For the control experiment with pBR322:
   a. Test transformants for tetracycline sensitivity by toothpicking (or replica plating) colonies from the selection plates to an LB/+amp/+tet plate and to another LB/+amp plate. Incubate plates at 37°C overnight.
   b. Score colonies for drug resistance phenotypes. Tet^S, Amp^R colonies are likely to contain deletion plasmids. The efficiency of mutagenesis is estimated by dividing the total number of colonies growing on the LB/+amp plate by the number of Tet^S, Amp^R colonies (i.e., colonies that do not grow on LB/+amp/+tet medium). The efficiency is expected to be >90% if the mutagenesis has been performed successfully. (*See* Fig. 3 for an example of nested deletions generated in the *tet*^{r} gene of pBR322 using the deletion method described here.)
2. For mutagenesis experiments that do not involve a visible phenotype, such as colony color, nutrition requirement, or resistance to another antibiotic, it may be necessary to isolate plasmid DNA to characterize the deletions. A quick estimate of relative deletion sizes can be obtained using a rapid lysis procedure *(7)*.
   a. With a sterile loop, transfer each transformant colony to be analyzed to 60 µL of TE buffer and vortex to disperse the cells. (Alternatively, use 100 µL of an overnight culture of each individual clone.)
   b. Add 50 µL of phenol:chloroform (1:1 [v/v]) and 10 µL of 10X gel-loading buffer (containing 4% glycerol).
   c. Vortex vigorously for 1 min.
   d. Pellet cellular debris by centrifugation at top speed for 3 min in a microcentrifuge.
   e. Load 10–30 µL of each supernatant to separate wells on a 0.8% agarose/EtBr gel. Estimate sizes of putative mutant plasmids by comparison with supercoiled marker DNA and parental plasmid.
3. Deletions can be further characterized by PCR screening or restriction analysis of plasmid DNA isolated from individual transformant colonies.
4. The exact length of deletions in individual clones should be verified by directly sequencing the mutagenized regions.

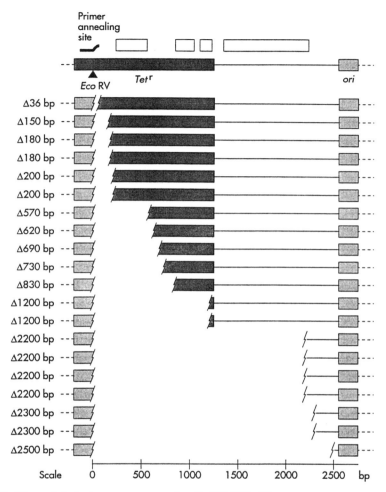

Fig. 3. Nested deletion mutagenesis of pBR322. The target sequence was the tetracycline-resistance (*tet*) gene of pBR322, and the deletion primer was a 29-mer oligonucleotide including a 4-mer arbitrary sequence (GGCG) at the 3' end. The *Eco*RV site of pBR322 was used to select against plasmids that were not mutated. Some 49 of 50 ampicillin-resistant transformants were also tetra-cycline-sensitive, and thus were candidates for carrying deletion plasmids. Plasmid DNA was isolated from 20 randomly chosen Amp^R, Tet^S transformants. The deletions were sized and ordered by restriction mapping, as shown in the figure; the deleted portions are represented by gaps in the DNA sequence. The open bars at the top of the figure represent regions longer than 150 bp in which the sequence GGCG is predicted not to occur in pBR322.

4. Notes

1. The 3' tail of the primer will typically consist of an arbitrary sequence of four or five nucleotides, primarily Gs and Cs. As and Ts may be used within the tail sequence; however, a G or C doublet should be at the 3' end of the tail to ensure proper annealing to the template. The exact length and sequence of the mismatched tail will determine the number and location of semi-random annealing sites within the cloned sequence in the target plasmid (Table 1). For example, a mismatched tail of three nucleotides will statistically find a match in the target sequence every 64 bases, thus generating deletions that are, on the average, multiples of 64 bp. Similarly, mismatched tails with lengths of four, five, and six nucleotides will generate deletions with average sizes that are multiples of 256, 1024, and 4096 bp, respectively.

    The average sizes of deletions can be further modified by making one or more nucleotide positions in the mismatched primer tail partially degenerate. For example, if one of the nucleotides in a five-nucleotide tail is doubly degenerate (e.g., synthesized as an equimolar mixture of G and C), the average deletion sizes will be multiples of 512 bp. Furthermore, altering the specific sequence in the mismatched primer tail, while keeping the length fixed, will generate deletions in roughly the same average size categories, but with endpoints in different regions of the target sequences. Although the majority of deletions generated in a given experiment will fall into discrete size categories, a few exceptions can be expected; the odd-sized deletions most likely result from imperfect annealing of the arbitrary tail.

2. A typical deletion primer consists of a 20-mer that anneals to a complementary sequence upstream (i.e., 5') of the MCS in a specific plasmid, and a short (e.g., 4-mer) 3' tail that anneals semirandomly to complementary sequences within the cloned gene. See Table 2 for sequence information.

3. The success of this mutagenesis procedure is directly correlated with the success of the restriction enzyme digestions used for mutant enrichment. Thus, it is important to obtain complete digestion of the parental plasmid before each transformation. The chances of obtaining complete digestion will be maximized if the plasmid DNA is purified before the digestion steps as explained in Note 13, and if you make sure that the target plasmid at low concentrations can be efficiently digested with the selection enzyme before beginning the mutagenesis experiment (*see* Note 14). The selection enzyme should also be tested for the presence of exonuclease—or nonspecific endonuclease—contaminants (*see* Note 14). Such contaminating nuclease activities can lead to a preponderance of large deletions thereby, reducing the desired deletion size range.

4. T4 DNA polymerase is used to extend the primers and to synthesize the mutant strand. Unlike the Klenow fragment of DNA polymerase I (an enzyme commonly used in in vitro mutagenesis), T4 DNA polymerase does not have strand displacement activity *(13,14)*. Thus, with T4 DNA polymerase, the primer (along with the desired nested deletions) will be incorporated into the newly synthesized strand. T4 DNA ligase is used to ligate the newly synthesized DNA strand to the 5' (phosphorylated) end of the oligonucleotide primer, a step that is necessary to obtain covalently closed circular DNA with high transforming ability. A specialized *E. coli* strain, BMH 71-18 *mutS*, defective in mismatch repair *(8)*, is used in the first transformation to prevent undesirable repair of the mutant DNA strand. The first transformation step also serves to amplify the entire deletion mutagenesis process.

5. *E. coli* strain BMH 71-18 *mutS* carries a Tn10 insertion in *mutS*; this Tn10 insertion causes a repair-deficiency phenotype as well as tetracyline resistance. For the repair-deficiency phenotype and Tn10 insertion to be maintained, this strain must be grown on medium containing 50 µg/mL tetracycline.

6. It is recommended to run a control deletion mutagenesis in advance of—or concurrently with—the experimental mutagenesis. The control experiment should be designed to result in a series of nested deletions that can be easily detected, for example, by a change in colony phenotype. The control system described here is designed to generate nested deletions in the gene conferring tetracycline resistance (*tet^r*) in the control plasmid (pBR322). The Quantum Leap Nested Deletion Kit (Clontech #K1610-1) includes control materials.

7. The control plasmid, pBR322, carries the gene for ampicillin resistance, which is used as the bacterial selectable marker. *E. coli* cells transformed by pBR322 are selected by plating on medium containing 50 µg/mL ampicillin. pBR322 also carries a tetracycline-resistance gene (*tet^r*), which is the region targeted for nested deletions in the control experiment. A deletion of any size from the 5' end into the coding region of this gene will render the bacteria sensitive to tetracycline. Thus, most of the deletions can be easily checked by replica plating the final transformants onto LB/+amp plates with and without tetracycline. The efficiency of mutagenesis is estimated by dividing the number of Tet^S, Amp^R colonies (i.e., colonies that do not grow on LB/+amp/+tet medium) by the total number of colonies growing on the LB/+amp plates.

8. Use of the control deletion primer with pBR322 will delete a unique *Eco*RV restriction site, thus allowing for selection against parental (unmutated) plasmids by digestion with *Eco*RV. The four-base, arbitrary 3' tail of the control primer will find a complementary sequence in the template every 256 bp, on average.

9. Restriction enzyme *Eco*RV is used for selection against the parental pBR322 plasmid in the control experiment. There is a unique *Eco* RV site immediately downstream from the control deletion primer binding site. Since the *Eco*RV recognition site is AT-rich, the possibility for any deletion mutants to regenerate a new *Eco*RV site is low.

10. Length of deletion primer: In most cases, 20 nucleotides of uninterrupted sequence complementary to a region flanking the deletion site should give sufficient annealing stability, provided that the GC content of the primer is >50%. If the GC content is <50%, the length of the complementary region on the primer should be extended accordingly *(12)*. For optimum primer annealing, the complementary region should start with a G or C (5' end) and end with a G or C doublet (3' end).

11. Primers for generation of precise large deletions: With a modification in deletion primer design, the nested deletion method can be used to generate specific, large deletions. In this case, the deletion primer should have regions of at least 15 bp of complementary sequences flanking both sides of the segment to be deleted. Using such a primer, we have generated deletions up to 6.6 kb. The upper limit on the size of deletions has not been determined, but it is presumed to be quite large, provided that no genes required for replication or selection of the plasmid are incapacitated.

12. Plasmids with tetracycline as the only selection marker are not suitable for mutagenesis since the bacterial strain BMH 71-18 *mutS* has a Tn10 transposon that confers tetracycline resistance.

13. Because proteins and other impurities in the plasmid pool can significantly affect the degree of digestion obtained, it is important to use purified target plasmid DNA in the mutagenesis procedure. To achieve the maximum efficiency of cutting in the first digestion, the target plasmid should be purified by CsCl banding or a method that yields plasmid of comparable purity.

14. Restriction enzyme digestion is the sole selection mechanism operating in this nested deletion procedure. Therefore, before using a particular restriction enzyme in a mutagenesis experiment, check to make sure that the target plasmid at low concentrations can be efficiently digested with the selection enzyme. We have found that the enzyme unit definition of 1 μg/h under defined buffer and temperature conditions does not necessarily correspond to the enzyme's ability to cut very low concentrations of DNA. The selection enzyme should also be checked for the presence of contaminating exonuclease activities. We have found significant lot-to-lot variation from the same manufacturer.

    a. Set up two digestions, each using 0.1–0.2 μg of the target plasmid with 5–20 U of the chosen restriction enzyme in a 30-μL (final vol) reaction. In one of the digestions, use the annealing buffer described in Section

2.1.; in the other digestion, use the buffer recommended by the enzyme manufacturer. The mutagenesis procedure is simpler if you can perform the first digestion in the annealing buffer used in the step preceding the digestion; the annealing buffer (with BSA added) is functionally similar to *Eco*RV buffer. If the glycerol concentration is >5% (v/v) after adding the restriction enzyme, the reaction volume should be increased proportionally to avoid undesirable star activity. The same amount of DNA should be maintained.

  b. Incubate for 1 h at 37°C.

  c. Transform an appropriate *E. coli* strain separately with the two plasmid digests and with an equivalent amount of undigested plasmid. Plate out cells on appropriate selection medium and incubate overnight.

  d. Compare the number of colonies obtained in each transformation. Ideally, you should see a 1000-fold reduction in transformation efficiency using the plasmid samples that have been restriction digested, compared to using undigested plasmid. If digestion of the target plasmid does not reduce the number of transformants to ≤1% of the control transformation, the final mutation efficiency may be less than expected. If this is the case, consider choosing a different restriction enzyme.

  e. To check for the presence of contaminating exonucleases or nonspecific endonucleases in the selection enzyme, isolate plasmids (minipreps) from 10–20 colonies derived from the transformation with restriction digested DNA. Electrophorese 5.0-µL samples on a 0.8% agarose minigel, in parallel with the parental plasmid. If the plasmids isolated from the transformant clones are smaller than the parental plasmid, this could indicate that the restriction enzyme is contaminated with other nuclease activities. If this is the case, try to find a new batch of enzyme—or a different enzyme—that is free of undesirable nucleases.

15. Alternatively, a 5' phosphate group can be added (with 100% efficiency) to an oligonucleotide during automated DNA synthesis using an appropriate CE-phosphoramidite reagent, such as 5'-Phosphate-ON (#5210-1). These phosphorylated synthetic oligonucleotides are stable for more than 6 mo at –20°C.

16. An alternative denaturing and annealing protocol that completely denatures the double-stranded DNA template is especially recommended when mutating large (i.e., >10 kb) plasmids. However, when a small amount (<1 µg) of plasmid DNA is used, care must be taken to avoid losing the DNA pellet during the ethanol wash (step f). In general, it is safer to use larger quantities (1–2 µg) of DNA with this annealing procedure.

  a. Mix at least 100 ng of plasmid (1–2 µL) in 16 µL of water with 4 µL of 2*M* NaOH in a microcentrifuge tube.

b. Incubate at room temperature for 10 min.

c. Neutralize with 4 μL of 3M NaOAc (pH 4.8).

d. Add 70 μL of ethanol and cool to −70°C.

e. Centrifuge for 10 min to pellet the precipitated DNA.

f. Carefully wash pellet with 70% ethanol. Collect pellet by centrifugation. Allow pellet to air dry.

g. Resuspend DNA in water to a concentration of 0.05 μg/μL. The resuspended DNA may be stored at 4°C for a few days.

h. For annealing, mix 100 ng of the control plasmid and 200 ng of primer. Adjust the volume to 18 μL with water and add 2 μL of annealing buffer.

i. Incubate at 37°C for 10 min and then place on ice for another 10 min.

j. Proceed with synthesis and ligation.

17. Complete denaturation of the template DNA must occur. To achieve this, it is necessary to boil the DNA at 100°C. Lower temperatures do not suffice.

18. The recommended concentration of the plasmid is 0.05–0.1 μg/μL. To ensure saturated annealing of the deletion primer, the primer should be present in a 200–400-fold molar excess over the single-stranded template DNA.

19. The concentration of NaCl in the synthesis/ligation mixture is 37.5 mM in a total volume of 30 μL. If the NaCl concentration must be increased for optimal digestion, the 10X annealing buffer (which contains 500 mM NaCl) can be used to make the adjustment. If the NaCl concentration must be reduced (or other undesirable components eliminated), the DNA mixture can be ethanol precipitated or passed through a spin column (e.g., Clontech's Chroma Spin-30 Column, #K1301-1). The desalted DNA can then be resuspended in the new buffer. BSA (100 μg/mL) may be added to the reaction if necessary to obtain optimal digestion.

20. Unlike in the original USE site-directed mutagenesis procedure, we do not recommend overnight liquid culture here. Growth of a mixed plasmid population in liquid culture favors growth of smaller plasmids (i.e., those having larger deletions) at the expense of larger plasmids (i.e., those having smaller deletions). To avoid competition among the deletion mutants—and thus to obtain an unbiased spectrum of deletion sizes—we utilize growth on solid medium; in this way, all deletion mutants have an equal opportunity to grow and form colonies.

Acknowledgments

We thank Anne Scholz for helpful discussions, John Ledesma and John Stile for technical assistance, and Kristen Mayo for editing the manuscript.

References

1. Legerski, R. J., Hodnett, J. L., and Gray, H. B., Jr. (1978) Extracellular nucleases of *Pseudomonas* BAL 31. III. Use of the double-strand deoxyriboexonuclease activity as the basis of a convenient method for the mapping of fragments of DNA produced by cleavage with restriction enzymes. *Nucleic Acids Res.* **5,** 1445.
2. Henikoff, S. (1987) Unidirectional digestion with exonuclease III in DNA sequence analysis. *Methods Enzymol.* **155,** 156–165.
3. Shen, W. and Waye, M. M. (1988) A novel method for generating a nested set of unidirectional deletion mutants using mixed oligodeoxynucleotides. *Gene* **70,** 205–211.
4. Deng, W. P. and Nickoloff, J. A. (1992) Site-directed mutagenesis of virtually any plasmid by eliminating a unique site. *Anal. Biochem.* **200,** 81–88.
5. Conley, E. C. and Saunders, J. R. (1984) Recombination-dependent recircularization of linearized pBR322 plasmid DNA following transformation of *Escherichia coli. Mol. Gen. Genet.* **194,** 211–218.
6. Holmes, D. S. and Quigley, M. (1981) A rapid boiling method for the preparation of bacterial plasmids. *Anal. Biochem.* **114,** 193–197.
7. Akada, R. (1994) Quick-check method to test the size of *Escherichia coli* plasmids. *BioTechniques* **17,** 58.
8. Zell, R. and Fritz, H. (1987) DNA mismatch repair in *Escherichia coli* counteracting the hydrolytic deamination of 5-methyl-cytosine residues. *EMBO J.* **6,** 1809–1815.
9. Chung, C. T., Niemela, S. L., and Miller, R. H. (1989) One-step preparation of competent *Escherichia coli*: Transformation and storage of bacterial cells in the same solution. *Proc. Natl. Acad. Sci. USA* **86,** 2172–2175.
10. *Protocol for Transformer™ Site-Directed Mutagenesis Kit.* (1994) Clontech Laboratories, Inc., PT1130-1, Palo Alto, CA.
11. Sambrook, J., Fritsch, E. F., and Maniatis, T. (1989) *Molecular Cloning: A Laboratory Manual,* 2nd ed., Cold Spring Harbor Laboratory Press, Cold Spring Harbor, NY.
12. Zhu, L. (1992) Highly efficient site-directed mutagenesis of dsDNA plasmids. *CLONTECHniques* **VII(1),** 1–5.
13. Masumune, Y. and Richardson, C. A. (1971) Strand displacement during deoxyribonucleic acid synthesis at single-strand breaks. *J. Biol. Chem.* **246,** 2692–2701.
14. Nossal, N. G. (1974) DNA synthesis on a double-stranded DNA template by the T4 bacteriophage DNA polymerase and the T4 gene 32 DNA unwinding protein. *J. Biol. Chem.* **249,** 5668–5676.

CHAPTER 12

Ordered Deletions Using Exonuclease III

Denise Clark and Steven Henikoff

1. Introduction

An important manipulation in molecular genetics is to make ordered deletions into a cloned piece of DNA. The most widely used application of this method is in DNA sequencing. Ordered deletions can also be used in delineating sequences that are important for the function of a gene, such as those required for transcription. The principle behind using deletions for sequencing is that consecutive parts of a fragment cloned into a plasmid vector are brought adjacent to a sequencing primer site in the vector. Deletions are generated by digesting DNA unidirectionally with *Escherichia coli* exonuclease III (ExoIII) *(1)*. ExoIII digests one strand of double-stranded DNA by removing nucleotides from 3' ends if the end is blunt or has a 5' protrusion. A 3' protrusion of 4 bases or more is resistant to ExoIII digestion.

We present two procedures, outlined in Fig. 1, for preparation of the template for ExoIII digestion. Procedure I begins with double-stranded plasmid DNA. The DNA is digested with restriction endonucleases A and B, where A generates a 5' protrusion or blunt end next to the target sequence and B generates a 3' protrusion next to the sequencing primer site. The linearized plasmid DNA is digested with ExoIII, with aliquots taken at time points that will yield a set of deletions of the desired lengths. Procedure II *(2)* begins with single-stranded phagemid DNA. A nicked double-stranded circle is generated by annealing a primer to the phagemid

From: *Methods in Molecular Biology, Vol. 57: In Vitro Mutagenesis Protocols*
Edited by: M. K. Trower Humana Press Inc., Totowa, NJ

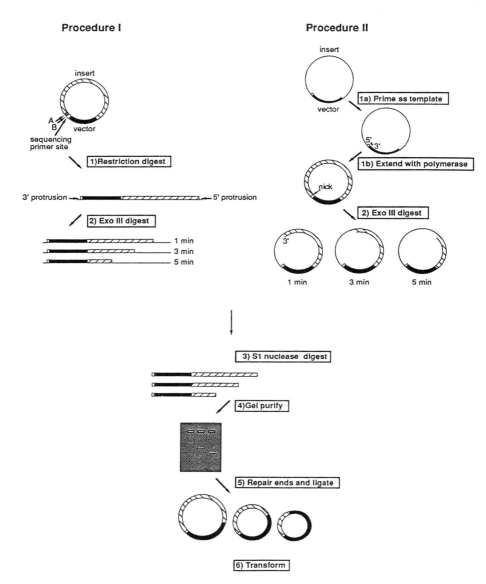

Fig. 1. Outline of the method.

so that its 5' end is adjacent to the insert and synthesizing the second strand with T4 DNA polymerase.

The 3' end of the nicked strand is then digested with ExoIII. The remaining undigested single strands are digested with S1 nuclease. The deletion reactions are examined by electrophoresis in a low melting point agarose gel and the desired deletion products are isolated in gel slices *(3,4)*. This step serves to eliminate DNA products that do not contain the desired deletion. Repair of ends with Klenow DNA polymerase and ligation to circularize are performed on the DNA in diluted agarose. Following transformation into *E. coli*, clones are selected for sequencing.

An advantage of Procedure I is that deletions can be made into the insert from either end, so that both strands of the insert can be sequenced starting with a single plasmid clone. However, the requirement for multiple unique restriction sites in the vector polylinker cannot always be met, and this is where Procedure II is advantageous, since no restriction sites are necessary. This also means that, with Procedure II, a set of nested deletions can be made from any fixed point using a custom primer. A disadvantage of Procedure II is that, to sequence both strands of an insert, two clones with the insert in either orientation are required. Nevertheless, the two procedures can be used together to obtain the sequence of both strands from a single parent clone, reducing the need for multiple unique restriction sites. When planning a sequencing strategy, it is important to realize that although either single- or double-stranded templates for sequencing are possible for Procedure I, only double-stranded templates are possible for Procedure II. The reason is that for most phagemid vectors, the primer for synthesis of the second strand of the nicked circle anneals to a site on the other side of the insert from the primer site that would be used for sequencing a single-stranded template.

2. Materials

2.1. General

Solutions are made with distilled water that when used for enzyme buffers is sterilized by autoclaving. Store solutions at room temperature, unless otherwise specified. Store enzymes as directed by the manufacturer.

2.1.1. Restriction Enzyme Digestion

1. 10 µg of double-stranded DNA: The fragment should be cloned into the multiple cloning site (polylinker) of a plasmid or phagemid vector such as Bluescript (Stratagene, La Jolla, CA). DNA can be prepared using an alkaline lysis procedure *(5; see* Note 1*)*. A 10-mL liquid culture incubated overnight in LB media with the appropriate selection (e.g., ampicillin) should yield a sufficient amount of DNA.

2. Restriction enzymes and buffers as supplied by manufacturer. Select a restriction enzyme (A in Fig. 1) that cuts the plasmid only in the polylinker adjacent to the insert and yields a 5' protrusion or blunt end. Restriction enzyme B must also cut at a unique site in the polylinker and yield a 4 base 3' protrusion to make the end of the linearized fragment nearest the sequencing primer site resistant to ExoIII. If such a site is not available, a 5' protrusion can be generated that is filled in with α-phosphorothioate nucleotides using Klenow fragments *(6)*.
3. Phenol:chloroform solution: 1:1 mix; store at 4°C.
4. 10M Ammonium actetate.
5. Ethanol: both 95 and 70% (v/v).
6. 10X ExoIII buffer: 660 mM Tris-HCl, pH 8.0, 6.6 mM MgCl$_2$.

2.1.2. Procedure II: Synthesis of a Nicked Circular Plasmid

7. Template: 2.5 μg single-stranded phagemid DNA, 0.2–2.0 μg/μL. A small-scale preparation (2–3 mL culture) should yield a sufficient amount of DNA *(5)*.
8. Primer: α-T3 20-mer (5' CCCTTTAGTGAGGGTTAATT 3'), or the equivalent, e.g., reverse hybridization 17-mer (5' GAAACAGCTATGACCAT 3') at 4 pmol/μL; store at –20°C.
9. T4 DNA polymerase: 1–10 U/μL, cloned or from T4-infected cells.
10. 10X TM: 660 mM Tris-HCl, pH 8.0, 30 mM MgCl$_2$.
11. 2.5 mM dNTPs: 2.5 mM each of the 4 deoxynucleoside triphosphates; store at –20°C.
12. BSA: 1 mg/mL bovine serum albumin (nuclease-free); store at –20°C.

2.2. Exonuclease III and S1 Nuclease Digestion

13. *E. coli* exonuclease III: 150–200 U/μL (1 U = amount of enzyme required to produce 1 nmol of acid-soluble nucleotides in 30 min at 37°C).
14. S1 buffer concentrate: 2.5M NaCl, 0.3M potassium acetate (titrate to pH 4.6 with HCl, not acetic acid), 10 mM ZnSO$_4$, 50% (v/v) glycerol.
15. S1 nuclease: e.g., 60 U/μL from Promega (1 U = amount of enzyme required to release 1 μg of perchloric acid-soluble nucleotides per minute at 37°C). Mung bean nuclease may also be used.
16. S1 mix: 27 μL S1 buffer concentrate 173 mL of H$_2$O, 1 μL (60 U) of S1 nuclease. Prepare just before use and store on ice.
17. S1 stop: 0.3M Tris base (no HCl), 50 mM EDTA.

2.3. Gel Purification, End Repair, Ligation, and Transformation

18. Agarose: Low melting point agarose. Use a grade appropriate for cloning, e.g., Seaplaque GTG agarose (FMC).

19. Ethidium bromide: 10 mg/mL; store in a dark container.
20. 50X TAE gel running buffer: 1 L = 242 g Tris base, 57.1 mL glacial acetic acid, 100 mL 0.5M EDTA (pH 8). When diluted this gives a 1X buffer of 40 mM Tris-acetate, 1 mM EDTA.
21. 10X Gel-loading buffer: 0.25% bromophenol blue, 50% (v/v) glycerol in distilled water.
22. 10X Klenow buffer: 20 mM Tris-HCl, pH 8.0, 100 mM MgCl$_2$.
23. Klenow enzyme: the large fragment of the *E. coli* DNA polymerase (2 U/μL). Store at –20°C.
24. Klenow mix: For every 10 μL 10X Klenow buffer, add 1 U of Klenow enzyme. Prepare just before use and store on ice.
25. dNTPs: 0.125 mM of each deoxyribonucleoside; store at –20°C.
26. 10X Ligase buffer: 0.5M Tris-HCl, pH 7.6, 100 mM MgCl$_2$, 10 mM ATP; store at –20°C.
27. PEG: 50% (w/v) polyethylene glycol 6000–8000 fraction, store at 4°C.
28. DTT: 0.1M dithiothreitol; store at –20°C.
29. T4 DNA ligase: (1 U/μL). Store at –20°C.
30. Ligation cocktail (1 mL): 570 μL H$_2$O, 200 μL ligase buffer, 200 μL PEG, 20 μL 0.1M DTT, 10 U of T4 ligase. Prepare just before use and store on ice.
31. Host *E. coli* cells: Competent recA⁻ cells, e.g., DH5α.
32. Growth media: LB medium *(5)*.

3. Methods
3.1. Preparation of Exonuclease III Substrate
3.1.1. Procedure I: Restriction Enzyme Digestion

1. Digest 10 μg of plasmid to completion in a 100 μL volume. At least 200 ng is required for each ExoIII digestion time point (*see* Note 1).
2. To extract the DNA, vortex in 100 μL of phenol:chloroform and remove the aqueous layer to a fresh tube.
3. Add 25 μL of 10M ammonium acetate and 200 μL of 95% ethanol. Chill on ice for 15 min and pellet the DNA in a microfuge (12,000g) for 5 min.
4. Wash pellet with 70% ethanol and air dry. Resuspend the DNA pellet in 90 μL of distilled H$_2$O and 10 μL of 10X ExoIII buffer (i.e., 100 ng/μL).

3.1.2. Procedure II: Synthesis of a Nicked Circular Phagemid

1. Mix in a volume of 22 μL: approx 2.5 μg single-stranded phagemid DNA, 4 μL of 10X TM, 1 μL (4 pmol) of α-T3 primer (or equivalent).
2. Heat to 75°C for 5 min, then cool slowly over 30–60 min. Evaporation and condensation can be minimized by placing a piece of insulating foam over

the tube in an aluminum tube-heating block. Remove a 2-μL aliquot for subsequent gel analysis.

3. Mix in a volume of 20 μL: 2 μL of DTT, 4 μL of 2.5 m*M* dNTPs, 4 μL of BSA, and 5 U of T4 DNA polymerase.

4. Prewarm to 37°C and add to the primed DNA at 37°C. Incubate 2–8 h. An example of a nicked circle is shown in Fig. 2. When the plasmid is as large as this one, we recommend supplementing the extension reaction with an additional 0.4 m*M* dNTPs and 0.1 U/μL polymerase after 4–6 h, and then incubation overnight. Extension can be monitored by removing a 0.5-μL aliquot and electrophoresing it on an agarose gel.

5. Inactivate polymerase by heating for 10 min at 70°C and store on ice.

3.2. Exonuclease III Digestion

Deletions separated by 200–250 bases are required for obtaining contiguous sequence with some overlap, therefore to sequence a 4-kb insert, 16–20 time points are desirable (*see* Note 2). The following protocol is written to give 16 time points.

1. Prepare 16 7.5-μL aliquots (*see* Note 3) of S1 nuclease mix on ice, one for each time point.

2. Place 40 μL of DNA (from Section 3.1.1., step 4 or 3.1.2., step 5) into a single tube. Warm the DNA to 37°C in a heating block (*see* Note 3). Add 1–2 μL of ExoIII (5–10 U/μL), mix rapidly by pipeting up and down.

3. Remove aliquots of 2.5 μL at 30-s intervals and add into the S1 mix tubes on ice. Mix by pipeting up and down and hold on ice until all aliquots are taken.

4. Remove samples from ice and incubate at room temperature for 30 min.

5. Add 1 μL of S1 stop and heat to 70°C for 10 min to inactivate the enzymes.

3.3. Gel Purification, End Repair, Ligation, and Transformation

1. Add 1 μL of 10X gel loading buffer to each sample and load onto a 0.7% low melting point agarose gel in 1X TAE gel running buffer containing 0.5 μg/mL ethidium bromide. Electrophorese for about 2 h at 3–4 V/cm until the deletion time points can be resolved (*see* Note 4). Using a 300-nm wavelength ultraviolet light source, remove the desired bands from the gel with a small spatula or scalpel.

2. Dilute gel slices in approx 2 vol of distilled water and melt at 68°C for 5 min. Transfer 1/3 of the diluted DNA to a new tube containing 0.1 vol Klenow mix at room temperature and mix by pipeting up and down. Incubate at 37°C for 3 min. Add 0.1 vol of dNTPs and mix. Incubate for 5 min at 37°C (*see* Note 5).

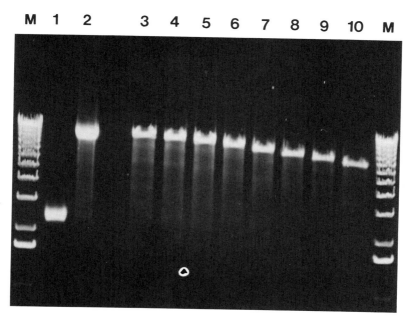

Fig. 2. Low melting point agarose gel electrophoresis of a set of deletions prepared following Procedure II. The size of the phagemid is 9.5 kb. Lane 1: Single-stranded phagemid. Lane 2: Double-stranded nicked circle after overnight extension with T4 DNA polymerase. Depending on the gel, one occasionally sees a minor band below the nicked circle that may be the result of extension of single-stranded linear molecules that are primed by their own 3' end *(2)*. Lanes 3–10: ExoIII digestion of the material in Lane 2 for 1, 2, . . ., 8 min. Lane M: 1-kb ladder (BRL), with the 7-kb band comigrating with the 8 min time point.

3. Add an equal volume of ligation cocktail, mix, and incubate at room temperature for at least 1 h. The yield of transformants is greatest if ligations are incubated overnight.

4. Transform *E. coli* by combining 1/2 of each ligation with 2–3 vol of competent cells that have been thawed on ice. Incubate for 30 min on ice, heat shock at 42°C for 90 s and further incubate the cells in 0.2 mL LB medium for 60 min at 37°C. Plate using the appropriate selection and incubate at 37°C overnight. The yield from each transformation can be up to 500 colonies, depending on ligation time and competence of the cells. Store the remaining ligation mixtures at −20°C.

5. Set up cultures to prepare plasmid DNA from one colony from each time point and verify that each one contains a deletion of expected size before sequencing.

4. Notes

1. ExoIII digestion occurs at nicks in the DNA as efficiently as at ends. This gives rise to a background of undesired clones. Nicks can be introduced by impurities in the DNA and by restriction enzymes. Gel purification eliminates this background. As a result of the gel purification step, plasmid DNA can be prepared with a standard alkaline lysis procedure, including a phenol:chloroform extraction *(4)*. If nicking proves to be a problem, supercoiled DNA may be column purified using the premade columns from Qiagen, Inc. (Chatsworth, CA). Restriction enzymes can also occasionally have excessive nicking or "star" activity. Often this problem can be overcome by trying different suppliers.

2. At 37°C, ExoIII digests 400–500 bases/min, with the rate changing directly with temperature about 10%/1°C in the 30–40°C range *(7)*. It is advisable to perform a test run of the ExoIII digestion on your DNA, picking a few time points. The three reasons for this are:
   a. You can confirm that both enzymes cut to completion if using Procedure I (*see also* Note 4);
   b. You can get an accurate rate of digestion for your particular batch of ExoIII; and
   c. You can confirm that there is not excessive nicking of your DNA (*see* Note 3).

3. When processing a large number of time points, it is much more efficient to use a conical bottom microtiter plate with a lid rather than microfuge tubes. These plates can be used for the S1 nuclease step, collecting and diluting gel slices, end repair, ligation, and transformation.

4. Occasionally, an ExoIII resistant fragment is seen. This results from incomplete digestion by enzyme A (Fig. 1). Provided this is not a dominant band, the gel isolation of the digested fragment should eliminate this as a problem. Alternatively, a second fragment that digests at a higher rate may be present. This results from incomplete digestion by enzyme B and subsequent ExoIII digestion of the fragment from both ends. Again, if this is not a dominant product, gel isolation should alleviate this problem.

5. An alternative method for in-gel ligation incorporates end repair and ligation into one step. For 1 mL of cocktail, mix 560 µL of water, 200 µL of ligation buffer, 200 µL PEG, 20 µL DTT, 20 µL each of dNTP (2.5 m*M*), 1 U of T4 DNA polymerase, and 10 U of T4 DNA ligase. Mix 1/3 of the DNA in the diluted gel slice with an equal volume of the cocktail. Incubate at room temperature 1 h to overnight. Transformation is done following step 6.

References

1. Henikoff, S. (1984) Unidirectional digestion with exonuclease III creates targeted breakpoints for DNA sequencing. *Gene* **28,** 351–359.
2. Henikoff, S. (1990) Ordered deletions for DNA sequencing and in vitro mutagenesis by polymerase extension and exonuclease III gapping of circular templates. *Nucleic Acids Res.* **18,** 2961–2966.
3. Nakayama, K. and Nakauchi, H. (1989) An improved method to make sequential deletion mutants for DNA sequencing. *Trends Genet.* **5,** 325.
4. Steggles, A. W. (1989) A rapid procedure for creating nested sets of deletions using mini-prep plasmid DNA samples. *Biotechniques* **7,** 241,242.
5. Sambrook, J., Fritsch, E. F., and Maniatis, T. (1989) *Molecular Cloning: A Laboratory Manual.* Cold Spring Harbor Laboratory, Cold Spring Harbor, NY.
6. Putney, S. D., Benkovic, S. J., and Schimmel, P. R. (1981) A DNA fragment with an α-phosphorothioate nucleotide at one end is asymmetrically blocked from digestion by exonuclease III and can be replicated in vivo. *Proc. Natl. Acad. Sci. USA* **78,** 7350–7354.
7. Henikoff, S. (1987) Unidirectional digestion with exonuclease III in DNA sequence analysis. *Methods Enzymol.* **155,** 156–165.

CHAPTER 13

Ligase Chain Reaction
for Site-Directed In Vitro Mutagenesis

Gerard J. A. Rouwendal, Emil J. H. Wolbert,
Lute-Harm Zwiers, and Jan Springer

1. Introduction

Before the advent of polymerase chain reaction (PCR) technology, many methods for site-directed mutagenesis basically relied on enzymatic extension of a mutagenic oligonucleotide annealed to a single-stranded template and amplification of the ligase-sealed double-stranded heteroduplex in an *Escherichia coli* host *(1)*. Several techniques have been employed to enhance the frequency of clones containing the desired mutation by selecting against the parental strand through biological means or by in vitro manipulations *(2–4)*.

PCR technology allowed for alternative ways of in vitro selection of the mutant strand in the classic single-stranded DNA-based strategies and made it possible to develop novel approaches to site-directed mutagenesis *(5–7)*. Various methods have been adopted to incorporate mutations, which through necessity are present only at the termini of PCR products, into cloned genes *(5,6,8,9)*.

The ligase chain reaction (LCR) is based on the ligation of exactly juxtaposed oligonucleotides annealed to a single-stranded DNA template by a DNA ligase *(10)*. Exponential amplification of the ligation product is achieved by making the ligation product itself act as a template through thermal cycling of a reaction mixture in which the complementary oligonucleotides have also been included *(11)*. The use of a thermostable DNA ligase greatly enhanced the utility of such an approach.

From: *Methods in Molecular Biology, Vol. 57: In Vitro Mutagenesis Protocols*
Edited by: M. K. Trower Humana Press Inc., Totowa, NJ

Extending the application of this technique for joining immediately adjacent oligonucleotides to the joining of long single-stranded DNA molecules derived from denatured PCR fragments, allowed ordered coupling of three PCR fragments. Moreover, as these PCR fragments were generated using mutagenic primers, the LCR yielded a readily clonable product containing the desired internal mutations *(12)*.

In this chapter the principle of LCR-mediated in vitro mutagenesis is outlined in Fig. 1 for the introduction of one mutation via coupling of two PCR fragments. The PCR fragments are generated in separate reactions using *Pfu* DNA polymerase to avoid the presence of 3' nontemplate additions *(13)*. Both internal primers II and III have to be phosphorylated at their 5' ends prior to the PCR or the PCR fragments have to be phosphorylated with T4 polynucleotide kinase to obtain ligation products in the LCR. The fragment with the mutation was obtained following PCR with primer I and the mutagenic primer II. The second primer set consisting of primers III and IV was used to amplify the remaining part of the gene. Heat denaturation of (a small amount of) template and equimolar amounts of the two fragments followed by cooling to the annealing/reaction temperature results in the formation of complexes consisting of two PCR-derived DNA strands annealed to the template in immediately adjacent positions. The nick separating the two strands is then closed by DNA ligase and the ligation product is released in the subsequent denaturation step. In the following cycles, both the original template and the ligation products may act as template leading to an exponential increase in amount of mutant ligation product. Thus, starting the experiment with amounts of PCR fragment that are readily visible on an agarose gel yields amounts of ligation product that are also readily visible on agarose gel and amenable to further manipulations such as cloning.

To facilitate cloning of the ligation product it may be helpful to include (unique) restriction enzyme recognition sites into the flanking primers I and IV. However, it is quite likely that in many cases existing primers for sequences flanking the multiple cloning sites could be used instead of gene-specific primers.

2. Materials
2.1. PCR

1. Cloned *Pyrococcus furiosus (Pfu)* DNA polymerase (Stratagene, La Jolla, CA) (*see* Note 1).

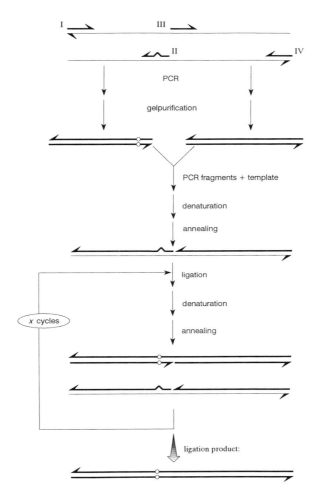

Fig. 1. Diagram of LCR-mediated site-directed mutagenesis. The primers I, II, III, and IV are indicated by arrows annealed to a double-stranded template with primer II containing the mismatch(es). The LCR procedure has been depicted for only one of the two strands of the template (thin line). The white dot indicates the position of the mutation in a homoduplex.

2. 10X PCR buffer: 200 mM Tris-HCl, pH 8.75, 100 mM KCl, 100 mM $(NH_4)_2SO_4$, 20 mM $MgCl_2$, 1% Triton X-100, 1 mg/mL bovine serum albumin.
3. Primers I, II, III, and IV at a concentration of 0.3–1.0 μM; primers II and III chemically 5' phosphorylated in the final round of synthesis (*see* Notes 2 and 3).

4. DNA template.
5. dNTPs: 1.25 mM stock.
6. Paraffin oil.
7. Tris-acetate-EDTA (TAE) electrophoresis running buffer: 40 mM Tris-acetate, pH 7.8–8.0, 1 mM EDTA, 0.125 µg/mL ethidium bromide.
8. 5X Loading buffer: 15% Ficoll 400, 0.05% bromophenol blue, 0.05% xylene cyanole.
9. 100 bp Ladder (Pharmacia, Roosendaal, The Netherlands).
10. QIAEX (Qiagen, Hilden, Germany).

2.2. LCR

1. *Taq* DNA ligase (New England Biolabs, Beverly, MA).
2. 10X LCR buffer: 200 mM Tris-HCl, pH 7.6, 250 mM KAc, 100 mM MgAc$_2$, 100 mM DTT, 10 mM NAD$^+$, 0.1% Triton X-100.
3. Two nonoverlapping PCR fragments that together comprise a contiguous, DNA sequence (*see* Fig. 1).
4. Single- or double-stranded DNA template comprising the PCR fragments to be joined (*see* Notes 4 and 5).
5. Paraffin oil.
6. Agarose gel and buffer (*see* Section 2.1.).
7. Suitable restriction enzymes and appropriately cut vector.

3. Methods
3.1. PCR Design

In designing primers for this step it should be remembered that the efficiency of the LCR may also be affected by some of the choices made in this process. But first of all, for the PCR step it should be taken into account that the optimal annealing temperature when using *Pfu* DNA polymerase is lower than with *Taq* DNA polymerase owing to the lower salt concentration in the reaction buffer. The following LCR requires, in addition to the PCR, not merely that the 3' end of the oligonucleotide should be able to bind efficiently to the template, but also that the 5' end is able to bind stably to the template. Therefore, it may be advisable to check both 5' and 3' terminal ends of the sequences at either side of the nick for potential instabilities (*see* Note 6). Naturally, this also implies that the mutation(s) in the mutagenic oligonucleotide should be positioned in the middle.

3.2. PCR

1. Set up both PCR reactions as follows:
   a. 10 µL of 10X PCR buffer;
   b. 16 µL of 1.25 mM dNTP solution;

c. 10–250 ng of template DNA;
d. 30–100 pmol of either primers I + II or primers III + IV;
e. 2.5 U *Pfu* DNA polymerase;
f. Sterile water to a final volume of 100 μL and mix by pipeting up and down several times; and
g. Overlay sample with paraffin oil.

2. Amplify by PCR using 35 cycles with the following cycle parameters: denaturation, 94°C, 1 min; annealing, 50–55°C, 1 min; synthesis, 72°C, 2 min with 3-s extension each cycle.
3. After thermocycling is completed, transfer 80 μL of the PCR reaction mix into a fresh Eppendorf tube containing 20 μL of 5X loading buffer and mix by pipeting up and down several times.
4. Load samples onto a gel with an agarose concentration depending on the sizes of the fragments to be obtained using 0.5 μg of a 100-bp ladder as molecular weight marker (*see* Note 7).
5. Visualize the DNA by UV transillumination with the gel lying on Saran wrap and cut the agarose containing the desired fragments from the gel using a fresh scalpel and transfer the gel pieces to a fresh Eppendorf tube.
6. Recover the DNA by QIAEX-extraction exactly as described by the manufacturer.

3.3. LCR

1. Set up the LCR as follows:
a. 2 μL of 10X LCR buffer;
b. 10 fmol of double-stranded template;
c. 50 fmol of each of the two PCR fragments (*see* Note 8);
d. 4 U *Taq* DNA ligase;
e. Sterile water to 20 μL and mix by pipeting up and down several times; and
f. Overlay the sample with paraffin oil.
2. Ligate by LCR using 15–30 cycles with the following cycling parameters (*see* Note 9): denaturation, 94°C, 1 min; annealing/ligation, 65°C, 4 min.
3. After the reaction is completed, transfer the 20-μL reaction mix to a fresh Eppendorf tube containing 5 μL loading buffer (*see* Section 3.2., step 3).
4. Run a gel with the ligation products, visualize the separated DNA, and recover the ligation products as described in Sections 3.2., steps 4–6 and Notes 7, 10, and 11).
5. Cut the fragment with appropriate restriction enzymes and clone into a suitable vector according to standard procedures.

4. Notes

1. *Taq* DNA polymerase could also be used to synthesize the PCR fragments provided these are blunt-ended by another treatment prior to the LCR.

However, this is not advisable, as the use of thermostable DNA polymerases with proofreading activity does not only avoid 3' nontemplated
additions, but it also improves the reliability of DNA replication.

2. The efficiency of the ligation depends heavily on the quality of the internal
oligonucleotides and the extent of phosphorylation of their 5' ends. Especially in the case of long oligonucleotides a significant fraction of the
preparation may consist of shorter oligos, which will lead to shorter PCR
fragments that cannot be coupled in the LCR. Similarly, a PCR fragment
containing a nonphosphorylated end can not be coupled to the immediately adjacent 3' end of the other PCR fragment. One way of obtaining an
almost pure preparation of the desired oligo is to use the hydrophobicity of
the terminal dimethoxytrityl-group to purify it away from shorter or
nonphosphorylated oligo's with reverse-phase Pure-Pak cartridges (Perkin-
Elmer Cetus, Norwalk, CT).

3. Although phosphorylation of the internal primers II and III may be carried
out very efficiently during oligonucleotide synthesis using a phosphorylat-
ing amidite in the final round of synthesis, it also tends to be rather expensive. Alternatively, either the oligos or the PCR fragments may be
phosphorylated using T4 polynucleotide kinase.

4. In our original paper describing the use of the LCR for site-directed
mutagenesis we employed a single-stranded template. However, it is obvious that the nature of the method implies that double-stranded templates
may be used as well. The only drawback to the use of double-stranded
template may be that one should be more careful about the amount of template added to the LCR; very high concentrations will reanneal (too) fast.

5. We have often found it to be unnecessary to add template to the LCR! It
would seem therefore, that the trace amount of template contaminating the
gel-purified PCR fragments is already sufficient to drive the reaction. This
ligation product is produced in a template-dependent way as can be shown
by agarose gel electrophoresis of the LCR reaction products indicating a
lack of self-ligated products. In fact, special precautions have to be taken
to demonstrate template-dependent ligation and to suppress the formation
of ligation product in control reactions where the template is left out.

6. It may be helpful to optimize the binding of 5' and 3' ends using nearest
neighbor analysis as available through software for oligonucleotide design
(14). In addition, this type of software gives reliable estimates of the
annealing temperature of primers.

7. Separation of small PCR (or LCR) fragments is conveniently carried out
using Nusieve GTG agarose (FMC Bioproducts, Rockland, ME)

8. High concentrations of the participating PCR fragments in the LCR (more
than 150 fmol of a particular fragment in 20 µL) may completely inhibit

ligation, possibly because of a strong enhancement of the rate of reannealing at the expense of (potentially) productive annealing to the template.

9. The number of cycles required for obtaining a readily visible amount of ligation product on agarose gel electrophoresis will depend on many factors. We have obtained good yields with only 15 cycles of 1 min denaturation at 94°C and 4 min annealing and ligation at 65°C. In this case, using 30 cycles did not improve the yield and was even found to be slightly counterproductive, possibly owing to thermal degradation. In our hands both *Taq* DNA ligase (NEB, Beverly, MA) and *Pfu* DNA ligase (Stratagene) gave similar results.

10. In our lab, DNA fragments with sizes ranging from 250–760 bp have been coupled successfully.

11. If coupling of more than two fragments is the goal then chances are that the yields will be suboptimal. This would hinder an approach in which the ligation product is purified from an agarose gel and cloned directly into a suitable vector. In that case it may be advisable to design flanking primers with mutant strand-specific tags that would allow PCR amplification following inefficient LCRs.

Acknowledgments

This work was funded by Eurpoean Chips and Snacks Association Research Ltd. and the European Union.

References

1. Zoller, M. J. and Smith, M. (1983) Oligonucleotide directed mutagenesis of DNA fragments cloned into M13 vectors, in *Methods in Enzymology* (Wu, R., Grossman, L., and Moldave, K., eds.), Academic, New York, pp. 468–500.
2. Kunkel, T. A. (1985) Rapid and efficient site-specific mutagenesis without phenotypic selection. *Proc. Natl. Acad. Sci. USA* **82**, 488–502.
3. Vandeyar, M. A., Weiner M. P., Hutton, C. J., and Batt, C. A. (1988) A simple and rapid method for the detection of oligodeoxynucleotide-directed mutants. *Gene* **65**, 129–133.
4. Taylor, J. W., Ott, J., and Eckstein, F. (1985) The rapid generation of oligonucleotide-directed mutations at high frequency using phosphorothioate-modified DNA. *Nucleic Acids Res.* **13**, 8765–8785.
5. Higuchi, R., Krummel, B., and Saiki, R. (1988) A general method of *in vitro* preparation and specific mutagenesis of DNA fragments: study of protein and DNA interactions. *Nucleic Acids Res.* **16**, 7351–7367.
6. Ho, S. N., Hunt, H. D., Horton, R. M., Pullen, J. K., and Pease, L. R. (1989) Site-directed mutagenesis by overlap extension using the polymerase chain reaction. *Gene* **77**, 51–59.
7. Lundberg, K. S., Shoemaker, D. D., Adams, M. W. W., Short, J. M., Sorge, J. A., and Mathur, E. J. (1991) High-fidelity amplification using a thermostable DNA polymerase isolated from *Pyrococcus furiosus*. *Gene* **108**, 1–6.

8. Perrin, S. and Gilliland, G. (1990) Site-specific mutagenesis using asymmetric polymerase chain reaction and a single mutant primer. *Nucleic Acids Res.* **18,** 7433–7438.
9. Sarkar, G. and Sommer, S. S. (1990) The "megaprimer" method of site-directed mutagenesis. *BioTechniques* **8,** 404–407.
10. Landegren, U., Kaiser, R., Sanders, J., and Hood, L. (1988) A ligase-mediated gene detection technique. *Science* **241,** 1077–1080.
11. Barany, F. (1991) Genetic disease detection and DNA amplification using cloned thermostable ligase. *Proc. Natl. Acad. Sci. USA* **88,** 189–193.
12. Rouwendal, G. J. A., Wolbert, E. J. H., Zwiers, L.-H., and Springer, J. (1993) Simultaneous mutagenesis of multiple sites: application of the ligase chain reaction using PCR products instead of oligonucleotides. *BioTechniques* **15,** 68–75.
13. Clark, J. M. (1988) Novel non-templated nucleotide addition reactions catalyzed by prokaryotic and eukaryotic DNA polymerases. *Nucleic Acids Res.* **16,** 9677–9686.
14. Rychlik, W. and Rhoads, R. E. (1989) A computer program for choosing optimal oligonucleotides for filter hybridization, sequencing and *in vitro* amplification of DNA. *Nucleic Acids Res.* **17,** 8543–8551.

CHAPTER 14

PCR-Based Site-Directed Mutagenesis

Atsushi Shimada

1. Introduction

Protocols for site-directed mutagenesis are widely used in molecular biology and include many polymerase chain reaction (PCR)-based methods that have been developed in order to achieve efficient mutagenesis of a target DNA sequence *(1–4)*. However, some of these methods described require two or more specific-oligonucleotides for each round of mutagenesis, making the cost of such procedures expensive. This chapter describes an efficient and economic PCR-based site-directed mutagenesis method, which is designed to introduce a series of mutations into DNA cloned into pUC vectors (pUC 18, 19, 118, 119). The protocol uses a combination of a primer designed for introducing a mutation at the target sequence, with primers that may be reused for each mutagenesis reaction (Fig. 1). By using this method, a series of site-directed mutations may be undertaken that only require a single primer for each desired change, and furthermore, no reiterative transformation steps are necessary.

2. Materials

1. *Taq* DNA polymerase, 5 U/µL (TaKaRa Shuzo Co. Ltd., Kyoto, Japan).
2. 10X PCR buffer: 100 mM Tris-HCl, pH 8.3, 500 mM KCl, 15 mM MgCl$_2$, 0.01% (w/v) gelatin.
3. dNTP Stock: 2.5 mM each of dATP, dCTP, dGTP, and dTTP (TaKaRa Shuzo).
4. Oligonucleotides: MUT 1-6 (5 pmol/µL), M13 M4 (5 and 20 pmol/µL), M13 RV (5 and 20 pmol/µL), and R1 (5 pmol/µL) *(see* Fig. 2 on p. 160).

From: *Methods in Molecular Biology, Vol. 57: In Vitro Mutagenesis Protocols*
Edited by: M. K. Trower Humana Press Inc., Totowa, NJ

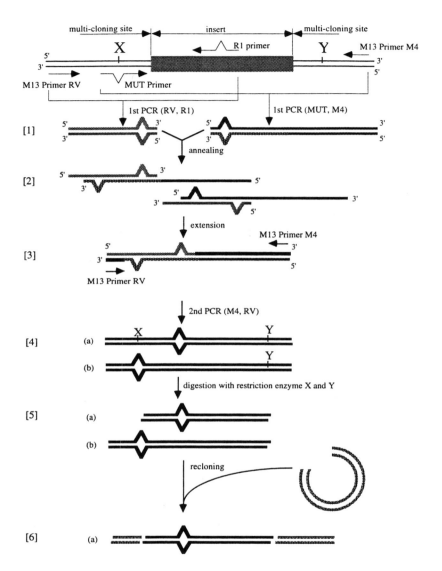

Fig. 1. Principle of PCR in vitro mutagenesis. [1] First round PCR of target DNA following cloning of sequence into multicloning site of one of the pUC series of vectors. One of the MUT primers is chosen to destroy a restriction site, based on both the direction of R1 primer (primer for introducing a mutation) and the restriction site used for cloning the target DNA sequence. The first round PCR is carried out by the combination of R1 primer and M13 primer RV (or M13 primer M4), MUT primer, and M13 primer M4 (or M13 primer RV)

MUT 1	5' CATGATTACGAGTTCTAGCT 3'
MUT 2	5' GATCATCTATAGTGGACCTG 3'
MUT 3	5' TGATTACGCCTAGCTTACAT 3'
MUT 4	5' GGCCAGTGCCTAGCTTACAT 3'
MUT 5	5' CAGGTCCACTATAGATGATC 3'
MUT 6	5' ACGGCCAGTGAGTTCTAGCT 3'
M13 M4	5' GTTTTCCCAGTCACGAC 3'
M13 RV	5' CAGGAAACAGCTATGAC 3'

For the design of Primer R1, *see* Note 1.

5. Plasmid DNA, into which the target sequence is cloned, prepared using standard protocols *(5)*.
6. Phenol saturated in TE buffer.
7. Chloroform.
8. 3M Sodium acetate, pH 4.8–5.2.
9. Appropriate restriction enzymes.
10. SUPREC-01. Filter cartridge for rapid recovery of DNA from agarose gels (TaKaRa Shuzo).
11. SUPREC-02. Filter cartridge for rapid purification and/or concentration of DNA samples (TaKaRa Shuzo).
12. T4 DNA ligase (350 U/μL) with 10X reaction buffer (660 mM Tris-HCl, pH 7.6, 66 mM MgCl$_2$, 100 mM DTT, and 1 mM ATP) (TaKaRa Shuzo).
13. Competent *Escherichia coli* cells.
14. TE Buffer: 10 mM Tris-HCl, pH 8.0, 1 mM EDTA.

3. Methods

The procedure requires that the target DNA sequence is cloned into a pUC vector (pUC 18, 19, 118, 119).

---

separately in two tubes. [2] After DNA purification to remove excess primers, the amplified products are mixed, heat denatured, and annealed. [3] *Taq* DNA polymerase is added to complete the DNA heteroduplex. [4] The second round PCR is performed using M13 primer M4 and M13 primer RV flanking oligonucleotides, which will result in two types of amplified products, (a) and (b). [5] The amplified products are digested with two restriction enzymes, one of which shall recognize the site (X) that had been destroyed by the MUT primer and the other which recognizes the appropriate site (Y) within the multicloning site. [6] Reclone the digested fragment into the vector digested with the same two restriction enzymes. Only the fragment (a) that contains the mutation introduced by R1 primer sequence will be recloned.

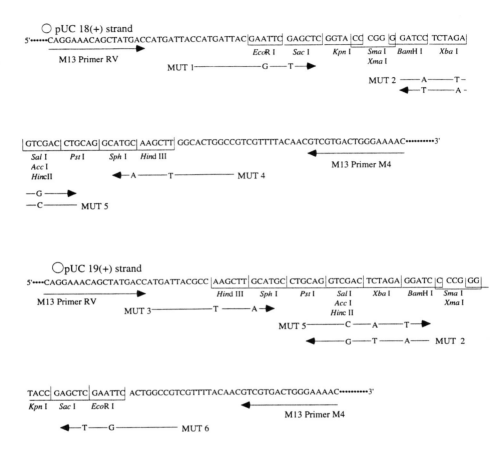

Fig. 2. Position of MUT primers, M13 primer M4 and RV. The MUT primers are designed to anneal within the multicloning site of pUC vectors; each has a single base mismatch in the recognition sequence of the restriction enzymes with which it is associated. M13-M4 and M13-RV primers also bind to sequences within the multicloning site, but flank the MUT series of oligonucleotides.

3.1. Preparation of First Round PCR Products

1. Design and prepare the mutagenic primer (R1) to introduce the desired change into the target DNA sequence (*see* Note 1).
2. Prepare the first round of PCR reactions using the primer combinations described in a and b (*see* Fig. 3 and Note 2):

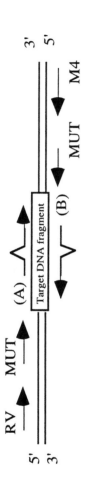

pUC 18(pUC118)

Insertion site of target DNA	Direction of R1 primer	Applicable MUT primers
EcoR I, Sac I	(A)	MUT 4 or MUT 5
Kpn I, Sma I	(A)	MUT 4 or MUT 5
	(B)	MUT 1
Acc I, BamH I	(A)	MUT 4
Hinc II, Sal I, Xba I	(B)	MUT 1
Pst I	(A)	MUT 4
	(B)	MUT 1 or MUT 2
Sph I, Hind III	(B)	MUT 1 or MUT 2

pUC 19(pUC119)

Insertion site of arget DNA	Direction of R1 primer	Applicable MUT primers
Hind III, Sph I	(A)	MUT 6 or MUT 2
Pst I	(A)	MUT 6 or MUT 2
	(B)	MUT 3
Acc I, BamH I	(A)	MUT 6
Hinc II, Sal I, Xba I	(B)	MUT 3
Kpn I, Sma I	(A)	MUT 6
	(B)	MUT 3 or MUT 5
EcoR I, Sac I	(B)	MUT 3 or MUT 5

Fig. 3. Selection of MUT primer.

a. Combination of R1 primer and M13 primer M4* (or M13 primer RV): 10 pg–1 ng plasmid template DNA, 1 μL R1 primer, 1 μL M13 primer (5 pmol/μL), 10 μL 10X PCR buffer, 8 μL dNTP stock, 0.5 μL *Taq* DNA polymerase, make up to 100 μL with distilled sterilized water.

b. Combination of a MUT primer (MUT 1–6) and M13 primer RV* (or M13 primer M4): 10 pg–1 ng plasmid template DNA, 1 μL MUT primer, 1 μL M13 primer (5 pmol/μL), 10 μL 10X PCR buffer, 8 μL dNTP stock, 0.5 μL *Taq* DNA polymerase, make up to 100 μL with distilled sterilized water.

3. Overlay each tube with mineral oil (approx 100 μL) and perform first stage PCR using the following program for 25 cycles: denaturation, 94°C for 30 s; primer annealing, 55°C for 2 min; primer extension, 72°C for 1 min (*see* Note 3).

4. Remove a small aliquot (5 μL) from 2a and 2b for analysis by agarose gel electrophoresis (1.5% gel) to determine if the PCR reactions were successful (*see* Note 4).

5. Purify the PCR products using standard phenol–chloroform extraction/ ethanol precipitation. Alternatively, products available commercially such as SUPREC-02 filter cartridges may be used. Each of the purified PCR products should be resuspended in 100 μL TE.

3.2. Heteroduplex Formation and Second Round PCR

1. Prepare the following reaction mixture and then overlay with 100 μL of mineral oil: First round PCR product a, 1 μL; first round PCR product b, 1 μL; 10X PCR buffer, 10 μL; dNTP stock, 8 μL; make up to 97.5 μL with distilled sterilized water.

2. Perform the following annealing/extension step with the mix in step 1 using a thermal cycler with the program: denaturation, 94°C for 30 s; cool to 37°C over a period of 30 min; maintain at 37°C over 15 min.

3. Add 0.5 μL *Taq* and mix gently. Spin down any droplets on the tube wall and then incubate at 72°C for 3 min.

4. To this reaction mix add: 1 μL M13 primer M4 (20 pmol/μL), 1 μL M13 primer RV (20 pmol/μL).

5. Carry out PCR using the following program for 5–10 cycles: denaturation, 94°C for 30 s; primer annealing, 55°C for 2 min; primer extension, 72°C for 1 min.

6. Remove an aliquot (5 μL) following the amplification reaction and confirm that a specific DNA product of the correct size has been generated.

*Different M13 primers must be used in a and b.

7. Purify the remaining amplified DNA by phenol/chloroform extraction followed by ethanol precipitation. Resuspend in 10 μL distilled sterilized water.

3.3. Recloning of the Mutated Target DNA Sequence

The second round PCR product is then digested with two restriction enzymes (X and Y in Fig. 1), which are dictated by the MUT primer/M13 primer combination used in the first round PCR reaction (*see* Note 2).

1. To 10 μL of the purified second round PCR product, add 2 μL of appropriate 10X restriction buffer, 6 μL of distilled sterilized water, mix, and then add 1 μL of each specified restriction enzyme. Mix gently and then incubate at 37°C for at least 1 h.
2. Restrict the DNA of an appropriate cloning vector with identical enzymes. Take 1 μg vector DNA, add 5 μL of appropriate 10X restriction buffer, 1 μL of each restriction enzyme, and make up to an appropriate volume with distilled water. Mix gently and incubate as before.
3. Purify the restricted PCR product and cloning vector by phenol/chloroform extraction and ethanol precipitation. Resuspend each purified DNA in 2 μL TE or water.
4. Separate the restricted cloning vector by agarose gel electrophoresis. Excise the desired band from the gel and recover the DNA using a SUPREC-01 filter cartridge. Purify the eluted DNA by phenol/chloroform extraction and ethanol precipitation. Resuspend the DNA pellet in 20 μL TE or distilled sterilized water.
5. To 1 μL of restricted cloning vector add 2 μL PCR product (*see* Note 5), 1 U (cohesive end) or 100 U (blunt-end) T4 DNA ligase, 2 μL 10X ligation buffer, and then make up to 20 μL with sterile distilled water. Mix gently and incubate at 16°C for 16 h.
6. Transform 20 μL (maximum) of the ligation reaction into 100 μL competent *E. coli* cells using standard protocols.

Following transformation at least three clones should be submitted for DNA sequencing to confirm that the desired mutation has been introduced.

An example of the utility of this PCR in vitro mutagenesis method can be demonstrated by site-directed mutagenesis of codon 12 of the protoncogene c-ki-ras, changing the usage from glycine to alanine (G12A). The first stage involved cloning a 108 bp PCR fragment containing c-ki ras codon 12 into the *Hinc*II site of pUC 18. This was followed by the first round PCR reactions using a combination of: a, R1 primer (c-ki-ras/12 Ala type, "5'-GTTGGAGCTGCTGGCGTAGG-3'") and M13-RV primer; b, MUT1 primer (which flanks the *Hinc*II cloning site) and M13-M4 primer. After the heteroduplex formation, the second round PCR was performed with M13 primer M4 and M13 primer RV. The resulting PCR fragment was purified and digested with *Eco*RI and *Hin*dIII. Only DNA fragments containing the c-ki-ras codon G12A mutation were recloned, which was confirmed by DNA sequencing.

4. Notes

1. For the design of the mutagenic primer R1, the following should be considered to ensure the oligonucleotide will anneal efficiently to the specified target: If a single- or double-point mutation is to be introduced, then 10 flanking bases should be incorporated into the primer sequence either side of the mutation site. If the flanking regions are A + T rich or substantial alterations are involved, this can be extended to 15 bases or more. Ensure that the designed R1 primer does not have significant complementarity to itself or to its possible partners for PCR, particularly at their 3' ends. This will avoid "primer dimer" formation in which two primers hybridize to each other forming a very effective substrate for PCR. If possible keep the G + C composition of the primer to about 50–60% and avoid long stretches of the same base.

2. The choice of the MUT primer used when designing the reaction will be dependent on: the cloning site used for insertion of the target DNA sequence (*see* Fig. 3); the direction of the R1 primer; the mutated fragment must be recloned following mutagenesis, which should be undertaken with unique restriction sites (enzymes X and Y in Fig. 1), i.e., that neither of these enzymes should have sites within the cloned target DNA sequence.
   a. For enzyme X (*see* Fig. 1), any of the restriction endonuclease recognition sequences mutated by the particular MUT primer used in the first round PCR reaction (*see* Fig. 2) may be chosen. The choice of enzymes that may be selected for by a particular MUT primer are:

MUT 1	*Eco*RI, *Sac*I
MUT 2	*Bam*HI, *Xba*I, *Sal*I, *Acc*I, *Hin*cII
MUT 3	*Sph*I, *Hin*dIII
MUT 4	*Sph*I, *Hin*dIII
MUT 5	*Bam*HI, *Xba*I, *Sal*I, *Acc*I, *Hin*cII
MUT 6	*Eco*RI, *Sac*I

   b. For enzyme Y (*see* Fig. 1), any of the restriction enzymes with sites in the multicloning site on the side flanking both the inserted DNA fragment and the recognition sequence for enzyme X may be utilized.

3. MUT 2 and MUT 5 primers are sometimes difficult to anneal to the template at 55°C. In such cases lower the annealing temperature to 45°C.

4. If any nonspecific bands appear on the agarose gel following electrophoresis of the first and second round PCR products, the desired band in each case should be excised from the gel and purified. This may be achieved by electroelution or by using commercial products such as SUPREC-01 filter cartridges.

5. Recommended amounts of DNA are vector:insert = 0.03 pmol:0.1–0.3 pmol (0.03 pmol of pUC 18 DNA corresponds to about 50 ng).

References

1. Ito, W., Ishiguro, H., and Kurosawa,Y. (1991) A general method for introducing a series of mutations into cloned DNA using the polymerase chain reaction. *Gene* **102,** 67–70.

2. Hemsley, A., Arnheim, N., Toney, M. D., Cortopassi, G., and Galas, D. J. (1989) A simple method for site-directed mutagenesis using the polymerase chain reaction. *Nucleic Acids Res.* **17,** 6545–6551.

3. Higuchi, R., Krummel, B., and Saiki, R. (1988) A general method of *in vitro* preparation and specific mutagenesis of DNA fragments: study of protein and DNA interactions. *Nucleic Acids Res.* **16,** 7351–7367.

4. Ho, S. N., Hunt , H. D., Horton, R. M., Pullen, J. K., and Pease, L. R. (1989) Site-directed mutagenesis by overlap extension using the polymerase chain reaction. *Gene* **77,** 51–59.

5. Sambrook, J., Fritsch, E. F., and Maniatis, T. (1989) *Molecular Cloning. A Laboratory Manual,* 2nd ed., Cold Spring Harbor Press, Cold Spring Harbor, NY.

CHAPTER 15

In Vitro Recombination and Mutagenesis by Overlap Extension PCR

Robert J. Pogulis, Abbe N. Vallejo, and Larry R. Pease

1. Introduction

The polymerase chain reaction (PCR) *(1,2)* is now a fundamental tool of molecular biology. Although PCR provides the basis for a variety of sensitive analytical techniques, it can also be used in a synthetic capacity to generate large quantities of specific DNA fragments. The alteration of amplified DNA sequences is also possible, since synthetic oligonucleotide primers become incorporated into the final PCR product. Although the 3' ends of these primers must match the target DNA sequence, the 5' ends may contain modifications. Sequence modifications in the primers will therefore be present in the ends of the amplified DNA fragment, offering a straightforward, although limited, ability to introduce site-directed mutations during PCR.

The "overlap extension" technique *(3,4)* provides a means of introducing mutations into the center of a PCR fragment. In this case, primers are designed to provide two different PCR products with a region of common sequence. The two overlapping fragments are then fused in a subsequent PCR amplification. Depending on the choice of primers and templates, mutant or chimeric DNA molecules can be generated. Overlap extension represents a simple and versatile approach to genetic engineering. Subcloning of the wild-type sequence into a single-stranded vector is unnecessary and mutagenic efficiency approaches 100%. In

From: *Methods in Molecular Biology, Vol. 57: In Vitro Mutagenesis Protocols*
Edited by: M. K. Trower Humana Press Inc., Totowa, NJ

addition, "splicing by overlap extension" (SOE) allows segments from different genes to be recombined without relying on restriction sites.

1.1. Mechanism of Overlap Extension

The general mechanism of overlap extension, as applied to site-directed mutagenesis, is illustrated in Fig. 1. In separate reactions, two overlapping sub-fragments of the target sequence are amplified. Each reaction uses one flanking primer (a or d) and one internal primer containing the desired mutation (b or c). Since the two internal primers overlap, the overlapping fragments generated in the first PCRs can be fused in a second round of PCR. When fragments AB and CD are mixed, denatured, and reannealed, the 3' end of the upper strand of fragment AB and the 5' end of fragment CD's lower strand can hybridize. In the presence of a DNA polymerase, each of the overlapping strands acts as a primer on the other, and extension of the overlap results in a full-length mutant product (AD). Even if overlap extension occurs at relatively low frequency, only the fusion product will be amplified with primers a and d.

The flexibility of the overlap extension technique is illustrated in Figs. 2 and 3. Insertional mutations can be generated by simply adding the sequence to be inserted to the 5'-ends of primers b and c (Fig. 2A). Deletions are created by designing b and c primers that contain sequence on either side of the deletion (Fig. 2B). Last, Fig. 3 depicts the mechanism of SOEing. In this case, sequence from gene II is added to the 5'-end of primer b, and the first two reactions utilize different templates. Thus, the intermediate products overlap and can be fused by overlap extension to generate the recombinant product AD. It is also possible to perform recombination and mutagenesis simultaneously, by combining the strategies shown in Figs. 1 and 2C *(5)*.

2. Materials

1. A thermocycler ("PCR machine").
2. *Taq* DNA polymerase (*see* Note 1 and Note 2).
3. 10X PCR buffer: 100 mM Tris-HCl, pH 8.3, 500 mM KCl, and 15 mM MgCl$_2$ (*see* Note 3).
4. 10X dNTP solution: 2 mM each, dATP, dCTP, dGTP, and dTTP, pH 7.5 (prepared from commercially available aqueous stocks).
5. Oligonucleotide primers (*see* Section 3.1. and Notes 4 and 5).
6. DNA template(s) (*see* Section 3.2.).
7. Light mineral oil.

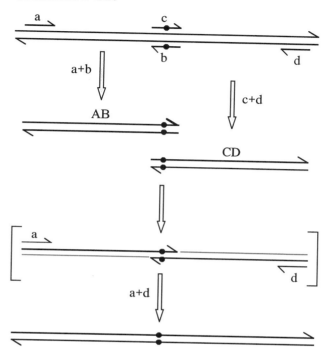

Fig. 1. Mutant product AD. Site-directed mutagenesis by overlap extension. DNA strands and synthetic oligonucleotide primers are represented by lines, with arrows indicating the 5'–3' orientations. The mutation is depicted by a solid circle. Primers are labeled with lowercase letters. PCR products are named by pairs of uppercase letters corresponding to the primers used to generate them. The intermediate species enclosed in brackets is formed by annealing at the overlap region. The overlap is extended from the 3'-end of each strand (gray dotted line) by *Taq* polymerase to generate a fusion product that can be amplified with primers a and d.

8. Microfuge tubes that fit precisely into the heating block of the thermocycler (usually 0.5 mL).
9. Agarose gel electrophoresis supplies and apparatus.
10. A method for purifying amplified fragments from agarose gels—the authors use GeneClean and/or Mermaid kits (Bio 101, La Jolla, CA), depending on the size of the fragment(s) to be isolated.

3. Methods
3.1. Primer Design (see Notes 4 and 5)

1. All of the standard considerations in PCR primer design *(6)* apply to SOE primers as well. For example, they must not be complementary to one

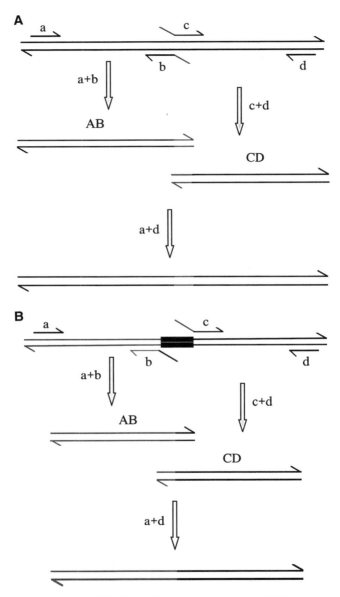

Fig. 2. Insertion product AD. Use of overlap extension PCR to generate insertion and deletion mutations. **(A)** Insertional mutation. The 5' ends of primers b and c contain the inserted sequence, which also serves as the region of overlap. **(B)** Deletion mutation. The sequence to be deleted is represented by heavy lines. The sequences on either side of the deletion are represented by gray and solid lines. Primers b and c contain sequence from each side of the region to be deleted.

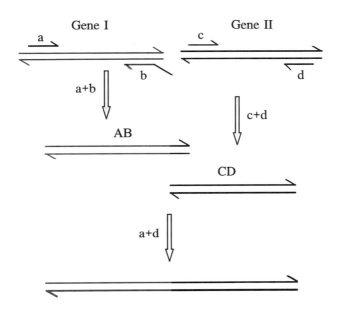

Fig. 3. Fusion product AD. Splicing by Overlap Extension (SOEing). PCR products AB and CD are derived from different genes. The overlap region is provided by the addition of CD sequence to primer b.

another (except for primers b and c, which are complimentary by design), or capable of any obvious secondary structure formation.

2. The internal primers used in an overlap extension protocol (primers b and c in Figs. 1–3) serve two functions. They must contain sequences complementary to the template in order to serve as PCR primers ("priming regions"), as well as sequences that provide a region of overlap between the two intermediate PCR products ("overlap regions"). In the case of site-directed mutagenesis (Fig. 1), the priming and overlap regions may completely coincide. The mismatched bases should, however, be positioned near the middle of each internal primer to ensure proper priming. In the case of gene SOEing (Fig. 3), the 3' end of an internal primer serves as the priming region and its 5' end contains the overlap region.

3. We routinely design our internal primers so that the region of overlap in the fusion reaction has an estimated melting temperature (T_m) of 50°C, according to the following formula *(7)*:

$$T_m(°C) = [4(G + C) + 2(A + T)]$$

The priming region of an internal primer should also have a T_m of at least 50°C.

4. The flanking primers (a and d) do not contribute to the region of overlap. Since they serve only to amplify the intermediate products and the recombinant product, no special considerations apply to their design. In some cases, restriction sites may be added to the 5' ends of these primers to facilitate cloning of the final product (*see* Note 6). The flanking primers should be capable of annealing at 50°C.

3.2. Source and Preparation of Template(s)

Most often, the starting template is a cloned version of the gene(s) to be modified, although other types of PCR templates, such as first-strand cDNA (reverse-transcribed from RNA) can also be used *(8)*. However, if the initial template is a complex mixture of DNA molecules, the risk of obtaining the wrong product and/or introducing mutations in the first amplification is increased. The advantage of using cloned DNA is that high concentrations of a defined, specific template can be used. This allows for generation of the expected final product in fewer cycles of amplification, which decreases the chance of misincorporation by *Taq* polymerase *(3)*. Since the reaction plateaus after the production of some maximum amount of product, it is not necessary to minimize the actual number of heating/cooling cycles to obtain the benefit derived from high template concentrations. The authors have successfully used plasmids prepared by cesium chloride gradient centrifugation or "miniprep" methods based on the alkaline lysis procedure.

3.3. Production of Intermediate Products AB and CD

1. Set up two separate amplification reactions to generate the intermediate products AB and CD, as illustrated in Fig. 1:

Component	PCR #1	PCR #2
10X PCR buffer	10.0 µL	10.0 µL
10X dNTP solution	10.0 µL	10.0 µL
100 pmol 5' primer	a	c
100 pmol 3' primer	b	d
Template	0.5 µg	0.5 µg
Taq polymerase	2.5 U	2.5 U
H$_2$O	to 100 µL	to 100 µL

For information regarding Mg^{2+} concentration in PCR buffer, *see* Note 3. For mutagenesis, the same template is used in both reactions; for SOEing, two different templates are used (*see* Figs. 1 and 2).

2. Overlay the reaction mixtures with two to three drops of light mineral oil, and amplify by PCR using the following cycle profile (*see* Note 7): 20–25 cycles: 94°C, 1 min (denaturation); 50°C, 2 min (annealing); 72°C, 2 min (extension).

3.4. Purification of Intermediate Products AB and CD

Gel purification of the intermediate products leads to a cleaner overlap extension reaction and increased product yield. Most important, gel purification removes the starting templates, which could be amplified to generate wild-type product if carried over into the overlap extension PCR.

1. Run each reaction mixture (100 μL) on an agarose gel. Usually, there is only one major product, so 1% agarose works well in most situations. If greater resolution is required, NuSieve agarose (FMC Bioproducts, Rockland, ME) can be used at concentrations up to 4%. It is often helpful to analyze a 5-μL sample of each intermediate PCR product by gel electrophoresis first—this can aid in estimating the approximate yield and choosing the best conditions for the preparative gel.
2. Excise the bands of interest (products AB and CD), and recover the DNA. This can be accomplished by a variety of methods, including "freeze-squeeze" *(9)* and electroelution *(10)*. We typically employ either the GeneClean or Mermaid kits (Bio 101), depending on the size of the fragment to be isolated: Mermaid is specifically designed for the purification of fragments ≤300 bp, whereas GeneClean works well for fragments larger than this.

3.5. Production of Fusion Product, AD

1. Set up the overlap extension PCR as follows. Component: 10.0 μL 10X PCR buffer; 10.0 μL 10X dNTP solution; 100 pmol 5' primer, a (*see* Note 3); 100 pmol 3' primer, d (*see* Note 8). Templates: intermediate AB, 1/4 of product from Section 3.4.; intermediate CD, 1/4 of product from Section 3.4.; *Taq* polymerase, 2.5 U; H₂O to 100 μL.
2. Overlay the reaction mixtures with two to three drops of light mineral oil, and amplify as before: 20–25 cycles: 94°C, 1 min (denaturation); 50°C, 2 min (annealing); 72°C, 2 min (extension).
3. Analyze a 5-μL sample of the final PCR product by agarose gel electrophoresis. A single fragment, representing the mutant product AD, of the anticipated size should be present.
4. Clone the fusion product AD for further analysis.

It is usually necessary to sequence the cloned mutant gene, since even a single unanticipated nucleotide change could affect the structure and function of the encoded protein. A "cassette" approach can reduce the amount of sequencing required: PCR-mediated mutagenesis is performed on a 300–500-bp gene segment, which is subsequently ligated back into a vector containing the remainder of the gene. As DNA sequencing technology advances, the need to sequence the products of overlap extension PCR is becoming less of a limitation. We sequence "miniprep" plasmid DNA (Wizard Minipreps, Promega, Madison, WI) directly using the Sequenase kit (US Biochemical, Cleveland, OH) or via an automated sequencing system (Applied Biosystems [Foster City, CA] Sequencer Model 373A).

Although the concept of overlap extension PCR is straightforward, the power of this approach to genetic engineering is significant. It enables gene sequences to be altered quickly and easily with nearly 100% efficiency. Complex constructs involving the fusion of multiple gene segments have been generated by SOEing *(4,5)*. In another extension of SOE, mixed populations of internal (b and c) primers have been used to effect random mutagenesis in the overlap region *(11,12)*.

4. Notes

1. The *Taq* polymerase error frequency associated with the overlap extension protocol outlined here is approx 1/4000 nucleotides *(3)*. A slightly higher error frequency (approx 1/2000) may be observed during complex constructions involving multiple SOE reactions *(4)*. Although these error frequencies are sufficiently low to make overlap extension practical for routine use, several precautions are in order. As indicated in Section 3.2. and Note 3, template and Mg^{2+} concentrations are important considerations.

2. It has been reported that other thermostable DNA polymerases (*Vent* polymerase, New England Biolabs, Beverly, MA; *Pfu* DNA polymerase, Stratagene, La Jolla, CA) with higher fidelity than *Taq* can be used for overlap extension *(13–16)*.

3. Mg^{2+} concentration is a critical parameter in PCR, and overlap extension PCR is no exception. "Standard" reaction conditions include 1.5 mM (final concentration) $MgCl_2$. In cases where standard conditions either do not yield significant amounts of product, or result in a high background of nonspecific products, we titrate $MgCl_2$ concentration over a range of 0.5–2.5 mM, in 0.5 mM increments. Also, since *Taq* polymerase error rates increase with increasing Mg^{2+} concentration, it is desirable to use the lowest $MgCl_2$ concentration possible. We find that many amplifications from cloned templates will tolerate a drop to 1.0 mM $MgCl_2$.

4. Oligonucleotides used in our laboratory are synthesized with an Applied BioSystems DNA Synthesizer. The final step in the synthesis involves treatment with concentrated NH_4OH, which is subsequently evaporated

away under vacuum. The dried DNA pellet is resuspended in water, and desalted over a Sephadex G-25 column (NAP-10 columns, Pharmacia, Uppsala, Sweden).

5. On a few occasions we have found several clones derived from the same overlap extension reaction that contain a deoxythymidine (T) residue at the nucleotide (same strand) immediately 5' of a mutagenic primer. This may be explained by the fact that *Taq* polymerase can add untemplated deoxyadenosine (A) residues to the 3' ends of amplified DNA fragments *(17)*. An additional A residue at the 3' end of one of the overlapping DNA strands (Fig. 1: upper strand of AB, lower strand of CD) would result in a T on the opposite strand, immediately 5' to the mutagenic primer. In our experience, this is a rare event (observed in less than 1 in 10 constructions), probably because a mismatch at the 3' terminal nucleotide significantly inhibits priming efficiency. However, others have reported that unwanted mutations owing to untemplated 3' nucleotide addition pose a significant problem *(18,19)*. If this type of mutation does become a problem, design of primers b and c to begin immediately 3' to T residues in their respective strands ensures that an untemplated 3' A residue would simply become part of the overlap region.

6. Cloning of SOE-generated DNA fragments is facilitated by the use of flanking primers (a and d) designed to include one or more restriction sites at their 5' ends. The restriction site sequences should be three to nine bases from the 5' termini for optimal digestion of the overlap extension product. We have successfully used *Bam*HI, *Bgl*II, *Cla*I, *Eco*RI, *Hind*III, *Sal*I, and *Xho*I (20 bp from 5' end).

7. The exact PCR cycle profile used does not seem to be critical. In addition to the profile suggested in Sections 3.3. and 3.5., profiles using a shorter (30-s) denaturation step or an extension step ranging from 1–3 min also work.

8. If the yield of fragments AB and CD from the first PCRs is good, but the fusion product AD is being amplified inefficiently, withholding the primers (a and d) for two to three cycles sometimes results in more efficient formation of fragment AD by overlap extension. Addition of PCR primers after this reaction has been allowed to begin may prevent undesirable side reactions that compete for the available reagents.

References

1. Mullis, K., Faloona, F., Scharf, S., Saiki, R., Horn, G., and Erlich, H. (1986) Specific enzymatic amplification of DNA in vitro: the polymerase chain reaction. *Cold Spring Harbor Symp. Quant. Biol.* **51**, 263–273.
2. Saiki, R. K., Gelfand, D. H., Stoffel, S., Scharf, S. J., Higuchi, R., Horn, G. T., Mullis, K. B., and Erlich, H. A. (1988) Primer-directed enzymatic amplification of DNA with a thermostable DNA polymerase. *Science* **239**, 487–491.

3. Ho, S. N., Hunt, H. D., Horton, R. M., Pullen, J. K., and Pease, L. R. (1989) Site-directed mutagenesis by overlap extension using the polymerase chain reaction. *Gene* **77,** 51–59.

4. Horton, R. M., Hunt, H. D., Ho, S. N., Pullen, J. K., and Pease, L. R. (1989) Engineering hybrid genes without the use of restriction enzymes: gene splicing by overlap extension. *Gene* **77,** 61–68.

5. Horton, R. M., Cai, Z., Ho, S. N., and Pease, L. R. (1990) Gene splicing by overlap extension: tailor-made genes using the polymerase chain reaction. *Biotechniques* **8,** 528–535.

6. Rychlik, W. (1993) Selection of primers for polymerase chain reaction, in *PCR Protocols: Current Methods and Applications* (White, B.A., ed), Humana, Totowa NJ, pp. 31–40.

7. Suggs, S. V., Hirose, T., Miyake, T., Kawashima, E. H., Johnson, M. J., Itakura K., and Wallace, R. B. (1981) Use of synthetic oligo-deoxyribonucleotides for the isolation of cloned DNA sequences, in *Developmental Biology Using Purified Genes* (Brown, D. D. and Fow, C. F., eds.), Academic, New York, pp. 683–693.

8. Davis, G. T., Bedzyk, W. D., Voss, E. W., and Jacobs, T. W. (1991) Single chain antibody (SCA) encoding genes: one-step construction and expression in eukaryotic cells. *Biotechnology* **9,** 165–179.

9. Tautz, D. and Renz, M. (1983) An optimized freeze-squeeze method for the recovery of DNA fragments from agarose gels. *Anal. Biochem.* **132,** 14–19.

10. Sambrook, J., Fritsch, E. F., and Maniatis, T. (1989) *Molecular Cloning: A Laboratory Manual,* 2nd ed., Cold Spring Harbor Laboratory, Cold Spring Harbor, NY

11. Morrison, H. G. and Desrosiers, R. C. (1993) A PCR-based strategy for extensive mutagenesis of a target DNA sequence. *Biotechniques* **14,** 454–457.

12. Kirchhoff, F. and Desrosiers, R. C. (1993) A PCR-derived library of random point mutations within the V3 region of simian immunodeficiency virus. *PCR Methods Appl.* **2,** 301–304.

13. Hanes, S. D. and Brent, R. (1991) A genetic model for interaction of the homeodomain recognition helix with DNA. *Science* **251,** 426–430.

14. Cease, K. B., Potcova, C. A., Lohoff, C. J., and Zeigler, M. E. (1994) Optimized PCR using Vent polymerase. *PCR Methods Appl.* **3,** 298–300.

15. Juncosa-Ginestra, M., Pons, J., Planas, A., and Querol, E. (1994) Improved efficiency in site-directed mutagenesis by PCR using a *Pyrococcus* sp. GB-D polymerase. *Biotechniques* **16,** 820–823.

16. Picard, V., Ersdal-Badju, E., Lu, A., and Bock, S.C. (1994) A rapid and efficient one-tube PCR-based mutagenesis technique using *Pfu* DNA polymerase. *Nucleic Acids Res.* **22,** 2587–2591.

17. Clark, J. M. (1988) Novel non-templated nucleotide addition reactions catalyzed by prokaryotic and eukaryotic DNA polymerase. *Nucleic Acids Res.* **17,** 3319.

18. Landt, O., Grunert, H. P., and Hahn, U. (1990) A general method for rapid site-directed mutagenesis using the polymerase chain reaction. *Gene* **96,** 125–128

19. Kuipers, O. P., Boot, H. J., and de Vos, W. M. (1991) Improved site-directed mutagenesis method using PCR. *Nucleic Acids Res.* **19,** 4558.

CHAPTER 16

Site-Directed Mutagenesis
Using Overlap Extension PCR

Ashok Aiyar, Yan Xiang, and Jonathan Leis

1. Introduction

Site-directed mutagenesis and the polymerase chain reaction (PCR) represent two powerful techniques that have led to rapid advances in our understanding of gene expression and function. Early protocols for site-directed mutagenesis depended on the production of single-stranded DNA containing the gene of interest *(1)*, using M13 phage, or phagemids such as pBluescript. One limitation with this method is the presence of inverted repeat sequences and other complementary regions, which form extensive secondary structures within single-stranded DNA, which often severely decrease the ability to extend annealed primers containing the mutation of interest.

Recently, several groups have described PCR-based site-directed mutagenesis techniques that avoid this problem by using thermal stable DNA polymerases and high temperatures to melt secondary structure *(2–4)*. Although several variations of these techniques have been reported, this chapter focuses on a derivative of the Sarkar and Sommer *(4)* megaprimer method termed Overlap Extension Mutagenesis, which is schematically depicted in Fig. 1. In the first round of PCR, primer A and mutagenic primer B are used to amplify the region of interest as well as introduce the desired mutation. This amplified product is then used as a primer in the second round of PCR and, as such, is referred to as a megaprimer. In the second round of PCR, megaprimer A/B and primer C

From: *Methods in Molecular Biology, Vol. 57: In Vitro Mutagenesis Protocols*
Edited by: M. K. Trower Humana Press Inc., Totowa, NJ

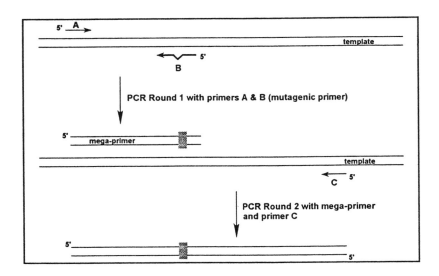

Fig. 1. Schematic representation of PCR mutagenesis as described by Sarkar and Sommer *(4)*. Oligodeoxynucleotide B is the mutagenic primer. The mutation is indicated by the stippled box.

are used to amplify the entire region of interest. The purified PCR product can then be restriction digested and cloned as desired.

Although this technique is elegantly simple in principle, there are often problems with amplifying a final PCR product of a specific size. In many cases, amplified products are found to be heterogeneous in size and migrate as smears on agarose gels. Even increasing the amount of template DNA as suggested by Barik and Galinski *(5)*, does not reliably improve the yield of the final PCR product.

An alternative method in which two overlapping PCR fragments are amplified in separate PCR reactions, each of which contains the mutation of interest, has been described by Ho et al. *(3)*. In this method, the overlapping fragments are mixed, and a full length DNA containing the desired mutation is amplified, using two outer primers. The amplification depends on strand switching using the regions of overlap between the different oligodeoxynucleotides. Although this method is effective, it requires two mutagenic primers for every mutation. In addition, three separate rounds of PCR are needed, which increases the probability of introducing undesired mutations owing to misincorporation of deoxynucleotides during DNA synthesis.

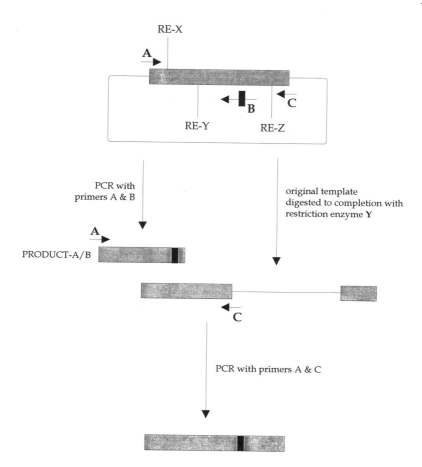

Fig. 2. Schematic representation of overlap extension mutagenesis as described in the Introduction of this chapter. Oligodeoxynucleotide B is the mutagenic primer. RE-X and RE-Z are restriction enzymes sites used to clone the final PCR product into the vector. RE-Y is a restriction site that lies between primers A and B.

The overlap extension method described herein improves the mutagenesis technique of Ho et al. *(3)* by using only a single mutagenic oligodeoxynucleotide and two rounds of PCR. The method is outlined in Fig. 2. At the top of this figure, the gene of interest is shown as a shaded box within a plasmid vector. Primers A and C flank the region to be amplified, and primer B contains the desired mutation. Restriction enzymes sites X and Z are used to subclone the mutated PCR product back into the plasmid vector. Ideally, these sites should be unique to avoid partial restriction digests.

For the simplified overlap extension method to work, one needs an additional restriction enzyme site (or sites) Y, that lies between primers A and B but not between primers B and C (*see* Note 1). Restriction site Y may be present elsewhere in the template DNA without interfering with mutagenesis. In the first round of the mutagenesis, product A/B, which contains the desired mutation, is amplified using primers A and B. Concurrently, a separate aliquot of the original template plasmid is digested to completion with restriction enzyme Y. If there is an additional unique restriction enzyme site outside of primers A and C, it is recommended that the template DNA be digested in combination with restriction site Y. This will produce a smaller fragment of template DNA that is more efficient in the overlap extension mutagenesis reaction. Both DNA products are then purified by agarose gel electrophoresis.

In the second round of PCR, the mutagenic product A/B and the plasmid fragment are used as templates in a reaction that employs two outer oligodeoxynucleotides (A and C in Fig. 2) as primers. The ratio of megaprimer and cut plasmid is of importance. A molar ratio of 5:1 to 10:1 in favor of the megaprimer consistently results in mutagenesis efficiencies in the range of 70–80%. The product of the second PCR is then gel purified and cloned using restriction enzymes X and Z. The yield of the overlap extension PCR is sufficiently high that it is not necessary to reamplify any of the products.

The overlap between the mutagenic product A/B and the cut plasmid, in successful mutagenesis procedures, has varied from <100 deoxynucleotides to a few hundred deoxynucleotides. An example of this mutagenic technique is shown in Fig. 3 where lane 1 shows the first round of PCR mutagenic product A/B, lane 2 the cut plasmid, lane 3, the second round of PCR product using DNAs from lanes and 2 as template.

The modified protocol described significantly improves the efficiency and reliability of mutagenesis and has been successfully used to introduce mutations into both the 5' noncoding and the *gag* region of Rous sarcoma virus RNA (6; unpublished data). Both regions are predicted t contain considerable secondary structure.

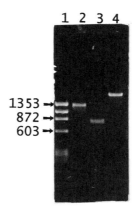

Fig. 3. Agarose gel electrophoresis of overlap extension mutagenesis. Lane 1, 100 ng of ΦX174 DNA digested with *Hae*III; lane 2, purified 1.25-kb PCR product from the first round of overlap extension mutagenesis; lane 3, purified 0.8-kb plasmid produced by *Sac*I and *Sca*I digestion of the template DNA; lane 4, purified 1.7-kb final product from the second round PCR using the DNAs from lanes 2 and 3 as templates.

2. Materials

1. Wild type and mutant plasmid DNAs propagated in *Escherichia coli* stains DH5α, XL1-Blue, or MC1061 and purified by cesium chloride isopynic gradient centrifugation, alkali lysis miniprep procedures, or commercially available columns such as QiaQUICK (Qiagen, Chatsworth, CA).
2. Restriction enzymes are used according to the manufacturer's instructions.
3. PCR primers and mutagenic oligodeoxynucleotides (25 pmol/µL) are chemically synthesized and need not be purified. (*See* Notes 2–5 for advice on primer design and Notes 6 and 7 on oligonucleotide quantitation and purification.)
4. 10X Deoxynucleotide stock solutions containing 2.5 mM each of dATP, dCTP, dGTP, and TTP.
5. *Vent* DNA polymerase (2 U/µL) (New England Biolabs, Beverly, MA) (*see* Note 8). 10X *Vent* buffer: 100 mM KCl, 200 mM Tris-HCl, pH 8.8, 100 mM ammonium sulfate, 20 mM magnesium sulfate, 1% Triton-X100.
6. Light mineral oil (Sigma, St. Louis, MO, cat. no. M-5904).
7. Chloroform:isoamyl alcohol (24:1).
8. Phenol equilibrated with TE, pH 8.0.
9. 10 mg/mL Ethidium bromide solution.
10. 10X Agarose gel-loading buffer: 50% glycerol, 50 mM EDTA, 0.4% bromophenol blue, 0.4% xylene cyanole.

11. 1X TBE: 89 mM Tris-borate and 2 mM EDTA *(7)*.
12. High salt gel elution buffer: 1.08M NaCl, 50 mM Tris-HCl, pH 8.0, 5 mM EDTA.
13. DE-81 paper (Whatmann, Maidstone, UK).
14. Millipore UltraFree MC 0.45-μm spin filter (Millipore cat. no. UFC3 OHV NB).
15. 10 mg/mL Glycogen (Boehringer Mannheim, Mannheim, Germany).
16. 70% Ethanol.
17. TE: 10 mM Tris-HCl, pH 8.0, 1 mM EDTA.
18. T4 DNA ligase (5 Weiss U/μL) (Boehringer Mannheim). 10X ligase buffer: 500 mM Tris-HCl, pH 7.8, 100 mM magnesium chloride, 100 mM dithioerythritol, 10 mM ATP, 250 μg/mL bovine serum albumin.
19. Competent *E. coli* cells.

3. Method

In this section we describe in detail the procedures used for the mutagenesis reactions shown in Fig. 3.

1. Round I PCR. Mix the following components in a clean 500-μL microfuge tube (*see* Note 9):

Linearized plasmid template (25 ng/μL)	2 μL
Primer A (25 pmol/μL)	2 μL
Primer B (25 pmol/μL)	2 μL
10X dNTP stock	10 μL
10X *Vent* buffer	10 μL
ddH$_2$O	73 μL

Top the reaction with 50 μL of light mineral oil. Heat the tube to 94°C for 5 min, and then add 1 μL of *Vent* DNA polymerase (2 U/μL). Start the following temperature cycling program for 18 cycles: 94°C for 2 min, 55°C for 1 min, and 72°C for 1 min.

2. During the PCR reaction, restrict an aliquot of the same plasmid as follows:

Uncut plasmid DNA (200 ng/μL)	20 μL
10X buffer for restriction enzyme Y	5 μL
Restriction enzyme Y (10 U/μL)	2 μL
ddH$_2$O	23 μL

The 10X buffer for the restriction enzyme is provided by the supplier of the enzyme. The reaction is normally carried out at 37°C for 1 h.

3. Extract the completed PCR reaction mixture containing product A/B (*see* Note 10) with 100 μL of chloroform:isoamyl alcohol (24:1). Transfer the upper layer of the extraction to a new tube and add 10 μL of 10X agarose gel-loading buffer.

4. Raise the volume of the restriction digestion to 100 μL by adding 100 μL of ddH$_2$O. Extract the restriction digestion once with 100 μL of phenol, followed by a further extraction with 50 μL of chloroform:isoamyl alcohol. Transfer the upper layer of the final extraction to a new tube and add 10 μL of 10X agarose gel-loading buffer.
5. Submit both reactions to gel electrophoresis using a 1% agarose gel with 0.5X TBE as the gel running buffer. The progress of the electrophoresis can be periodically monitored by UV illumination for very short lengths of time (<30 s). To facilitate this, include ethidium bromide (0.2 μg/mL) in the gel and running buffer.
6. After electrophoresis, cut slits into the gel immediately in front of and behind each band of interest from the two reactions (the desired plasmid DNA fragment and the correct sized PCR product). Insert strips of DE-81 paper (2 × 1 cm) into both sets of holes and then continue the electrophoresis until the DNAs have migrated onto the DE-81 papers in the slits in front of the original bands. Remove the papers from these slits and gently rinse them in 0.5X TBE to remove any agarose, and then trim and discard the excess paper.
7. Transfer the trimmed papers to separate 1.5-mL microfuge tubes; to each add 330 μL of high-salt buffer and mix the contents vigorously using a Vortex mixer for 30 s. Incubate the tubes at 65°C for 60 min, then spin them for 5 min at maximum speed in an Eppendorf microfuge.
8. Pass each supernatant through a Millipore UltraFree MC 0.45-μm spin filter; add 1 μL of glycogen (10 mg/mL) to the filtrate, together with 900 μL of cold ethanol, mix, and then incubate on crushed dry-ice for 5 min. Spin the tubes for 20 min at maximum speed in an Eppendorf microfuge at 4°C.
9. Wash the precipitates twice with 500 μL of 70% ethanol, and then dry the pellets in a SpeedVac, before suspending each in 20 μL of TE. Remove 2 μL to quantitate the amount of DNA present in each tube (typically between 15 and 30 ng/μL).
10. Setup the second round of PCR as follows:

Purified round I PCR product (product A/B) (25 ng/μL)	6 μL
Purified fragment from cut plasmid (25 ng/μL)	2 μL
Primer A (25 pmol/μL)	2 μL
Primer C (25 pmol/μL)	2 μL
10X dNTP stock	10 μL
10X *Vent* buffer	10 μL
Vent DNA polymerase (2U/μL)	1 μL
ddH$_2$O	67 μL

Add, mix, and cycle these components as described in step 1.

11. Purify the final PCR product by gel electrophoresis as described in steps 3 and 5–9 (*see* Notes 11 and 12).
12. Digest 500 ng of the purified PCR product, with either restriction enzymes X and Z (*see* Fig. 2) or restriction sites incorporated into the 5' ends of primers A and C, in two sequential steps. Purify the products by phenol/chloroform extraction and ethanol precipitation using standard protocols. Ligate 20 ng of the digested product into an appropriately restricted recipient vector, and transform into a competent strain of *E. coli* (*see* Notes 13–16).

4. Notes

1. In the event that a suitable internal restriction enzyme site Y cannot be found, a reliable variant of the aforementioned procedure (8) is schematically depicted in Fig. 4. This procedure uses three PCRs, and four primers, and, in that respect, is similar to the technique described by Ho et al. (3). However, only one of the four primers is mutagenic. As shown in Fig. 4, two products are independently amplified in the first round. Product I, which contains the desired mutation, is amplified using primers A and B. Product II, which is wild type in sequence, is amplified using primers C and D. Both these products are gel purified and mixed in a ratio similar to that described in the previous section, and a third PCR is performed using the two outer oligodeoxynucleotides (A and D in Fig. 4). The product of this final PCR is gel purified and cloned.

   An example of this procedure is shown in Fig. 5. Product I is 112 nucleotides long (lane 2) while product II is 190 nucleotides long (lane 3). The overlap between the two DNAs is 15 bp and the final PCR product is 287 nucleotides long (lane 4).

2. As with other protocols for site-directed mutagenesis, it is important that attention be paid to the design of the mutagenic oligodeoxynucleotide. Its size is dependent on the nature of the mutation being introduced. For a single point mutation, it is recommended that a primer of at least 25 deoxynucleotides in length be used, with 15 bases from the 3' side being complementary to the template DNA. Insertions, deletions, or substitutions as large as 70 deoxynucleotides in length have been constructed with this method, but need primers which have as much as 30 deoxynucleotides complementary to the template on each side of the mutation. Larger mutations will require primers with correspondingly larger complementary regions flanking the desired change.

3. Care should be taken to ensure that the designed primer is not self-complementary forming stable hairpins. Wherever possible, it is helpful to incorporate a unique restriction site into the mutagenic primer, as this considerably simplifies screening for the mutation. The commercial program

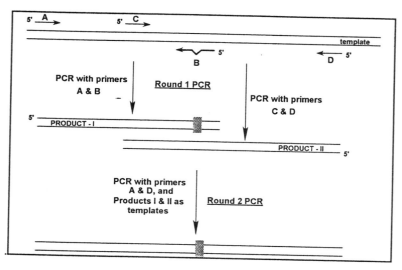

Fig. 4. Schematic representation of mutagenesis by overlap extension using four primers as described by Aiyar and Leis *(8)*. Two short regions are separately amplified by two independent PCRs. Product I is amplified using primers A and B, and product II is amplified using primers C and D. The products of both these PCRs are then purified and used as templates for a third PCR with the two outer oligos, A and D, used as primers. Oligodeoxynucleotide B is the mutagenic primer. The mutation is indicated by the stippled box. From ref. *7* with permission.

Gene Runner (Hastings Software, Inc., Hastings, NY) is very useful in designing the mutagenic PCR primers. Two freeware alternatives, which provide most of the versatility of *Gene Runner*, are *Oligo* and *SilMut*. Both programs can be found at the IUBIO molecular biology software repository (ftp.bio.indiana.edu) at Indiana University (Bloomington, IN).

4. It is also important to take melting temperature of the desired oligodeoxy-nucleotide into consideration The "%GC − T_m" formula described by Baldino et al. *(9)* provides an estimate of T_m for any given PCR primer. This formula, corrected for salt and formamide concentrations, is:

$$81.5 + 16.6 \log[\text{Na}^+] + 0.41(\%G + \%C) - 0.65(\%\text{formamide}) - 675/\text{length} = T_m \qquad (1)$$

For purposes of calculation of the T_m of a primer, set the salt concentration to 100 m*M* and the %formamide concentration to 0. This simplifies the equation to:

1   2 3 4

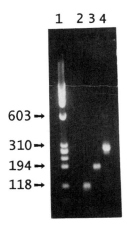

603 →

310 →
194 →
118 →

Fig. 5. Agarose gel electrophoresis of DNA products from mutagenesis by overlap extension using four primers. Lane 1, 600 ng of ΦX174 *Hae*III digested and used as size markers. Lanes 2 and 3, purified 112- and 190-bp fragments produced by PCR. The 112-bp fragment contains the mutation. Lane 4, PCR amplification done using the PCR products shown in lanes 2 and 3 as templates.

$$64.9 + 0.41(\%G + \%C) - 675/\text{length} = T_m \qquad (2)$$

It is recommended that designed oligodeoxynucleotides have predicted T_ms in the range of 50–60°C. The actual annealing temperature used in the PCRs is 2–3°C lower than the smaller of the two melting temperatures. While calculating T_ms, readers may wish to avail themselves of the freeware program MELT. To obtain this program, send mail to "Netserv@EBI.AC.UK." The body of the message should contain the text "GET DOS_SOFTWARE:MELT.UUE". For a considerably more detailed examination of annealing temperatures used during amplification, the reader is referred to the work of Rychlik et al. *(10).*

5. The nonmutagenic flanking primers can be considerably shorter than the mutagenic primers. These are typically in the range of 15–20 deoxynucleotides in length. While their size is not critical, care should be taken that these primers have a sufficiently high annealing temperature (~50–60°C).

6. It is also important that the concentration of the two primers used in each PCR be close to each other. The following formula can be used to estimate the primer concentrations.

$$(\text{OD}_{260}/\text{mL})/10/(\text{length} \times 1000) \approx [\text{primer}] \ \mu M \qquad (3)$$

This formula is more accurate for longer oligodeoxynucleotides of heterogeneous sequence.

7. Unlike single-stranded mutagenesis, it is not crucial that the mutagenic oligodeoxynucleotide be OPC-cartridge purified or gel purified. Since most mutagenic primers are used only once, it is recommended that only small amounts be synthesized.

8. The first thermostable polymerases widely used for PCR mutagenesis were *Taq* or *Pyrostase* DNA polymerases. Both of these polymerases have high processivity, but lower fidelity as they lack a 3' to 5' editing exonuclease activity. In addition, these DNA polymerases have been observed to add a single 3' nontemplated deoxynucleotide (usually dAMP) to the amplified product. If present in the mutagenic product A/B, this additional deoxynucleotide interferes with the final PCR reaction. In addition, 3' nontemplated overhangs interfere with blunt end cloning.

   An effective alternative to *Taq* or *Pyrostase* is either *Vent* or *DeepVent* DNA polymerases (New England Biolabs), which contain 3' to 5' exonuclease activities. The presence of the exonuclease permits *Vent* DNA polymerase to repair 3' terminal mismatches as determined by direct sequencing of numerous clones (data not shown). Also, 5' phosphorylated PCR products prepared with *Vent* or *DeepVent* can be self-ligated to form multimers up to heptamers and can be efficiently ligated into plasmid cut with restriction enzymes *Sma*I or *Eco*RV, both of which leave blunt ends. In contrast, the *Taq* or *Pyrostase* products are ligated with poor efficiency into *Eco*RV cut vector and do not self-ligate efficiently. Moreover, the presence of the proofreading exonuclease in *Vent* DNA polymerase, leads to DNA products with very low rates of misincorporation, again detected by sequencing of many clones.

   Other thermostable polymerases with proofreading exonuclease activity include *Pwo* DNA polymerase (Boerhinger Mannheim), and *Pfu* DNA polymerase (Stratagene, La Jolla, CA).

   If the mutagenic or final PCR product is longer than 2 kb, it may be useful to use a combination of *Taq* or *Pyrostase* along with *Vent* (New England Biolabs) or *Pfu* (Stratagene) DNA polymerase as has been described by Barnes *(11)*.

9. The PCR conditions used are dependent on the primer sequence. The following conditions have worked for a variety of primers and may represent a good starting set of conditions to optimize the use of different combinations of primers and templates. In addition, the PCR products are much cleaner when the template plasmid is linear rather than supercoiled. This is especially true if the mutagenic product A/B in Fig. 2, or product I or product II in Fig. 4 are >500 deoxynucleotides in length. The products of PCR are also cleaner and obtained in higher yields if the reactions are "hot-started." In this technique, all the components of the PCR reaction are

mixed with the exception of the thermostable DNA polymerase. The mixture is heated to 94°C for 5–10 min, the DNA polymerase is added, and then the temperature cycling is begun.

For all amplifications, PCR reactions contain 10–20 ng of cut plasmid template DNA, 25–50 pmol of primers A and B, and 2 U of DNA polymerase in a final reaction volume of 100 µL. *Vent* and *DeepVent* polymerase were used in buffer conditions suggested by the vendor. For amplifications in the size range of 0.5–2 kb, reaction conditions include 0.25 m*M* dNTPs, 10 m*M* KCl, 20 m*M* Tris-HCl, pH 8.8 (at 25°C), 10 m*M* ammonium sulfate, 0.1% Triton X-100, and 2 m*M* magnesium sulfate. Longer extensions may require additional magnesium sulfate, as suggested by the manufacturer.

The cycling conditions are: 94°C for 2 min, 50°C for 1 min, and 72°C for 1.5 min for three cycles, followed by: 94°C for 2 min, 57°C for 1 min, and 72°C for 1.5 min for 15 cycles. It has routinely been found that 18 cycles provides a sufficient yield of product for all subsequent manipulations. It is recommended not to use more than 18 cycles, since this increases the risk of introducing unwanted mutations owing to deoxynucleotide misincorporation. If *Taq* or *Pyrostase* DNA polymerases are used, it is critical to optimize the concentration of Mg^{2+}, as this greatly decreases the amount of primer-dimer and other artifactual products in the reaction.

10. If no mutagenic product A/B is amplified or it is heterogeneous in size, try and optimize both the annealing temperature and the ratio of the two primers used in the PCR. If this does not increase the specificity of the reaction sequence the template DNA with each primer individually to ensure that the primers anneal at the correct position. It may also be prudent to radio label the primers with γ^{32}P-ATP and directly examine the labeled product on a 20% denaturing polyacrylamide sequencing gel to ensure that the vast majority of each oligodeoxynucleotide primer is of the expected size.

11. An alternative method of purification of the second round of PCR is as follows: submit one-third of the PCR reaction to gel electrophoresis employing 1–2% agarose gels in 45 m*M* Tris-borate, 1 m*M* EDTA. Detect the DNA products by ethidium bromide staining and then recover the desired fragments from the gels either by electroelution onto DEAE paper as described by Sambrook et al. *(7),* or by QIAQUICK spin column (Qiagen) or using QIAEX resin (Qiagen). If the latter two methods are used, care should be taken to ensure that the purified DNAs are free of guanidine hydrochloride, which may affect the efficiency of both cloning and PCR if carried over with the purified DNA.

12. If no product can be amplified from the second round of PCR, then attempt to establish amplification conditions using both external primers on a co

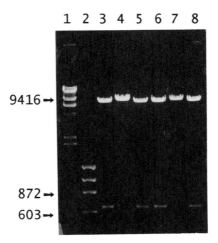

Fig. 6. Detection of mutations in DNA products by restriction digestion. Lane 1, 100 ng of λ DNA digested with *Hind*III; lane 2, 100 ng of Φ174 DNA digested with *Hae*III; lanes 3–8, miniprep plasmid DNA digested with *Kpn*I. The DNA in lanes 3, 5, 6, and 8 contain mutations, detected by the presence of the second *Kpn*I DNA product at the bottom of the gel.

tiguous DNA template. Pay careful attention to the annealing temperature and the Mg^{2+} concentration. Very often a Mg^{2+} titration is required, especially for amplifying fragments >1.5 kb in size with *Vent* DNA polymerase. If the overlap between the mutagenic product A/B and cut-plasmid is <100 deoxynucleotides, the annealing temperature for the second round of PCR might have to be decreased to 45°C.

13. Once the mutant PCR product is cloned, DNA minipreps of the colonies can be easily screened for the presence of the mutation by restriction digestion. An example of this is shown in Fig. 6, where the clones are screened for the presence of a second *Kpn*I site introduced during the mutagenesis. Four of six clones were found to contain the mutation.

14. If the mutagenic PCR product is cloned into a vector other than the original, one can use a rapid PCR-based screen to identify bacterial colonies containing plasmids with the desired inserts. In this method, each colony is suspended in 10 μL of 10 m*M* Tris-HCl, pH 8.3, 1 m*M* EDTA. A 1-μL aliquot of the bacterial suspension is brought to a volume of 25 μL using PCR reaction conditions and primers that can detect the insert. An example of such a screen in shown in Fig. 7. In the figure, colonies examined in lanes a–c and e–l contain plasmid with inserts, while the colony in lane d does not. The advantage of this PCR screen is that it is very quick, requir-

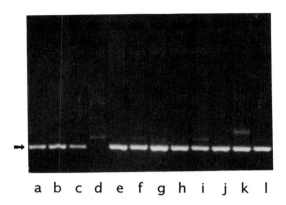

a b c d e f g h i j k l

Fig. 7. A rapid colony PCR screen for plasmid DNAs containing inserts.
Colonies obtained after transformation are suspended as described in Note 14
and used in PCRs to test for the presence of an insert in the plasmid DNA. The
products of amplification are subjected to 1% agarose gel electrophoresis. The
colonies used in reactions a–c and e–l contain the insert as shown by the presence of a 294-bp fragment marked by the arrow.

ing only 3 h to perform and avoids growing minipreps. If the mutation
introduces an unique restriction site, the PCR products can be restriction
digested to detect the presence of the mutation as in Fig. 6.

15. If the final PCR product can be amplified but cannot be efficiently
cloned, then ensure that the restriction enzymes being used can individually cut the amplified DNA segment. This can be ascertained by
digesting the DNA with each enzyme individually, purifying and
ligating the cut product. The cut products should form dimers but not
multimers since the other (blunt) end is not phosphorylated. It is also
important to note that several restriction enzymes do not efficiently cleave
if the cut site is close to an end of DNA. A detailed analysis of site size
requirements of different restriction enzymes has been described by
Kaufman and Evans *(12)*.

16. If the final PCR product can be cloned, but the clones do not contain the
desired mutation, then increase the ratio of mutagenic product A/B to the
cut plasmid template in the second round of PCR to 20:1. You can also
confirm that the mutagenic product A/B contains the desired mutation by
directly sequencing the purified product. If the mutant oligodeoxynucleotide introduces a restriction site, the efficiency of mutagenesis can
be examined by digesting the purified final PCR product with the appropriate restriction enzyme.

Acknowledgments

This work was supported by Public Health Service Grants CA38046 and CA52047 from the National Cancer Institute. A. Aiyar is supported in part by the Retrovirus and AIDS Training Grant AI07381 from the National Institutes of Health.

References

1. Vieira, J. and Messing, J. (1983) Production of single-stranded plasmid DNA. *Methods Enzymol.* **153,** 3–11.
2. Higuchi, R., Kurimmel, B., and Saiki, R. (1988) A general method of *in vitro* preparation and specific mutagenesis of DNA fragments: study of protein and DNA interactions. *Nucleic Acids Res.* **16,** 7351–7367.
3. Ho, S. N., Hunt, H. D., Morton, R. M., Pullen, J. K., and Pease, L. R. (1989) Site-directed mutagenesis by overlap extension using the polymerase chain reaction. *Gene* **77,** 51–59.
4. Sarkar, G. and Sommer, S. S. (1990) The "Megaprimer" method of site-directed mutagenesis. *BioTechniques* **8,** 404–407.
5. Barik, S. and Galinski, M. S. (1991) "Megaprimer" method of PCR: increased template concentration improves yield. *BioTechniques* **10,** 489,490.
6. Aiyar, A., Ge, Z., and Leis, J. (1994) A specific orientation of RNA secondary structures is required for initiation of reverse transcription. *J. Virol.* **68,** 611–618.
7. Sambrook, J., Fritsch, E. F., and Maniatis, T. (1989) *Molecular Cloning: A Laboratory Manual,* 2nd ed. Cold Spring Harbor Laboratories, Cold Spring Harbor, NY.
8. Aiyar, A. and Leis, J. (1993) Modification of the megaprimer method of PCR mutagenesis: improved implification of the final product. *BioTechniques* **14,** 366,367.
9. Baldino, F., Chesselet, M.-F., and Lewis, M. E. (1989) High resolution *in situ* hybridization histochemistry. *Methods Enzymol.* **168,** 761–777.
10. Rychlik, W., Spencer, W. J., and Rhoads, R. E. (1990) Optimization of the annealing temperature for DNA amplification *in vitro*. *Nucleic Acids Res.* **18,** 6409–6412.
11. Barnes, W. M. (1994) PCR amplification of up to 35 kb DNA with high fidelity and high yield from bacteriophage templates. *Proc. Natl. Acad. Sci. USA* **91,** 2216–2220.
12. Kaufman, D. L. and Evans, G .A. (1990) Restriction endonuclease cleavage at the termini of PCR products. *BioTechniques* **9,** 304–306.

CHAPTER 17

Modification
of the Overlap Extension Method
for Extensive Mutagenesis
on the Same Template

Ivan Mikaelian and Alain Sergeant

1. Introduction

Polymerase chain reaction (PCR) is a powerful and efficient method allowing enzymatic amplification of small quantities of DNA. This technology has also been widely used as a quick and efficient alternative for introducing mutations into specific DNA sequences. Various general methods for site-directed mutagenesis using the PCR have been described recently *(1–5)*. In the overlap extension method two pairs of primers are used to generate two DNA fragments with overlapping ends containing the desired mutation. These two DNA products are combined and subsequently annealed. Finally, the resulting hybrids are amplified by PCR to generate homogeneous products containing the mutation. This method has proved to be simpler, faster, and much more efficient than traditional methods for site-directed mutagenesis *(2)*. However, because synthesis of two complementary primers is required for each mutation, the overlap extension is not the method of choice for extensive mutagenesis of a target sequence.

The method described in this chapter is a modification of the overlap extension method that is particularly suitable when multiple mutations are to be made on the same DNA template. The major improvement of this procedure lies in the fact that only one primer is required for each

From: *Methods in Molecular Biology, Vol. 57: In Vitro Mutagenesis Protocols*
Edited by: M. K. Trower Humana Press Inc., Totowa, NJ

mutation once the initial mutation has been generated. Moreover, the procedure remains very efficient (90–100% efficiency) and very rapid (the whole protocol can be achieved in 2 d, from the template DNA to the cloning of the mutated fragment).

The principle of the method is illustrated in Fig. 1 (*see* pp. 196–197). The DNA template to be mutagenized is subjected to two simultaneous PCR reactions using two different sets of primers. Three of these primers (primers 1, 2, and 3) are constant and common to all mutations. Primer 2 is homologous to the DNA sequence but contains a "tail" of mismatch bases. The fourth primer (primer M) is specific for each mutation. Similar to the overlap extension method, this specific primer contains the mutation, which can be an insertion, a deletion, or a substitution.

Two overlapping DNA fragments are generated from these two independent PCR reactions. One fragment, product A, is identical to the original sequence but contains additional mismatch bases at one end because of the incorporation of primer 2. The second DNA fragment, product B, contains the expected mutation at one end. These two PCR products are then gel-purified, mixed in equimolar ratios, and finally subjected to another round of amplification using external primers (primers 1 and 3). In addition to the parental DNA fragments (products A and B), two types of DNA hybrids (hybrids a/b and b/a) are formed during the first hybridization step of this second PCR reaction (*see* Fig. 1). Among these DNA molecules, only hybrid a/b can be used as a template for amplification. Because of the mismatch at the 3' end, the "a" strand of this hybrid is not likely to be extended by the *Taq* DNA polymerase. However, the "b" strand is extended using the "a" strand as template. This elongated "b" strand that contains the mutation is then amplified with primers 1 and 3. Ultimately, the mutated DNA can be digested with appropriate restriction enzymes and subcloned into the original vector or any other cloning vector.

2. Materials

1. Cesium chloride purified DNA template in TE 10/1 buffer. Store at –20°C.
2. 10X *Taq* reaction buffer: 100 mM Tris-HCl, pH 8.3 (25°C), 500 mM KCl, 15 mM MgCl$_2$, 0.1% gelatine. Store at –20°C.
3. 20 mM dNTP mix: 20 mM each of dATP, dTTP, dCTP, and dGTP, pH 7.0. Store at –20°C.
4. Primers: Gel-purified synthetic oligonucleotides at 0.1 mM in water. Store at –20°C.

5. *Taq* DNA polymerase (5 U/µL) (supplied by Perkin Elmer Cetus, Norwalk, CT, *see* Note 1).
6. Mineral oil.
7. Thermal cycler.
8. Chloroform.
9. Loading dye: 0.4% bromophenol blue, 0.4% xylene cyanole FF, and 50% glycerol in water. Store at room temperature.
10. 3*M* Sodium acetate, pH 4.5. Autoclave and store at room temperature.
11. 100 and 70% Ethanol.
12. TAE 1X: 0.04 m*M* Tris-acetate pH 7.5, 1 m*M* EDTA. Store at room temperature.
13. TE 10/1 buffer: 10 m*M* Tris-HCl, pH 7.5, 1 m*M* EDTA. Autoclave and store at room temperature.
14. Geneclean kit (Bio 101, La Jolla, CA) (optional).

3. Methods
3.1. Design of PCR Primers

The choice of primers is critical and must be done with care. For an extensive mutagenesis, primers 1, 2, and 3 are identical for all mutations. Primer M is the mutagenic primer and is different for each mutation. If the mutated DNA fragment has to be ultimately subcloned into the original vector or any other cloning vector, primers 1 and 3 are chosen so that the amplified fragment contains unique restriction sites on both sides of the mutations allowing easy cloning (Fig. 1, *see* Notes 2 and 3). These primers should be 18–20 bases long with a GC content approaching 50% (*see* Note 4). Primer 2 lies between primer M and 3. This oligonucleotide is designed to contain 18–20 bases homologous to the sequence of interest and eight or more additional bases at its 5' end that do not allow pairing with the template DNA. These additional bases are designed to inhibit amplification of the wild-type sequence during the second round of PCR and by doing so will increase the efficiency of the procedure (Fig. 1, *see* Note 1).

Similar to M13 mutagenesis, primer M contains a region of mismatch flanked by sequences complementary to the template to ensure the oligonucleotide anneals efficiently to the specified target. The mutation carried by primer M can be an insertion, a deletion, or a substitution (*see* Note 5). For primer M the extent of the sequences flanking the mutation, or "feet," depends on the type of mutation. For single nucleotide changes, feet of 10 nucleotides on either side of the mutation are usually suffi-

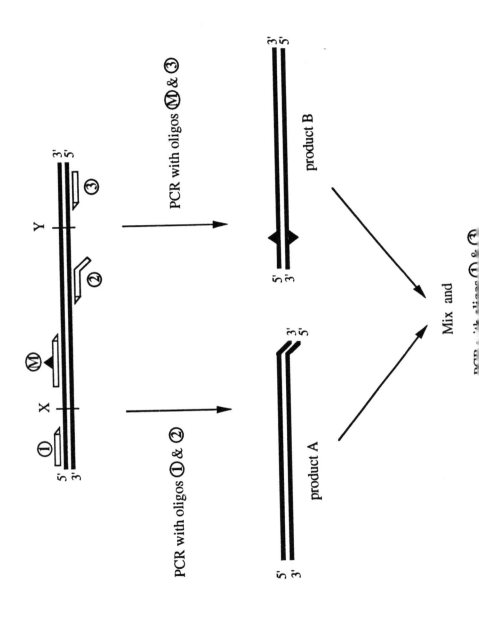

PCR with oligos ① & ②

PCR with oligos Ⓜ & ③

product A

product B

Mix and

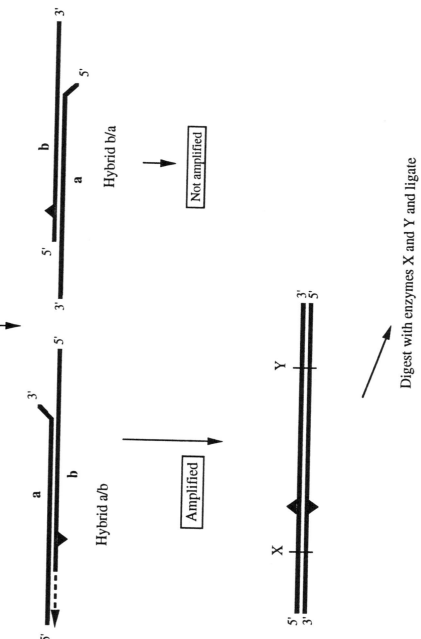

Hybrid a/b

Amplified

Hybrid b/a

Not amplified

X   Y

Digest with enzymes X and Y and ligate

Fig. 1. Schematic representation of the mutagenesis procedure.

198 *Mikaelian and Sergeant*

cient. Longer feet are required (up to 15 nucleotides) if bigger mutations are to be made, or if the flanking sequences are rich in A and T. Furthermore, in order to avoid problems with template-independent incorporation at 3' termini of amplified products (*see* Note 6), mutagenic primers have been designed as described by Kuipers et al. *(6)*, such that the first 5' nucleotide of the primer follows a T residue in the template sequence.

3.2. First Round of PCR

The first round of PCR is carried out simultaneously with two sets of primers on the same DNA template (*see* Fig. 1). Primers 1 and 2 are used in a first reaction to generate the PCR product A, which is the same for all the subsequent mutations. This product contains eight additional basepairs that do not match to the template. The second PCR reaction is performed with primer M and primer 3 to generate product B, which contains the appropriate mutation at one end (*see* Fig. 1). Reactions are performed in a final volume of 100 µL in 0.5-mL microfuge tubes.

1. Mix 20–100 ng of template DNA (*see* Note 7), 10 µL of 10X *Taq* reaction buffer, 1 µL of 20 m*M* dNTP mix, 1 µL of a 100-µ*M* solution of primer 1, 1 µL of a 100-µ*M* solution of primer 2, 2.5 U of *Taq* DNA polymerase (Perkin-Elmer Cetus), and water to 100 µL.
2. In a second tube, mix 20–100 ng of template DNA, 10 µL of 10X *Taq* reaction buffer, 1 µL of 20 m*M* dNTP mix, 1 µL of a 100-µ*M* solution of primer M, 1 µL of a 100-µ*M* solution of primer 3, 2.5 U of *Taq* DNA polymerase, and water to 100 µL.
3. Add three drops of light mineral oil (approx 100 µL) in both tubes to avoid evaporation.
4. Denature for 4 min at 94°C and perform 30 cycles of denaturation at 94°C for 20 s, annealing at 40–60°C for 1 min (*see* Note 8), and extension at 72°C for 2 min (*see* Note 9) in a thermal cycler. After the last cycle, incubate for a further 10 min at 72°C to allow extension to go to completion.

3.3. Purification of the PCR Products

After the first round of amplification, the PCR products are separated by electrophoresis on an agarose gel and subsequently purified by either Geneclean (Bio 101) or squeeze freeze. This step is necessary to eliminate traces of the original DNA template that would otherwise decrease the efficiency of the reaction (*see* Note 10).

1. To the reaction tubes, add 150 µL of chlorophorm to remove the mineral oil. Vortex briefly and centrifuge for 1 min in a microfuge at room temperature. Recover the upper aqueous phase into a new tube.

2. Check the success of the reaction by loading a 5-µL aliquot plus 0.5 µL of loading dye on a 1% agarose minigel (1X TAE). If the reaction is unsuccessful, try varying the hybridization temperature and the MgCl$_2$ concentration in the reaction (*see* Note 8).
3. Precipitate the remaining DNA by adding 10 µL of 3M sodium acetate pH 4.5 and 250 µL of 100% ethanol. Store for 30 min at –20°C. Centrifuge for 15 min in a microfuge at maximun speed. Wash the pellet with 500 µL of 70% ethanol, centrifuge for 2 min, and air dry the pellet by leaving the tubes open at room temperature for 5–10 min.
4. Resuspend the pellet in 20 µL of TE 10/1, add 2 µL of loading dye, and load on a 1–2% agarose gel (1X TAE), depending on the fragment length.
5. After electrophoresis, soak the gel for 10–20 min in a 0.5-µg/mL ethidium bromide solution. Visualize the gel under a UV light (320 nm) and cut out the DNA bands using a razor blade. Purify the DNA using either a Geneclean kit (Bio 101) or, if the fragment is small (<800 bp), by "squeeze freeze" as follows.
6. With a 19-gage needle, make a hole in a 0.5-mL Eppendorf tube and plug the bottom with siliconized glass wool. Put the agarose fragment in the tube and freeze by immersing for 1 min in liquid nitrogen. Warm at room temperature and put the tube in a second 2-mL capless Eppendorf tube. Centrifuge for 15 min in a microfuge at 12,000 rpm. Precipitate the eluent by adding 0.1 vol of 3M sodium acetate pH 4.5 and 2.5 vol of 100% ethanol. Store for 30 min at –20°C and centrifuge for 15 min in a microfuge at maximum speed. Wash the pellet with 500 µL of 70% ethanol. Centrifuge for 2 min and dry at room temperature for 5–10 min. Resuspend in 50 µL of TE 10/1.
7. Evaluate the DNA concentration by loading an aliquot of the sample and a known amount of a DNA weight marker on a minigel (1% agarose, 1X TAE). The DNA concentration can be roughly estimated by comparing the intensity of the band with the bands of the marker.

3.4. Second Round of PCR

The second PCR reaction is performed using a mixture of products A and B as templates. Neither of these DNA fragments can be amplified with primers 1 and 3. Strand "a" of hybrid a/b is theoretically the only template suitable for extension, allowing the amplification of the mutated DNA (*see* Fig. 1). Typically, 50 ng of both purified products are used, which represents roughly equimolar amounts of both the primary products (*see* Note 11).

1. In a 0.5-mL microfuge tube, mix 50 ng of each purified template DNA with 10 µL of 10X *Taq* reaction buffer, 1 µL of 20 mM dNTP mix, 1 µL of

a 100-μ*M* solution of primer 1, 1 μL of a 100-μ*M* solution of primer 3, 2.5 U of *Taq* DNA polymerase, and water to 100 μL. Add three drops of mineral oil to avoid evaporation.

2. Denature for 4 min at 94°C and perform 30 cycles of denaturation at 94°C for 20 s, annealing at 50°C for 30 s (*see* Note 8), and extension at 72°C for 1 min (*see* Note 9) in a thermal cycler. Incubate for another 10 min at 72°C to allow extension to go to completion.

3. Extract the PCR products with 150 μL of chloroform, vortex, and centrifuge for 1 min in a microfuge. Recover the upper phase into a new tube. Check the success of the reaction by loading a 5-μL aliquot on a mini agarose gel (1X TAE, 1% agarose).

4. Precipitate the DNA by adding 10 μL of 3*M* sodium acetate pH 4.5 and 250 μL of 100% ethanol. Store for 30 min at −20°C. Centrifuge for 15 min in a microfuge at 12,000 rpm. Wash the pellet with 500 μL of 70% ethanol, centrifuge for 2 min, and dry the pellet at room temperature for 5–10 min. Resuspend the pellet in 20 μL of TE 10/1.

3.5. Digestion, Purification, and Cloning of the Mutated DNA Fragment

The amplified mutated DNA is then either used crude or digested with restriction enzymes in order to be cloned into the original vector or any other cloning vector (*see* Notes 3 and 12).

1. Digest the amplified fragment for 2 h in 50 μL with the appropriate enzymes and buffer.

2. Purify DNA after separation on a 1% agarose gel as described earlier *(see* Section 3.3., step 5). The DNA is now ready to be subcloned into the appropriate vector.

3. Clones should be sequenced, both to confirm that the mutation is present and to check for spontaneous mutations that may occur owing to the high misincorporation rate of the *Taq* DNA polymerase.

We have used this procedure to generate multiple mutations (deletions and substitutions) in the Epstein-Barr virus early transcriptional activator EB1 (or Z) *(7)*. In our hands, the efficiency of the procedure is very high (>90%). Identification of the expected clone is routinely achieved by picking up two colonies for each mutation and sequencing the corresponding DNA.

4. Notes

1. Care should be taken in the choice of the DNA polymerase. *Taq* DNA polymerase has proved to be suitable for this method. Despite their

increased fidelity, we do not recommend the use of thermophilic DNA polymerases possessing 3'–5' proofreading exonuclease activity. However, genetically modified thermophilic DNA polymerases like *Vent* (exo-), Deep *Vent* (exo-) (New England Biolabs, Beverly, MA), or Exo-*Pfu* (Stratagene, La Jolla, CA) can be used.

2. One of the major problems associated with all PCR mutagenesis methods is that the amplified fragment has to be sequenced completely after cloning owing to the high misincorporation rate of the *Taq* DNA polymerase *(8)*. Consequently, restriction sites used during the cloning step should be chosen with care to allow easy sequencing.

3. The primers can also carry additional restriction sites at their 5' ends to allow cloning into the pBluescript or pUC series of cloning vectors. Alternatively, a "TA" cloning vector (InVitrogen, San Diego, CA) can be used.

4. Primers should have similar GC content so that their optimal annealing temperatures are similar (*see* Note 8). Primers with an average GC content of 50% are typically used so that their melting temperature is above 55°C. Primers with complementary 3' ends or potential secondary structure should be avoided.

5. Substitutions, deletions, and insertions can be generated by this method. However, because it is difficult to synthesize oligonucleotides longer than 120 bases efficiently, mutations larger than 80 nucleotides are not possible.

6. It is well documented that *Taq* DNA polymerase possesses a "terminal transferase-like" activity that incorporates an untemplated dA residue at the 3' ends of amplified sequences *(9)*.

7. Owing to the poor fidelity of the *Taq* DNA polymerase *(8)*, the use of more template DNA (up to 1 μg) and fewer amplification cycles has been suggested.

8. The optimal hybridization temperature for a PCR reaction depends greatly on the primers used. The melting temperature or T_m of short primers (up to about 30 nt) can be estimated using the following equation:

$$T_m = [4(G + C) + 2(A + T)]$$

where G + C is the number of G and C residues and A + T is the number of A and T residues. An annealing temperature chosen close to the T_m of both primers is usually right. However, it is worth trying different temperatures to obtain both a good yield and a high specificity. The MgCl$_2$ concentration can also be critical and values between 1 and 4 mM are worth trying.

9. The extension time essentially depends on the length of the fragment to be amplified. Because the polymerization rate of *Taq* DNA polymerase is close to 50 nucleotides per second, 2 min are usually sufficient to amplify

fragments shorter than 2000 bp. However, shorter or longer elongation times can be used, depending on the fragment length.
10. Care should be taken not to contaminate the amplified DNA with traces of the original DNA template. This will lead to preferential amplification of the wild-type sequence and will reduce greatly the efficiency of the procedure. The purity of the purified fragments can be verified easily by performing the second PCR with product A or product B alone.
11. It can be useful to try different product A/product B ratios. Ratios equivalent to 0.1, 0.5, 1, 5, and 10 can be tested and have been shown in some cases to greatly improve the efficiency of the second amplification step.
12. If a double mutation has to be made on the same fragment, the purified DNA can be used as template for another round of mutagenesis. However the efficiency will drop.

Acknowledgments

The authors thank Mark J. Churcher and Simon Thompson for critical reading of the manuscript and Laura Corbo for helpful discussions.

References

1. Higuchi, R., Krummel, B., and Saiki, R. K. (1988) A general method of *in vitro* preparation and specific mutagenesis of DNA fragments: study of protein and DNA interactions. *Nucleic Acids Res.* **16,** 7351–7367.
2. Ho, S. N., Hunt, H. D., Horton, R. M., Pullen, J. K., and Pease, L. R. (1989) Site directed mutagenesis by overlap extension using the polymerase chain reaction *Gene* **77,** 51–59.
3. Kammann, M., Laufs, J., Schell, J., and Gronenborn, B. (1989) Rapid insertion mutagenesis of DNA by polymerase chain reaction (PCR). *Nucleic Acids Res.* **1** 5404.
4. Sakar, G. and Sommer, S. S. (1990) The "Megaprimer" method of site-directed mutagenesis. *BioTechniques* **8,** 404–407.
5. Mikaelian, I. and Sergeant, A. (1992) A general and fast method to generate multiple site directed mutations. *Nucleic Acids Res.* **20,** 376.
6. Kuipers, O. P., Boot, H. J., and de Vos W. M. (1991) Improved site-directed mutagenesis method using PCR. *Nucleic Acids Res.* **19,** 4558.
7. Mikaélian I., Drouet, E., Marechal, V., Denoyel, G., Nicolas, J.-C., and Sergeant A. (1993) The DNA binding domain of two b-ZIP transcription factors, the Epstein Barr virus switch gene product EB1 and jun is a bipartite nuclear targeting sequence. *J. Virol.* **67,** 734–742.
8. Tindall, K. R. and Kunkel, T. A. (1988) Fidelity of DNA synthesis by the *Thermus aquaticus* DNA polymerase. *Biochemistry* **27,** 6008–6013.
9. Clark, J. M. (1988) Novel non-templated nucleotide addition reactions catalyzed by procaryotic and eucaryotic DNA polymerases. *Nucleic Acids Res.* **16,** 9677–9686

CHAPTER 18

Site-Directed Mutagenesis
In Vitro by Megaprimer PCR

Sailen Barik

1. Introduction

Among the various mutagenesis procedures based on polymerase chain reaction (PCR), the "megaprimer" method appears to be the simplest and most versatile. The method utilizes three oligonucleotide primers and two rounds of PCR performed on a DNA template containing the cloned gene to be mutated *(1–3)*. The basic megaprimer procedure is shown schematically in Fig. 1, where A and B represent the "flanking" primers that can map either within the cloned gene or outside the gene (i.e., within the vector sequence) and M represents the internal "mutant" primer containing the desired base change. The mutagenic primer may encode any of the following mutations or combinations thereof: a point mutation (single nucleotide change), a deletion, or an insertion *(1,4)*. The first round of PCR is performed using the mutant primer (e.g., M1 in Fig. 1) and one of the flanking primers (e.g., A). The double-stranded product (A-M1) is purified and used as one of the primers (hence the name "megaprimer") in the second round of PCR along with the other flanking primer (B). The wild-type cloned gene is used as template in both PCR reactions. The final PCR product (A-M1-B) containing the mutation can be used in a variety of standard applications, such as sequencing and cloning in expression vectors, or in more specialized applications, such as production of the gene message in vitro if primer A (or the template sequence downstream of primer A) also contains a transcriptional promoter (e.g., that of SP6 or T7 phage).

From: *Methods in Molecular Biology, Vol. 57: In Vitro Mutagenesis Protocols*
Edited by: M. K. Trower Humana Press Inc., Totowa, NJ

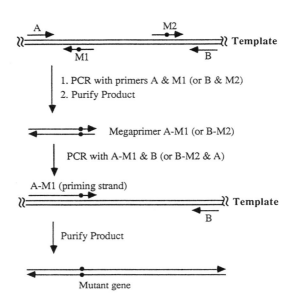

Fig. 1. The megaprimer PCR method of site-directed mutagenesis. Primers A, B, M1, and M2 (as well as the priming strand of the megaprimer, AM1) are indicated by single lines with arrowhead, whereas the double lines represent the template. The dots in M1 and M2 denote the desired mutations (substitution, insertion, or deletion) to be introduced into the product via the megaprimer. *See text* for details.

Primers A and B are usually designed to contain restriction sites so that the final mutant PCR product can be restricted and ligated to the same vector, thus retaining the original flanking sequences of the gene. This is especially important when sequences upstream of A (e.g., a Shine-Dalgarno sequence or an upstream activating sequence) or downstream of B (e.g., a polyadenylation site or a RNase processing site) are essential for gene expression or regulation, and therefore, must remain unaltered *(5,6)*.

It is quite common to mutagenize protein-coding genes, and studies of structure–function relationship require the generation of a battery of mutant proteins altered at specific amino acid residues *(5)*. In such cases, primers A and B can be kept constant and a variety of mutant primers (M1, M2, etc.) can be used to produce the various mutants. The reciprocal combination of primers (i.e., M2 and B in the first round of PCR; then A and megaprimer M2-B in the second round) can also be used provided primer M2 is of the opposite sense of B (Fig. 1). Choice of primer location is described in more detail in Note 1.

One unique feature of the megaprimer method is the use of double-stranded megaprimer directly in the second round of PCR, prior separation of the two strands being unnecessary. Melting of the megaprimer essentially is achieved in the denaturation step of the PCR cycle itself. Although both strands of the megaprimer will anneal to the respective, complementary strands of the template, the basic rules of PCR amplification automatically ensure that only the correct strand (one that extends to the other primer, B, in Fig. 1) will be amplified into the double-stranded product. Under some conditions, particularly with large megaprimers (1 kb and above), self-annealing of the megaprimer tends to reduce the yield of the product *(2)*. In order to avoid this, use of higher amounts of template (in the microgram range, as opposed to the nanogram quantities used in standard PCR) in the second PCR reaction has been recommended in the Methods section.

In general, since the megaprimer can be quite large (it may approach the size of the whole gene) and is incorporated within the gene sequence, successful and error-free PCR in the second round often requires special considerations. The reader is therefore strongly urged to browse through the whole chapter, including the Notes section, before proceeding with the actual experiment.

2. Materials

1. DNA template containing the cloned gene (e.g., in pUC or pGEM vector) to be mutated.
2. Oligonucleotide primers A, B, and mutant primer M: the "upstream" primer A in the message sense and the "downstream" primer B in the antimessage sense. Include restriction sites, preferably unique, in these primers so that the final product can be restricted and cloned. The mutant primer may be designed to contain a point mutation, or insertion, or deletion, as desired *(4)* (*see* Note 1).
3. Reagents needed for a basic PCR:
   a. 10X PCR buffer: 100 mM Tris-HCl, pH 8.0–8.3, 500 mM KCl, 15 mM MgCl$_2$, 0.01% gelatin.
   b. *Taq* DNA polymerase (5 U/µL) (Perkin-Elmer Cetus, Norwalk, CT).
   c. dNTP mix: Mixture containing 2.5 mM of each dNTP (dATP, dCTP, dGTP, dTTP). (We make it by mixing equal volumes of 10 mM stock solution of each nucleotide, available commercially.) Use autoclaved millipore water.

4. A system for purifying the PCR products; two choices, viz, membrane filtration and gel electrophoretic separation are described later in detail.
5. Reagents for agarose gel electrophoresis.
6. TE buffer: 10 mM Tris-HCl, pH 8.0, 1.0 mM EDTA.
7. TE saturated phenol.
8. Chlorophorm.
9. 70% and absolute ethanol.
10. TBE buffer (10X stock): 108 g Tris base, 55 g boric acid, 9.3 g Na$_2$EDTA, 2H$_2$O/L. Dissolve, filter through a 0.2-μM filter, and store at room temperature.
11. Ethidium bromide solution: 5 mg/mL stock in sterile water, store at 40°C in the dark.
12. 6X Gel loading dye: 0.25% bromophenol blue, 0.25% xylene cyanole, 30% glycerol.
13. DNA size markers: 100 bp ladder containing DNA fragments differing by 100 bp (Life Technologies, Gaithersburg, MD).
14. Electroelutor (Optional) (Kodak-IBI, New Haven, CT).
15. 3M Na-acetate, pH 4.8–5.2.
16. 8M Ammonium acetate, 0.01% bromophenol blue.
17. Carrier tRNA (Sigma, St. Louis, MO).

3. Methods
3.1. PCR1: Synthesis of Megaprimer

It is assumed that the readers are familiar with a standard PCR protocol. In brief, use the following recipe for the first PCR (PCR 1).

1. Make a 100-μL reaction mix in a 0.5-mL Eppendorf tube containing (*see* Note 2): 80 μL H$_2$O, 10 μL 10X PCR buffer, 8 μL dNTP mix (final concentration of each nucleotide is 200 μM), 0.5 μL *Taq* polymerase (2.5 U), 50 pmol of primer A (*see* Note 1), 50 pmol of primer M (*see* Note 1), 10–100 ng DNA template (usually a plasmid clone).
2. Vortex well to mix, then spin briefly in a microfuge. Reopen the tube, overlay the reaction mixture with ~100 μL mineral oil to cover the surface, then close cap. The tube is now ready for thermal cycling.
3. Amplify by PCR using the following cycle profiles (*see* Notes 3 and 4): Initial denaturation, 94°C, 2 min, 30–35 main cycles, 94°C, 1.5 min (denaturation); 45°C, 2 min (annealing); 72°C, appropriate elongation time (*n* min; *see* Note 3). Final extension, 72°C, 1.5 x *n* min.
4. After PCR, remove the oil overlay as follows: (It is important to remove the oil completely, otherwise the sample will float up when loaded into wells of a horizontal agarose gel.) Take out reaction tubes from the heating

block and add 200 µL of chloroform to each tube. The mineral oil overlay and chloroform will mix to form a single phase and sink to the bottom of the tube. Quick spin for 30 s in a microfuge. Collect ~80 µL of the top aqueous layer taking care not to touch the chloroform, and transfer to a fresh 1.5-mL Eppendorf tube.

3.2. Purification of Megaprimer

There is a choice of two procedures, membrane filtration and gel electrophoresis, both of which provide a recovery of >90% of the megaprimer and at the same time remove small primers (A, M) and salts; use whichever is more convenient.

3.2.1. Membrane Filtration

The author routinely uses Centricon 100 (Amicon, Beverly, MA) for this purpose, which safely retains DNA 100 bp or greater *(5,7)*. Thus, it works best when the megaprimer is >100 bp and the small primers are shorter than 30 nucleotides. Instructions for use are supplied by the manufacturer. In brief:

1. After assembling the unit, first wash the membrane by adding 1 mL H$_2$O and centrifuging at 2000 rpm (Beckmann J2-21, rotor JA 20, or an equivalent centrifuge) for 10 min.
2. Take out the assembly, discard the filtrate (from the bottom compartment), load the cleaned PCR1 product (*see* Section 3.1.), add another 1.5 mL H$_2$O, and spin as before. Repeat this step four times to completely remove the small primers as well as salts.
3. Collect the liquid from above the membrane by centrifuging briefly in an inverted position with the collector cup fitted at the bottom as per instructions.
4. The volume collected will be 150–200 µL; reduce it in a Speed-Vac evaporator (Savant Instruments, Farmingdale, NY) to <80 µL (takes ~10 min with a good vacuum pump) (*see* Note 5). This solution contains megaprimer and wild-type template. Use it in the PCR2 stage of the procedure (*see* Section 3.3.).

3.2.2. Gel Electrophoresis

1. Prepare a standard 0.7–0.8% agarose gel in 1X TBE containing ethidium bromide (1 µg/mL final concentration); use a midsize horizontal apparatus and a comb of well-volume >35 µL. Cover the gel with 1X TBE containing the same concentration of ethidium bromide.
2. Reduce the volume of the first stage PCR (PCR1) to ~25 µL by Speed-Vac.
3. Add 5 µL of 6X gel loading dye, mix, and load into the agarose gel well. Use DNA size markers in a parallel lane.

4. Electrophorese at appropriate voltage (~80 V) until desired resolution i achieved between megaprimer and the small primers (~1 h); monitor b hand-held UV light.
5. Following gel electrophoresis, excise the megaprimer band with a scalpe The megaprimer can now be recovered by either the freeze-squeeze metho or by electrophoretic elution (*see* Note 6).

3.2.2.1. FREEZE SQUEEZE *(8)* MEGAPRIMER DNA ISOLATION

1. Put the gel fragment (containing megaprimer) in an Eppendorf tube, freez for 5 min in a dry ice-ethanol bath (or 15 min in a −70°C freezer), spin fo 15 min in a microcentrifuge.
2. Collect the exudate by pipeting. Expect a recovery of 70–80% for DNA frag ments ~500 bp or smaller. Removal of ethidium bromide is not necessary

3.2.2.2. MEGAPRIMER DNA ISOLATION BY ELECTROELUTION

1. Place gel slice(s) (containing megaprimer) in one slot of the electroeluto which is already filled with TE or 1X TBE (*see* the instruction manual o the electroelutor).
2. Make sure that the apparatus is leveled, that buffers in the two chamber are connected, and that all buffer flow has stopped. Clear out any ai bubbles that may be trapped in the V-shaped grooves and put 75 µL of 8Λ ammonium acetate containing 0.01% bromophenol blue in each groove.
3. Electrophorese at 150 V for required period (approx 15–30 min), as judgec by the disappearance of the DNA band from the gel slice into the V groov (monitored by a hand-held UV light). Do not disturb the apparatus dur ing elution.
4. Discontinue electrophoresis, carefully drain buffer out of both chambers and collect 400 µL ammonium acetate solution containing DNA from eacl V groove. Add 2–4 µg carrier tRNA at this point to improve recovery.
5. Clean the DNA by standard phenol-chloroform, ethanol precipitation (dc not add extra salt) treatment. Wash the DNA pellet with prechilled 70% ethanol, air dry the pellet, and dissolve in 20 µL of water. Expect 30–60% recovery of DNA.

3.3. PCR2

1. In a 0.5-mL Eppendorf tube, make 100 µL PCR mix containing (*see* Note 7): 10 µL 10X PCR buffer, 8 µL dNTP mix, 50 pmol of primer B, all of the recovered megaprimer from the procedure in Section 3.2. (20–50 µL), 0.2 µg DNA template, 0.5 µL *Taq* polymerase (2.5 U); make up the volume to 100 µL with H_2O. Mix well.
2. Overlay the reaction mixture with ~100 µL mineral oil to cover the sur face, then close the cap. The tube is now ready for thermal cycling.

3. A representative set of thermal cycling parameters for a 1-kb long final product using a 400-bp long megaprimer: initial denaturation, 94°C, 5 min. Thirty-five cycles of denaturation, 94°C, 1 min 30 s; annealing, 2 min at appropriate temperature (*see* Note 3b); elongation, 72°C, 1 min (*see* Note 8). Final extension; 72°C, 1.2 min.

4. Remove the reaction tube from the heating block and add 200 µL of chloroform. The mineral oil overlay and chloroform will mix to form a single phase and sink to the bottom of the tube. Quick-spin for 30 s in a microfuge. Collect ~80 µL of the top aqueous layer taking care not to touch the chloroform, and transfer to a fresh 1.5-mL Eppendorf tube.

5. Analyze the PCR2 product by electrophoresis in an agarose gel. Run the gel long enough to resolve the full-length product (A-M-B) from the wild-type template. In a typical example, the 1-kb linear PCR product is to be resolved from a 3–5 kb supercoiled plasmid, which is easily achieved. Purify the PCR product by excising the band and recovering it from agarose by freeze-squeeze or electroelution (*see* Sections 3.2.2.1. and 3.2.2.2.).

6. If the DNA product is to be restricted for cloning, concentrate the DNA by precipitation with ethanol (*see* Note 5).

7. Restrict and ligate to appropriate cloning vectors using standard procedures (*see* Note 9).

4. Notes

1. Primer design (location and sequence): For technical reasons, avoid making megaprimers that approach the size of the final, full length product (gene) AB (Fig. 1). Briefly, if M1 is too close to B, it will make separation of AB and AM1 (unincorporated, leftover megaprimer) difficult after the second round of PCR. Ideally, the megaprimer should be shorter than the full length gene by more than 200–500 bp, depending on the exact length of the gene. (Example: If the gene [AB] is 2 kb, megaprimer [AM1] can be up to ~1.5 kb long, since 2 and 1.5 kb can be separated reasonably well in agarose gels. However, if the gene is 8 kb, the megaprimer should not be bigger than, say, 7 kb, since 8-kb and 7-kb fragments would migrate so close to each other.) As shown in Fig. 1, when the mutation is to be created near B, one should make an M primer of the opposite polarity, e.g., M2 and synthesize BM2 megaprimer (rather than AM2). Of course, when the mutation is at or very near the 5' or 3' end of the gene (say, within 1–50 nucleotides), there is no need to use the megaprimer method; one can simply incorporate the mutation in either A or B primer and do a straightforward PCR. In borderline situations, such as when the mutation is, say, 120 nucleotides away from the 5' end of the gene, incorporation of the mutation in primer A may make the primer too big to synthesize; or else, it will make the megaprimer AM1 too short to handle conveniently. In such a

case, simply back up primer A a few hundred bases further into the vector sequence in order to make the AM1 megaprimer longer. In general, remember that primers A and B can be located anywhere on either side of the mutant region, and try to utilize this flexibility as an advantage when designing these primers.

In addition to the standard rules of primer sequence (such as, a near 50% GC content, sequence specificity, extra "clamp" sequence for efficient restriction, absence of self-complementarity, etc), attention should be paid to the following aspects. As stated before, primers A and B should contain unique restriction sites for ease of cloning. With regard to the M primer, two things are important. First, the mutational mismatch (substitution, insertion or deletion) should not be too close to the 3' end of the primer. Mismatch at the very 3' nucleotide of the primer will virtually abolish amplification by *Taq* polymerase. For best results, the mismatch should be 10–15 bases away from the 3' end of the primer. Second, and most important, design M primer such that the problem of any 3' nontemplated base addition is solved (*see* Note 4).

2. If a number of PCRs are to be done using a common template and different mutagenic primers, make a "master mix" using the common reagents, distribute in different PCR tubes, then add one mutagenic primer into each tube.

3. General:
   a. Elongation time: As a rule, elongation time (at 72°C) in a PCR cycle should be proportional to the length of the product. An approximate guideline is 1 min of elongation per kb, i.e., 100 nt = 10 s; 500 nt = 40 s; 1 kb = 1 min, 10 s; 2 kb = 2 min, 20 s, and so on
   b. Annealing temperature: This is primarily governed by the base composition of the primers. A golden rule is to calculate the T_m of the primer as follows: add 2°C for each A or T, and 4°C for each G or C, then deduct 4 degrees. Example: for a 22-nt primer with 10 G + C and 12 A + T, T_m is $(10 \times 4 + 12 \times 2) = 64°C$; therefore, anneal at 60°C. However, the practical upper limit of the annealing temperature for any primer is 72°C, since it is the elongation temperature of the thermostable polymerases. In PCR2, the annealing temperature is dictated by the smaller primer B, since the T_m of the megaprimer is going to be too high.

4. The problem of 3' nontemplated base addition and its solution: *Taq* polymerase has a tendency to incorporate nontemplated residues, particularly A, at the 3' end of the daughter polynucleotide strand at a certain frequency *(9)*. These are then copied and amplified into the double-stranded product. This is generally not a problem in standard PCR where the termini of the

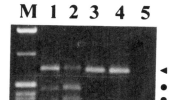

M 1 2 3 4 5

Fig. 2. The problem of nontemplated base addition and its solution (*see* Note 4). The following PCR products were analyzed by agarose gel electrophoresis: lanes 1 and 2, products from two different megaprimed reactions using *Taq* polymerase, digested with *Bgl*II; lane 3, product of megaprimed PCR using *Pfu* polymerase, digested with *Bgl*II; lane 4, product of megaprimed PCR using a "clever" primer design and *Taq* polymerase, digested with *Bgl*II; lane 5, standard PCR reaction using primer A and a 3'-end mismatched primer M1 (Fig. 1). M, size markers in kb (from top): 1.6, 1, 0.5, 0.39, 0.34, 0.29, 0.22.

product are usually cleaved off by restriction enzymes for cloning purposes. However, in the megaprimer method, the whole megaprimer is incorporated in the internal region of the final product. Therefore, nontemplated A residues in the megaprimer will eventually show up in a certain percentage of the final product and cause a mutation which may be undesirable. The frequency of such an "error" is usually low but may be appreciable in some cases (*see* Fig. 2).

There are two kinds of solution to this problem; one, exemplified by a, does not introduce the nontemplated base or remove it; the other, described in b, does not remove the nontemplated base, but tolerates the alteration.

a. Use a thermostable DNA polymerase with 3'-exonuclease (proofreading) activity; we have used the *Pfu* polymerase (Stratagene, La Jolla, CA) in standard PCR buffer with excellent results (Fig. 2). The temperature and time values of the thermal cycles are identical to those for *Taq* polymerase.

b. Tolerate the alteration ("If you can't beat 'em, join 'em"): *This is the method of choice.* It relies on clever primer design and does not require any extra steps (Fig. 2). There are two ways of achieving this. As an example, suppose the relevant region of the wild-type sequence is (the amino acids are shown at the bottom in single-letter codes):

```
5'— AAA CTG CCA ACT CCG TCA TAT CTG CAG —3'
3'— TTT GAC GGT TGA GGC AGT ATA GAC GTC —5'
      K    L    P    T    P    S    Y    L    Q
```

and the Ser (TCA) is to be mutated to Ala (GCA). A mutant primer in the message sense (like M2 in Fig. 1) may have the sequence 5' CA ACT CCG **G**CA TAT CTG CAG 3' (the boldface G being the mutant base). However, when this M2 primer and primer B is used in PCR, the nontemplated A incorporated at the M2 end of the product (megaprimer) will result in the sequence:

5'— <u>T</u>CA ACT CCG GCA TAT CTG CAG —
3'— <u>A</u>GT TGA GGC CGT ATA GAC GTC —

(the nontemplated A/T is underlined). When incorporated into the final product, this megaprimer will produce the following mutant (the underlined amino acids are altered from the wild-type sequence):

5'— AAA CTG TCA ACT CCG GCA TAT CTG CAG —3'
    K   L   <u>S</u>   T   P   <u>A</u>   Y   L   Q

resulting in an undesired Ala → Ser change (boldface). To avoid this, make the following M2 primer: 5' G CCA ACT CCG GCA TAT CTG CAG 3' so that there is a T residue upstream of the 5' end of M2 in the template sequence; any extratemplated T in this strand of the megaprimer will therefore match with the T residue in the wild-type sequence and will not cause any mutation.

When no T residues are available, use the wobble base of a codon. This is possible when the primary purpose of the clone is to produce a protein product; thus, substitution of a codon with another, synonymous codon is permissible (make sure that the resultant change in the nucleotide sequence is acceptable in terms of introduction or loss of restriction sites, etc.). Now, make the following M2 primer: 5' ACT CCG GCA TAT CTG CAG3', so that the codon upstream of it is CCA. The nontemplated T will change this codon to CCT; however, since they both code for proline, the protein will remain unaltered.

An experiment demonstrating nontemplated addition and its solution is presented in Fig. 2. In this case, the final product of a megaprimer procedure is 690-nt long (arrowhead in Fig. 2) and its correct sequence should not contain any *Bgl*II site (gene PPλ; 6). However, owing to misincorporation of a nontemplated A, an internal sequence AGCTCT is altered to AG<u>A</u>TCT, a *Bgl*II recognition sequence. Thus, the susceptibility of the product to *Bgl*II would serve as an indicator of misincorporation, and the product could then be cleaved with *Bgl*II to generate two fragments, 300- and 390-nt long (dots in Fig. 2). What fraction of the product will contain the misincorporation depends on how early in the PCR cycle the misincorporation took place. Thus, two separate PCRs (lanes 1 and 2) are seen to produce misincorporation to different extents, as judged by the different percentage of the 696 nt product that is sensitive to *Bgl*II restriction. Use of *Pfu* instead of *Taq* polymerase (lane 3) or a clever design of the M primer (lane 4) based on codon consideration (as just described) prevents this misincorporation, as shown by the insensitivity of the final product to *Bgl*II. When the same primer-template mismatch (i.e., A:G) was presented in the same position using a shorter "M1" (15-mer) primer with a deliberate 3'-end mismatch (instead of a megaprimer), and PCR was performed using A and M primers, no amplification of the 396-nt long AM sequence was observed (lane 5). In general, primer 3'-mismatch in standard PCR is known to abrogate amplification, although an A:C mismatch is more tolerable than A:G or A:A *(10,11)*. I presume that the large size of the megaprimer imparts an extraordinary stability to the primer–template duplex, which persuades *Taq* polymerase to prime synthesis, even when there is a mismatch at the growing (3') end of the primer strand.

5. As an alternative to Speed-Vac, concentrate DNA by precipitation with ethanol as follows: If the DNA is in, say, a volume of 50 µL, add 5 µL of 3*M* Na-acetate, 2–5 µg carrier tRNA, 150 µL absolute ethanol (–20°C), mix well, spin at 40°C in a microfuge at top speed. Add 500 µL of 70% ethanol (–20°C) and rinse the DNA pellet by inverting the tube a few times. Spin in the microfuge for 10 min and carefully remove the ethanol without losing the pellet. Dry DNA pellet under vacuum (Speed-Vac, 2–4 min). Dissolve in 20 µL H_2O.

6. The larger size of the megaprimer requires the use of a greater quantity of it to achieve the same number of moles as a smaller primer. Example: 0.3 µg of a 20-nt-long single-stranded primer will contain 50 pmol primer; however, 50 pmol of a 500 nt-long double-stranded megaprimer will equal 6 µg. This is why a good recovery of megaprimer is important. Procedures other than those suggested in the Methods section may work equally well. For example, various companies manufacture kits for DNA extraction from agarose gels; I have used the Qiaex gel extraction kit (Qiagen, Chatsworth, CA) with success. DNA fragments in low melting point agarose slices have been used in PCR reactions apparently without any problem *(12)*, which eliminated the need to recover the DNA from gel slices.

7. Final yield improvement (PCR2): One modification that I use routinely in my laboratory is the addition of a higher amount of template (100 ng or above) in the PCR2 stage, i.e., when the megaprimer is being used as a primer. Often, this dramatically improves the yield of the final mutant product *(2)*. This is probably owing to the fact that the template as well as the nonpriming strand of the megaprimer competes for the priming strand of

the megaprimer; at a higher concentration, the template may have a better chance to win the competition. Unfortunately, higher concentration of template tend to increase misincorporation (*see* Note 4) in some instances (*10*; unpublished observation).

On rare occasions, even higher concentrations of template may fail to improve yield; usually, this is also accompanied by the synthesis of spurious products of wrong lengths. In such cases, the best choice is to analyze PCR2 by electrophoresis in standard agarose gels, purify the product of the correct size (to recognize the product, do a standard PCR using A and B primers and run 5 μL of it in a parallel lane as a size marker) by electroelution, and use a portion of it as the template in a third PCR with A and B as primers.

8. Since the megaprimer is 400 bp long, you are only synthesizing another 600-nucleotide stretch in this PCR, therefore the extension time can be limited to 1 min.

9. As in any cloning procedure, the final mutants obtained by the megaprimer method must be confirmed by DNA sequencing. This may be done either directly with the PCR product *(13)* or after cloning the product in plasmid vectors by standard procedures *(14)*. When using the dideoxy method, PCR primer A or B may also be used as sequencing primers.

Acknowledgment

Research in the author's laboratory was supported in part by NIH grant AI37938.

References

1. Sarkar, G. and Sommer, S. S. (1990) The "megaprimer" method of site-directed mutagenesis. *BioTechniques* **8,** 404–407.
2. Barik, S. and Galinski, M. (1991) "Megaprimer" method of PCR: increased template concentration improves yield. *BioTechniques* **10,** 489,490.
3. Barik, S. (1993) Site-directed mutagenesis by double polymerase chain reaction. *Methods Mol. Biol.* **15,** 277–286.
4. Barik, S. (1995) Site-directed mutagenesis by PCR: substitution, insertion, deletion, and gene fusion. *Methods Neurosci.* **26,** 309–323.
5. Mazumder, B., Adhikary, G., and Barik, S. (1994) Bacterial expression of human respiratory syncytial viral phosphoprotein P and identification of Ser^{237} as the site of phosphorylation by cellular casein kinase II. *Virology* **205,** 93–103.
6. Barik, S. (1993) Expression and biochemical properties of a protein Ser/Thr phosphatase encoded by bacteriophage λ. *Proc. Natl. Acad. Sci. USA* **15,** 10,633–10,637.
7. Krowczynska, A. M. and Henderson, M. B. (1992) Efficient purification of PCR products using ultrafiltration. *BioTechniques* **13,** 286–289.

8. Stoflet, E.S., Koeberl, D. D., Sarkar, G., and Sommer, S. S. (1988) Genomic amplification with transcript sequencing. *Science* **239**, 491–494.
9. Clark, J. M. (1988) Novel nontemplated nucleotide addition reactions catalyzed by prokaryotic and eucaryotic DNA polymerases. *Nucleic Acids Res.* **16**, 9677–9686.
10. Sarkar, G., Cassady, J., Bottema, C. D. K., and Sommer, S. S. (1990) Characterization of polymerase chain reaction amplification of specific alleles. *Anal. Biochem.* **186**, 64–68.
11. Kwok, S., Kellogg, D. E., McKinney, N., Spasic, D., Goda, L., Levenson, C., and Sninsky, J. J. (1990) Effects of primer-template mismatches on the polymerase chain reaction: human immunodeficiency virus type I model studies. *Nucleic Acids Res.* **18**, 999–1005.
12. Zintz, C. B. and Beebe, D. C. (1991) Rapid re-amplification of PCR products purified in low melting point agarose gels. *BioTechniques* **11**, 158–162.
13. Meltzer, S. J. (1993) Direct sequencing of polymerase chain reaction products. *Methods Mol. Biol.* **15**, 137–142.
14. Maniatis, T., Fritsch, E. F., and Sambrook, J. (1982) *Molecular Cloning: A Laboratory Manual*, 2nd ed. Cold Spring Harbor Laboratory Press, Cold Spring Harbor, NY, pp. 113–119.

CHAPTER 19

Using PCR
for Rapid Site-Specific Mutagenesis
in Large Plasmids

Brynmor A. Watkins and Marvin S. Reitz, Jr.

1. Introduction

Using polymerase chain reaction (PCR) it is possible to amplify a segment of DNA by a factor of approx 2^{20} under standard conditions *(1)*. Any mutations present in the oligonucleotides used to prime the polymerization reactions will be incorporated in the resulting PCR products. Thus, a specific mutation can be introduced by designing mutagenic PCR primers. This principle has been used to introduce mutations into the DNA of bacterial plasmids *(2–4)*, or fragments of plasmids used for subcloning *(5–10)*. Until very recently, this technique has generally been limited by the size of fragments that can be amplified by a single PCR reaction, which in our hands was about 2700 bp (2.7 kb). When trying to introduce mutations into a plasmid of 3.9 kb, we found that methods for the site-specific mutagenesis by direct amplification of the entire plasmid did not produce amplification products.

To overcome the problems we were encountering, we developed a technique that relied on amplifying parts of the plasmid, such that none of the fragments to be amplified exceeded 2.7 kb *(11)*. To achieve this, two pairs of primers were designed in the vector so that these two pairs were approximately equidistant from each other. These were used with a group of four primers identical to those used in standard site-specific mutagenesis reactions. This gave us four sets of primers that could be

From: *Methods in Molecular Biology, Vol. 57: In Vitro Mutagenesis Protocols*
Edited by: M. K. Trower Humana Press Inc., Totowa, NJ

used to generate two plasmid fragments of approx 2.6 kb and two of approx 1.3 kb such that the two larger (2.6 kb) fragments overlapped by approx 1.3 kb, and the two smaller (1.3 kb) fragments filled the spaces to complete a plasmid of 3.9 kb *(11)*.

We have described the use of this technique to produce point mutations N463K and S465L in the fifth variable (V5) region of the HIV-1 major envelope glycoprotein, gp120 *(11)*. These mutants were then subcloned back into an infectious molecular of HIV-1 to investigate the role of a lost N-linked glycosylation site in neutralization escape. These studies showed that this mutation was not required for resistance to the selecting antiserum, but that a second mutation present in the same clone, A281V, was required *(12)*. A review of published HIV-1 sequences showed that four amino acids, A, V, T, and I, occur at position 281 *(13)*. As a result of this observation, we were interested in investigating the neutralization of 281T and 281I variants of HIV-1$_{HXB2}$, in order to assess the possible contribution of these variants to neutralization resistance by HIV-1. To generate these mutations, we have adapted our previous technique to a different template. This involved cloning a separate template, designing new mutagenic and flanking primers, and utilizing a different pair of primers in the cloning vector (*see* Fig. 1).

2. Materials

1. 1 mM dNTPs, store at –20°C in 500 μL aliquots: 1 mM dATP (5.35 mg/10 ml), 1 mM dGTP (5.07 mg/10 ml), 1 mM dCTP (5.11 mg/10 ml), 1 mM dTTP (4.66 mg/mL).
2. 10X PCR buffer, store at –20°C in 500 μL aliquots: 500 mM KCl, 100 mM Tris-HCl, pH 8.3, 15 mM MgCl$_2$, 0.1% (w/v) gelatin.
3. 10 μg/μL Ethidium bromide: Use at 1:1000 for staining gels.
4. Phenol/chloroform (1:1) stored under 50 mM Tris-HCl, pH 8.0.
5. Electromax DH10B competent *Escherichia coli* and the Cell-Porator electroporator were obtained from Life Technologies Inc. (Gaithersburg, MD). The use of electrocompetent cells and electrotransformation has been shown by us to increase the efficiency of transformation by a factor of more than 10 *(11,14)*.
6. Oligonucleotide PCR primers synthesized on an Applied Biosystems (Foster City, CA) 381A DNA synthesizer, dissolved in ultrapure water, concentration adjusted to 2.5 nM.
7. *Taq* DNA polymerase (5 U/μL) (Boehringer Mannheim, Indianapolis, IN).
8. SOC medium: Dissolve 20 g of bactotryptone, 5 g of yeast extract, and 0.5 g of NaCl in 950 mL of distilled water, autoclave, then add 10 mL of

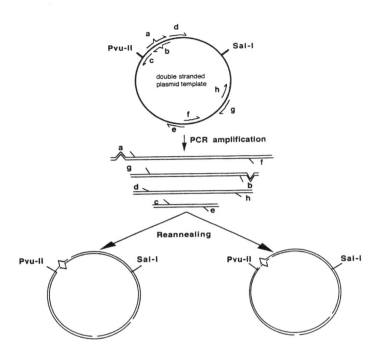

Fig. 1. Site-specific mutagenesis using partial plasmid PCR products. To produce a given mutation, four primers are designed: a and b contain the desired mutation, and c and d flanking primers a and b. To make several different mutants at the same site (like A281I and A281T), c and d are the same for all mutants, but a and b have to be synthesized specifically for each mutant (hence a1, a2, b1, b2). Additional primers e through h were designed within the vector, and generally remain constant for all mutations made to inserts cloned into that vector.

sterile 250 mM KCl and 10 mL sterile 2M D-glucose. Adjust pH to 7.0. (*See* ref. *14* for more detailed instructions. Commercially available from Life Technologies.)

3. Methods
3.1. Design of Oligonucleotide PCR Primers

Care in the design and positioning of the primers used for PCR is the key to the success of this technique. Figure 1 shows the basic strategy used for the placement of the primers, and Fig. 2 gives specific examples of primers used in the generation of two site-specific mutations (*see* Notes 1–3 for additional details on the design of mutagenic primers).

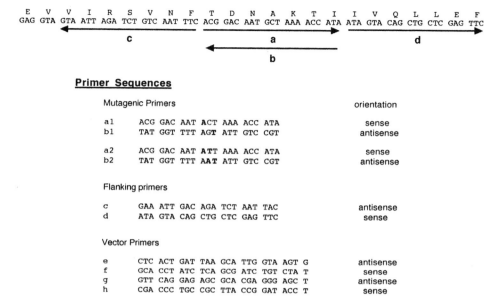

Fig. 2. Primer design and sequences. The sequence of the template plasmid is shown to illustrate the design of primers a–d, and the sequences of all primers described is given.

Our basic strategy for the design of a complete set of primers is as follows:

1. Identify the site of the desired mutation, and design and synthesize a sense and an antisense primer for each mutation that you wish to create (primers a and b in Fig. 1, a1 and b1 for mutation A281T, and a2 and b2 for mutation A281I in Fig. 2). Primer length should be 20–25 nucleotides, preferably sense and antisense should be completely complementary, with the mutation(s) in the middle.

2. Design and synthesize flanking primers (primers c and d in Figs. 1 and 2), paying close attention to the orientation (c must be antisense, d must be sense).

3. Design and synthesize two pairs of primers in the plasmid containing the sequence of interest (primers e through h in Figs. 1 and 2). These should be positioned to be approx equidistant from the mutation(s) being created, but still leave significant distance between each other, thereby creating a large overlap between the PCR fragments generated. Attention must again be given to orientation of these primers, ensuring that they are "back to back" (opposite orientations leading away from each other, 3' to 5').

3.2. Preparation of Template

Prepare plasmid DNA for use as PCR template using any one of a number of standard techniques *(3,14)*. Dilute to 1 pg/μL in ultrapure water.

3.3. PCR

1. Prepare four 50 μL PCR reactions in 500 μL microcentrifuge tubes by combining 5 μL of 10X PCR buffer, 8 μL of dNTPs, 1 μL of each primer, 1 μL of template, 0.5 μL of *Taq* DNA polymerase, and 23.5 μL of ultrapure water. Primer pairs for these reactions are shown in Fig. 1; a + f, b + g, d + h, c + e. If the template DNA consists of a sequence of interest cloned into a cloning vector, ensure that the relative orientations of vector and insert have been allowed for in pairing the primers.
2. Transfer PCR reactions to a thermal cycler, and run 25–30 cycles of 94°C/ 1 min, 45°C/2 min, and 72°C/2 min, followed by a final elongation step of 72°C/7 min (*see* Notes 4 and 5).
3. Analyze a small sample of each reaction (typically, 10 μL from a total of 50 μL) by electrophoresis on a 0.8% agarose gel *(17)*, stain with ethidium bromide, and view on a UV light box (*see* Fig. 3). If all four reactions have produced the expected size bands, proceed with denaturation and reannealing. If one or more of the reactions have failed it may prove beneficial to switch primer pairs, combining a + h and d + f (*see* Fig. 1) and/or b + e and c + g. If this approach is utilized, it is important to switch two pairs together (*see* Note 6).

3.4. Denaturation and Reannealing

1. For each mutation, combine the four PCR products in a 1.5-mL screwtop microcentrifuge tube. Generally, equal volumes of all four reactions can be used (typically, 25 μL of each), however, if one or two reactions are significantly weaker or stronger than the others when analyzed by agarose gel electrophoresis (*see* Section 3.3., step 3), it may be beneficial to compensate by adjusting the relative volumes accordingly. It is not necessary to purify the reaction products before combining.
2. Extract the combined PCR products with 100 μL of phenol/chloroform to remove proteins present in the reaction mix. Transfer upper layer to fresh 1.5 mL microcentrifuge tube.
3. Precipitate by adding of 1/10 vol 3*M* sodium acetate, pH 5.2 (10 μL) followed by two volumes of ethanol (approx 200 μL) stored at –20°C.
4. Centrifuge at 12,000*g* for 15 min at 4°C.
5. Decant supernatant, carefully remove any visible traces of liquid from the tube using a vacuum line or alternative, and allow pellet to air dry for approx 15 min.

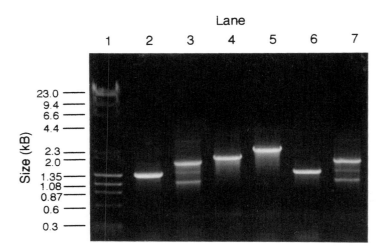

Fig. 3. Gel electrophoresis of PCR products used to generate mutants A281T and A281I. PCR and gel electrophoresis were performed as described in the Methods section and the primers are described in Fig. 2. Lane 1, molecular weight markers. Lanes 2–7, PCR products. Lane 2 primers a1 and h, lane 3 primers b1 and e, lane 4 primers c and g, lane 5 primers d and f, lane 6 primers a2 and h, and lane 7 primers b2 and e.

6. Resuspend dried pellet in 10 μL of ultrapure water.
7. Boil this mixture for 3 min, cool at room temperature, and centrifuge briefly to collect the contents at the bottom of the tube.

3.5. Transfection into **E. coli**

1. Add 1 μL of each reannealed PCR product mixture to 20 μL of Electromax DH10B competent *E. coli* (Life Technologies), and electroporate using the Cell-Porator electroporator (Life Technologies) set at 2.45 kV.
2. Add the transformed bacteria to 1 mL of SOC, shake at 37°C for 1 h, and plate onto agar plates containing selection medium (typically, LB/ ampicillin plates). The specific plates to use will be determined by the original plasmid used for the mutagenesis.
3. Incubate for 12–16 h at 37°C, 24 h at 30°C, or 48 h at room temperature.
4. Pick 6–10 colonies from the transformation plates and inoculate into selection medium (LB + ampicillin), and grow overnight.
5. Prepare plasmid DNA from each culture using Wizard Minipreps kits (Promega, Madison, WI) and screen for mutant clones.

Lane

1　2　3

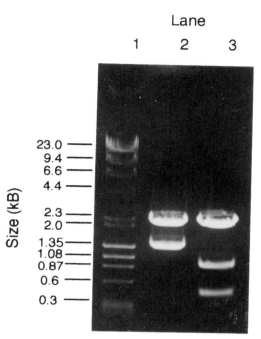

Fig. 4. Analysis of mutant A281I by restriction analysis. Screening of candidate clones is simplified if an additional restriction site is included in the site-specific mutagenesis, as was the case with variant A281I, which has an additional *Ssp*I site. Lane 1, molecular weight markers. Lane 2, pSP72/HXB2 *Pvu*II/*Sal*I, the template used for PCR, digested with *Ssp*I. Lane 3, A281I digested with *Ssp*I. Vector pSP72 and the HXB2 *Pvu*II/*Sal*II region each contain one *Ssp*I site, giving the two bands at 2.4 and 1.4 kb (Lane 2). The A281I mutation introduces another *Ssp*I site that divides the band of 1.4 into two bands of 0.9 and 0.5 kb (Lane 3).

If the mutation being screened for contains an additional restriction site (as with our A281I mutant), then this can be screened for by digesting miniprep DNA with the relevant restriction enzyme (for the A281I mutant this was Ssp-1; *see* Fig. 4). Mutants that do not contain additional restriction sites (such as our A281T mutant) can be screened for directly by sequencing clones that give the same restriction profile as the parent plasmid. Final verification in all cases should always be by sequencing (for this we generally use the dideoxy method *(15,16)* using Sequenase (USB, St Louis, MO). Additional screening techniques for finding clones that contain the desired mutation generally involve differential hybridization to radiolabeled oligonucleotide probes (*see* Note 7 and ref. *16*).

4. Notes

1. Design of oligonucleotide primers: In general, we try to design primers o about 25 nucleotides, with a positive G/C:A/T ratio (i.e., more Gs and C than As and Ts) and G or C at the 3' end. We try to put the mutations in th middle or toward the 5' end of the primers. We have also observed that an mutations in the eight nucleotides closest to the 3' end will effect the effi ciency of the primer; thus, designing primers that have mutations in thi region should be avoided if at all possible.
2. Multiple mutations: It is possible and relatively easy to design multipl mutations into a single pair of oligonucleotide primers in making a single multiple mutant. On the basis of our experience, the number of mutation in a single primer should not exceed 25% of the total number of nucle otides, and primers should not exceed about 45 nucleotides in length, o the efficiency will be severely effected. Any mutations within the eigh nucleotides at the 3' end of a primer will have a stronger effect on th efficiency of the primer than mutations elsewhere. When the number o mutations (mismatches) in a primer exceeds 20%, it may be necessar to reduce the annealing temperature of the PCR reaction to obtain a good reaction.
3. Primer overlap: Mistakes in the design of mutagenic primers have lead us to perform this procedure with overlap between the mutagenic primers (a and b), and the two primers that flank the mutagenic pair (c and d). We found that an overlap of three nucleotides with one primer on either side (refer to Fig. 2; primer a overlaps primer c and primer b overlaps primer d) significantly enhanced the number of colonies containing the mutation. Overlaps of six nucleotides on each side resulted in no colonies to screen (Watkins, unpublished observations). Any mutagenic reactions performed in this way should be carefully checked by sequencing to avoid clones with extra basepairs, and thereby an additional insertion mutation.
4. Cycle parameters: We generally start with a standard cycle of 94°C/1 min, 45°C/2 min, and 72°C/2 min for 25 cycles, followed by a final elongation step of 72°C/7 min. If problems are encountered with nonspecific reaction products (e.g., Fig. 3, lanes 3 and 7), it is sometimes necessary to increase the annealing temperature to 50° or 55°C. If, on the other hand, no product is observed, the number of cycles can be increased, up to a maximum of 40, preferably with the addition of more *Taq* polymerase after 20 cycles. As an alternative to increasing the number of cycles, the annealing temperature can be decreased or the amount of template used in the reaction can be increased. Each of these solutions has disadvantages; increasing cycle number will increase the chance of *Taq* polymerase error, and there-

fore, the creation of additional undesired mutations. Decreasing annealing temperature will increase the possibility of nonspecific reaction products and increasing the amount of template will increase the number of wild-type clones in the resulting transformation. It is important to consider all of these factors when making modifications to the cycle parameters.

5. Thermal cyclers: We have recently begun to use the Stratagene (La Jolla, CA) Robocycler for these reactions, and have found that it offers several advantages over conventional thermal cyclers. First, the time to complete a PCR reaction is significantly reduced as the use of three different hot blocks eliminates the time it takes for conventional thermal cyclers to "ramp" from one temperature to the next. This allows our standard program to be completed in a little over 2 h, compared with over 4 h in a conventional thermal cycler. Second, the Robocycler is available with a gradient block that allows reactions to be run at up to eight different annealing temperatures simultaneously. In addition, we have noticed that the Robocycler is more efficient at longer PCR amplifications (we have amplified bands of 4.3 kb), permitting the use of larger plasmids as templates for this and other PCR mutagenesis protocols.

6. Primer pairings: The method we have described also has the advantage of flexibility, in that primer combinations can be changed if a specific primer pair will not perform in PCR. The problem of certain PCR primer combinations failing to work has been noted, but not explained *(1)* and this problem was encountered in the construction of mutant V513E *(11)*, in which one primer pair (d and f) repeatedly failed to produce the 2.6 kb PCR product expected. We were, however, able to generate the 2.6-kb fragment with primers a and f, and produced the required 1.3-kb fill-in fragment by pairing primers d and h. Thus, if the initial primer pairings fail to produce the correct size reaction products, the first step in overcoming this problem should be to change the primer pairs (i.e., switch from pairing a with h and d with f to a with f and d with h or switch from b with g and c with e to b with e and c with g, depending on which reaction is not working; refer to Figs. 1 and 2).

7. Screening: Screening the clones resulting from transformations often can be the key to success with PCR mutagenesis. In this protocol, we have reduced the amount of plasmid used as template for PCR reactions to minimize screening, so that colonies can be picked randomly from plates and either diagnosed by restriction digestion or sequencing. This is easier if an additional restriction site can be inserted with the desired mutation, as in the A281I mutant, which contains an additional Ssp-I site (Fig. 4). This is not always possible, and sequencing a large number of clones is very labor intensive; therefore, we sometimes use differential hybridization to screen

the colonies from our transformations. To do this we use one of the two mutagenic primers labeled with [γ-32P]dATP by polynucleotide kinase (PNK). Hybridization is done using standard techniques *(16)* and the filters are washed initially in 6X SSC at 37°C for 1 h. We then use a Molecular Dynamics Phosphorimager to visualize and quantify the hybridization, and repeat the washing procedure at higher temperatures until a difference is noted between colonies on the resulting image. The stronger colonies are picked and minipreps are subject to restriction digest, followed by electrophoresis, blotting, and Southern hybridization to the same probe, then the same process of washing and imaging. The inclusion of wild-type plasmid with the minipreps in the restriction digest gel and blot greatly facilitates the diagnosis at this point. The washing temperature at which the difference becomes clear after a 10–15 min wash in 6X SSC is usually between 50° and 65°C, depending on the length of the primer (shorter = lower wash temperature) and the number of mutations (more mutations = lower wash temperature).

References

1. Saiki, R. K. (1989) The design and optimization of the PCR, in *PCR Technology* (Erlich, H. A., ed.), Stockton Press, New York, pp. 7–16.
2. Hemsley, A., Arnheim, N., Toney, M. D., Cortopassi, G., and Galas, D. J. (1989) A simple method for site-directed mutagenesis using the polymerase chain reaction. *Nucleic Acids Res.* **17**, 6545–6551.
3. Jones, D. H. and Howard, B. H. (1990) A rapid method for site directed mutagenesis and directional subcloning by using the polymerase chain reaction to generate recombinant circles. *BioTechniques* **8**, 178–183.
4. Jones, D. H., Sakamoto, K., Vorce, R. L., and Howard, B. H. (1990) DNA site-specific mutagenesis and recombination. *Nature* **344**, 793,794.
5. Jones, D. H. and Winsdorfer, S. C. (1992) Recombinant circle PCR for site-specific mutagenesis without PCR purification. *BioTechniques* **12**, 528–535.
6. Jones, D. H. and Howard, B. H. (1991) A rapid method for recombination and site-specific mutagenesis by placing homologous ends on DNA using polymerase chain reaction. *BioTechniques* **10**, 62–66.
7. Kadowaki, H., Kadowaki, T., Wondisford, F. E., and Taylor, S I. (1989) Use of polymerase chain reaction catalyzed by *Taq* DNA polymerase for site-specific mutagenesis. *Gene* **76**, 161–166.
8. Lee, N., Liu, J., He, C., and Testa, D. (1991) Site-specific mutagenesis method which completely excludes wild-type DNA from the transformants. *Appl. Environ. Microbiol.* **57**, 2888–2890.
9. Nassel, M. and Reiger, A. (1990) PCR-based site-directed mutagenesis using primers with mismatched 3'-ends. *Nucleic Acids Res.* **18**, 3077,3078.
10. Vallette, F., Mege, E., Reiss, A., and Adesnik, M. (1989) Construction of mutant and chimeric genes using the polymerase chain reaction. *Nucleic Acids Res.* **17**, 723–733.

11. Watkins, B. A., Davis, A. E., Cocchi, F., and Reitz, M. S. (1993) A rapid method for site-specific mutagenesis using larger plasmids as templates. *BioTechniques* **15,** 700–704.
12. Watkins, B. A., Reitz, M. S., Wilson, C. A., Aldrich, K., Davis, A. E., and Robert-Guroff, M. (1993) Immune escape by human immunodeficiency virus type-1 from neutralizing antibodies: evidence for multiple pathways. *J. Virol.* **67,** 7493–7500.
13. Meyers, G., Berzofsky, J. A., Korber, B., Smith, R. F., and Pavlakis, G. N. (1992) *Human Retroviruses and AIDS Meeting, 1992,* Los Alamos National Laboratory, New Mexico.
14. Sambrook, J., Fritsch, E. F., and Maniatis, T. (1989) Transformation of *E. coli* by high-voltage electroporation, in *Molecular Cloning: A Laboratory Manual,* 2nd ed., Cold Spring Harbor Laboratory Press, Cold Spring Harbor, NY, pp. 1–75.
15. Sanger, F., Nickien, S., and Coulsen, A.R. (1977) DNA sequencing with chain-terminating inhibitors. *Proc. Natl. Acad. Sci. USA* **74,** 5463–5467.
16. Sambrook, J., Fritsch, E. F., and Maniatis, T. (1989) Conditions for hybridization of oligonucleotide probes, in *Molecular Cloning: A Laboratory Manual,* 2nd ed. Cold Spring Harbor Laboratory Press, Cold Spring Harbor, NY, pp. 11.45–11.55.

CHAPTER 20

PCR-Assisted Mutagenesis for Site-Directed Insertion/Deletion of Large DNA Segments

Daniel C. Tessier and David Y. Thomas

1. Introduction

We present in this chapter a polymerase chain reaction (PCR)-based method to simultaneously introduce and remove large fragments of DNA in a single mutagenesis reaction without the need for restriction sites. We have favored the use of long single-stranded DNA primers synthesized by asymmetric PCR *(1,2)*, whereas others have used double-stranded PCR-amplified fragment directly *(3–5)* as primers in in vitro mutagenesis reactions.

Oligonucleotide-based mutagenesis has become the method of choice to correct or engineer small changes in cloned DNA sequences. As evident from other chapters in this book, single-base changes, multiple substitutions, deletions, small insertions, and random mutagenesis are among the most commonly used applications of oligonucleotide mutagenesis as developed by Zoller and Smith in 1982 *(6)*. More recently, the introduction of PCR technology *(7)* has revolutionized approaches to mutagenesis.

Replacement of DNA sequences requires the use of restriction enzymes to excise the DNA fragment of interest, remove the unwanted fragment, and replace it with the desired fragment. This method, generally referred to as "cassette mutagenesis," presents a major drawback since unique restriction sites are rarely found on both sides of the desired DNA fragment. Combining both oligonucleotide-based mutagen-

From: *Methods in Molecular Biology, Vol. 57: In Vitro Mutagenesis Protocols*
Edited by: M. K. Trower Humana Press Inc., Totowa, NJ

esis and PCR, it is possible to introduce convenient restriction enzyme cleavage sites (although not always!) in the recipient plasmid and amplify the desired DNA fragment to contain these newly created restriction sites. Even though this method works very well, it remains time consuming.

The principle of our procedure lies in the design of two oligonucleotide primers used to amplify the desired DNA fragment where the forward and the reverse primers perform two functions. First, they contain specific sequences at their 3' ends that are used in an initial PCR to amplify the desired DNA fragment. Second, at their 5' ends, they contain sequences that are complementary to the target plasmid in the region where insertion of the desired fragment will take place (Fig. 1). Therefore it is not only possible to insert but also simultaneously remove or substitute one fragment of DNA for another using this approach without the need for restriction enzymes or subcloning. Using this PCR-assisted mutagenesis method, the size of the DNA to insert is no longer limited to the size of the chemically synthesized oligonucleotide.

For this procedure, it will be necessary to prepare single-stranded DNA of the plasmid to be modified. Thus the plasmid requires the origin of replication of a filamentous phage like M13, fd, or f1 *(8)*. Amplification of the fragment of DNA to be introduced into this plasmid will make use of the specially designed primers and PCR. Then an excess of one of the two strands of this PCR fragment will be generated through asymmetric PCR. The product of this reaction will be used in a second-strand synthesis reaction to mutagenize the single-stranded plasmid DNA to yield a recombinant plasmid that will contain the desired DNA fragment exactly where wanted.

PCR-assisted large insertion/deletion (INDEL) mutagenesis allows the insertion and the exchange of large fragments of DNA for the study of DNA regulatory regions, protein domain function, polymorphism of evolutionarily related genes, and chimeric genes.

2. Materials
2.1. Preparation of Uracil-Containing Single-Stranded Template DNA

1. *Escherichia coli* strains CJ236 (*dut*-1, *ung*-1, *thi*-1, *rel*A-1; pCJ105 [Cmʳ]) (BioRad, Hercules, CA) and MC1061 (*ara*D139, Δ*[ara-leu]*7696, Δ*[lac]*174, *gal*K, *gal*U, *hsd*R, strA*[str¹]*) *(9)*.
2. M13KO7 helper phage *(8)*.

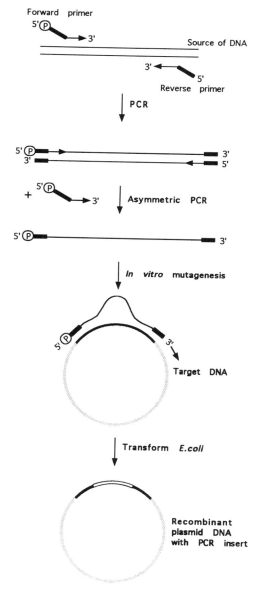

Fig. 1. Schematic representation of PCR-assisted large insertion/deletion mutagenesis. The thin lines in the forward and reverse primers represent sequences
complementary to the source DNA, the thicker blocks represent sequences complementary to the target DNA. The circled P on the forward primer indicates that it is
phosphorylated at its 5' end. The asymmetric PCR is carried out on the DNA fragment amplified in the initial PCR using only the phosphorylated forward primer.

3. 2YT medium: 16 g/L tryptone, 10 g/L yeast extract, 5 g/L NaCl, 0.2% glucose; sterilize by autoclaving *(10)*. For plates, add 15 g/L agar; autoclave to sterilize.
4. Ampicillin (Amp) stock: 100 mg/mL in sterile water; chloramphenicol (Cm) stock: 30 mg/mL in ethanol; kanamycin (Kan) stock: 70 mg/mL in sterile water. All stored at –20°C for months *(10)*.
5. PEG solution: 20% (w/v) polyethylene glycol 6000, 2.5M NaCl; filter sterilize, store at room temperature.
6. DNase/RNase buffer: 10 mM Tris-HCl, pH 7.5, 5 mM MgCl$_2$, 50 µg/mL DNase I, 10 µg/mL RNase A (Pharmacia Biotech, Uppsala, Sweden); prepared by adding fresh enzymes to filter-sterilized buffer.
7. Stop buffer: 50 mM EDTA, 1.5M sodium acetate pH 7.0; filter sterilize, store at room temperature.
8. TE: 10 mM Tris-HCl, pH 8.0, 1 mM EDTA; filter sterilize, store at 4°C.
9. Phenol saturated with TE; store at 4°C.
10. 7.5M Ammonium acetate; filter sterilize, store at room temperature.
11. 95% Ethanol.

2.2. PCR and Asymmetric PCR

1. C18 Sep-Pak reverse phase chromatography cartridges (Millipore [Bedford, MA] and Waters [Milford, MA]).
2. Enzymes: T4 polynucleotide kinase (Gibco/BRL, Life Technologies, Gaithersburg, MD); *Taq* DNA polymerase (Perkin Elmer-Cetus, Norwalk, CT).
3. 10X Kinase buffer: 700 mM Tris-HCl, pH 7.5, 100 mM MgCl$_2$, 50 mM DTT, 10 mM ATP.
4. 2X PCR buffer: 20 mM Tris-HCl, pH 8.3, 100 mM KCl, 3 mM MgCl$_2$, 0.02% (w/v) gelatin, 0.4 mM of each of the deoxyribonucleoside triphosphates (dNTPs).
5. All buffers should be filter-sterilized and stored at –20°C, stable for 3 mo.
6. GeneClean II Kit (Bio 101, La Jolla, CA).
7. 0.1X TE: 1 mM Tris-HCl, pH 8.0, 0.1 mM EDTA; filter sterilize and store at 4°C.

2.3. In Vitro Mutagenesis Reaction

1. Enzymes: T4 DNA polymerase, T4 DNA ligase and T4 Gene 32 protein (Pharmacia).
2. 10X Annealing buffer: 200 mM Tris-HCl, pH 7.4, 500 mM NaCl, 20 mM MgCl$_2$.
3. 10X Synthesis buffer: 250 mM Tris-HCl, pH 8.0, 350 mM NaCl, 50 mM MgCl$_2$, 15 mM DTT, 4 mM dNTPs, and 7.5 mM ATP.
4. All buffers should be filter-sterilized and stored at –20°C, stable for 3 mo.

3. Methods

3.1. Preparation of Uracil-Containing Single-Stranded Template DNA

The method that follows is merely an adaptation of the method described by Kunkel *(11,12)* that provides a strong selection against the parental or nonmutagenized strand of a double-stranded DNA molecule following an in vitro mutagenesis reaction.

1. Transform the plasmid for mutagenesis into CJ236 competent cells *(13)*.
2. Select transformants on 2YT plates containing 100 μg/mL Amp (assuming your plasmid carries the ampicillin resistance gene).
3. Inoculate a single colony in 10 mL 2YT + 30 μg/mL Cm (to maintain selection of the F' plasmid pCJ105 that carries the information for pili construction) and 100 μg/mL Amp, incubate at 37°C overnight with agitation.
4. Use 100 μL of the overnight culture to inoculate 10 mL of fresh medium, incubate at 37°C with agitation until OD_{600} = 0.5–0.8.
5. Infect 5 mL of culture with 10^8 M13KO7 helper phages, incubate at 37°C for 1 h with good agitation (300 rpm) in a sterilized 25-mL Erlenmeyer flask (*see* Note 1).
6. Use this 5-mL culture to inoculate 20 mL 2YT + 30 μg/mL Cm + 100 μg/mL Amp + 70 μg/mL Kan (to maintain selection of the helper phage) and incubate overnight at 37°C with good agitation (300 rpm) in a sterilized 125-mL Erlenmeyer flask.
7. Centrifuge culture at 8000*g* for 20 min.
8. Add 5 mL of PEG solution to 20 mL of supernatant culture medium and precipitate phage on ice for 15–30 min.
9. Centrifuge the phage at 12,000*g* for 20 min.
10. Gently decant the supernatant medium and remove excess liquid from the edges of the tube. Resuspend the white fluffy pellet in 400 μL of DNase/RNase buffer. Transfer to an Eppendorf tube. Incubate at 37°C for 30 min.
11. Stop the DNase/RNase digestions with 80 μL of stop buffer.
12. Extract once with an equal volume of phenol saturated with TE buffer. Vortex for 5 min and spin in a microfuge for 5 min.
13. Remove no more than 400 μL (*see* Note 2) of the aqueous layer (top layer) and add 1 mL of 95% ethanol. Precipitate at –80°C for 10 min and spin in a microfuge for 15 min.
14. Decant the ethanol, wash the pellet with 1 mL of 70% ethanol, spin for 1 min, decant the wash, air dry the pellet and resuspend the single-stranded DNA in 50 μL TE.
15. The quantity of uracil-containing single-stranded template DNA should be determined by spectrophotometry using the following for-

mula: $(OD_{260} \times 120)/y = $ pmol of ssDNA/μL, where y is the length of the plasmid in bases.

16. It is recommended to verify the quality of the single-stranded DNA by agarose gel electrophoresis. A good preparation of single-stranded DNA should show a major band of your plasmid and a minor band of M13K07 single-stranded DNA.

3.2. PCR and Asymmetric PCR

1. Following chemical synthesis using standard cyanoethyl phosphoramidites, each oligonucleotide primer is purified on a C18 Sep-Pak column *(14)*. For this, the column is fixed on the end of a 10-mL syringe and wetted with 10 mL of methanol by gravity flow. The column is then rinsed with 10 mL of sterile water. The oligonucleotide is diluted in 1 mL of sterile water and loaded into the syringe barrel and allowed to go through the column by gravity flow. The column is subsequently rinsed with 20 mL of sterile water and the oligonucleotide eluted with 1 mL of 50% methanol/water. The eluted material is then lyophilized and dissolved in 50–100 μL of sterile water. The quantity of oligonucleotide is determined spectrophotometrically using the same formula as in Section 3.1., step 15, where y should be taken as the length of the oligonucleotide in bases.

2. Phosphorylate 100 pmol of the forward primer in a final volume of 10 μL containing 1 μL of 10X kinase buffer and 10 U of T4 polynucleotide kinase. Incubate at 37°C for 45 min and inactivate the enzyme at 65°C for 15 min.

3. Denature 100 ng of linearized plasmid DNA (source of the desired DNA fragment; *see* Note 3) at 100°C for 10 min in the presence of 100 pmol each of the phosphorylated forward primer and the reverse primer in a final volume of 50 μL with an overlay of 50 μL of light paraffin oil. Transfer to an ice bath for 5 min.

4. Add 50 μL of ice-cold 2X PCR buffer containing 2.5 U of *Taq* DNA polymerase and take the reaction through 30 cycles of amplification as follows: denaturation at 94°C, 1 min; annealing at 50°C, 1 min, and polymerization at 72°C, 2 min.

5. Before proceeding with the asymmetric PCR, analysis of a 5-μL aliquot of the amplification by agarose gel electrophoresis is suggested (*see* Note 4).

6. For the asymmetric PCR, denature 5 μL of product from the initial amplification and 1 nmol of the phosphorylated forward primer only at 100°C for 10 min in a final volume of 50 μL with an overlay of 50 μL of light paraffin oil. Transfer to an ice bath for 5 min.

7. Add 50 μL of ice-cold 2X PCR buffer and give 20 cycles of amplification as in step 4.

8. Precipitate all 100 µL of the asymmetric PCR products by adding 50 µL 7.5*M* ammonium acetate and 375 µL of 95% ethanol, incubating at −80°C for 10 min and spinning in a microfuge for 15 min at 4°C.
9. Decant the ethanol, wash the pellet with 70% ethanol, spin for 1 min, decant the wash, air dry the pellet, and resuspend in 25 µL 0.1X TE.
10. Here it is also recommended to check an aliquot of the products from the asymmetric PCR amplification by agarose gel electrophoresis as it will become the source of mutagenic primer in the mutagenesis reaction to follow (*see* Note 5).

3.3. In Vitro Mutagenesis Reaction

1. Mix 5 µL of the mutagenic primer with 0.2 pmol of the uracil-containing single-stranded template DNA with 1 µL of 10X annealing buffer in a final volume of 12 µL. The mixture is incubated at 100°C for 3 min, 65°C for 2 min, 37°C for 5 min, and finally room temperature for 10 min. Transfer to an ice bath (*see* Note 6).
2. Mix on ice, 8 µL of the annealing reaction, 1 µL of 10X synthesis buffer, 1 U of T4 DNA polymerase, 2 U of T4 DNA ligase, and 100 µg/mL of T4 Gene 32 protein in a final volume of 12 µL. Leave on ice for 5 min, at room temperature for 5 min, and at 37°C for 90 min. All enzymes are then inactivated at 65°C for 20 min.
3. The mixture is diluted with 12 µL 0.1X TE, half is transformed into *E. coli* MC1061 competent cells and transformants selected on 2YT plates containing 100 µg/mL Amp.

The efficiency of a simple oligonucleotide-based mutagenesis using uracil-containing single-stranded templates *(11,12)* is generally around 80%. The method described in this chapter utilizes much longer and complex "oligonucleotides" to mutagenize the parental plasmid and will still yield a minimum of 10% recombinant clones. The 5' ends of the PCR primers, which are responsible for annealing to the single-stranded template DNA, should be carefully designed to have a melting temperature *(15)* above 50°C based on the following formula:

$$T_m(°C) = [(G + C) \times 4] + [(A + T) \times 2]$$

Every recombinant clones generated by this method, or by any method involving PCR for that matter, should be sequenced to verify the integrity of the junctions at the site of insertion of the desired fragment of DNA but also for the possibility of undesired mutations introduced during the amplification reaction. To reduce the risk of unwanted mutations, it is now possible to purchase thermostable polymerases with much better proofreading capabilities than that of *Taq* DNA polymerase *(16)*.

4. Notes

1. During the preparation of uracil-containing template, the volume of the culture vessel chosen and the vigorous agitation of the culture infected with the helper phage are strongly recommended as aeration will greatly improve the yield of single-stranded DNA.
2. The aqueous layer of the phenol extraction should be removed with great care during the purification of the template DNA as the quality of the single-stranded template is critical in any mutagenesis reaction.
3. Linearization of purified supercoiled plasmid DNA with any restriction enzyme that does not cut within the region to be amplified is recommended prior to PCR amplification as the molecules will not denature efficiently in a limited time at 94°C. If miniprep DNA is used, linearization is not necessary.
4. Electrophoretic analysis of the product of the initial PCR amplification should yield a single band. If the sample contains more than one band, you should repeat the amplification using a higher annealing temperature or purify the band corresponding to the DNA fragment of interest using GeneClean II Kit prior to the asymmetric PCR.
5. The single-stranded products of the asymmetric PCR are expected to migrate ahead of their double-stranded precursors on agarose gels *(17)*.
6. In case of failure to find clones, repeat the annealing of the mutagenesis reaction by heating a water bath to 85°C, placing the annealing mixture in the bath, and removing the bath from the heating surface leaving the temperature to return slowly to room temperature.

Acknowledgments

The authors thank Jean Chatellier for critical reading of this manuscript and Anne-Marie Sdicu for her help in the preparation of the figure. This chapter is issued as National Research Council of Canada publication No. 38524.

References

1. Tessier, D. C. and Thomas, D. Y. (1993) PCR-assisted large insertion/deletion mutagenesis. *BioTechniques* **15**, 498–501.
2. Wychowski, C., Emerson, S. U., Silver, J., and Feinstone, S. M. (1990) Construction of recombinant DNA molecules by the use of a single stranded DNA generated by the polymerase chain reaction: its application to chimeric hepatitis A virus/poliovirus subgenomic cDNA. *Nucleic Acids Res.* **18**, 913–918.

3. Clackson, T. and Winter, G. (1989) "Sticky feet"-directed mutagenesis and its application to swapping antibody domains. *Nucleic Acids Res.* **17**, 10,163–10,170.
4. Near, R. I. (1992) Gene conversion of immunoglobulin variable regions in mutagenesis cassettes by replacement PCR mutagenesis. *BioTechniques* **12**, 88–97.
5. Zhong, D. and Bajaj, S. P. (1993) A PCR-based method for site-specific domain replacement that does not require restriction recognition sequences. *BioTechniques* **15**, 874–878.
6. Zoller, M. J. and Smith, M. (1982) Oligonucleotide-directed mutagenesis using M13-derived vectors: an efficient and general procedure for the production of point mutations in any fragment of DNA. *Nucleic Acids Res.* **10**, 6487–6500.
7. Saiki, R. K., Gelfand, D. H., Stoffel, S., Scharf, S. F., Higuchi, R., Horn, R. T., Mullis, K. B., and Erlich, H. A. (1988) Primer-directed enzymatic amplification of DNA with a thermostable DNA polymerase. *Science* **238**, 487–491.
8. Vieira, J. and Messing, J. (1987) Production of single-stranded plasmid DNA. *Methods Enzymol.* **153**, 3–11.
9. Casadaban, M. and Cohen, S. N. (1980) Analysis of gene control signals by DNA fusions and cloning in *Escherichia coli. J. Mol. Biol.* **138**, 179–207.
10. Sambrook, J., Fritsch, E. F., and Maniatis, T. (1989) *Molecular Cloning: A Laboratory Manual.* Cold Spring Harbor Laboratory, Cold Spring Harbor, NY.
11. Kunkel, T. A. (1985) Rapid and efficient site-specific mutagenesis without phenotypic selection. *Proc. Natl. Acad. Sci. USA* **82**, 488–492.
12. Kunkel, T. A., Roberts, J. D., and Zakour, R. A. (1987) Rapid and efficient site-specific mutagenesis without phenotypic selection. *Methods Enzymol.* **154**, 367–382.
13. Hanahan, D. (1983) Studies on transformation of *Escherichia coli* with plasmids. *J. Mol. Biol.* **166**, 557–580.
14. Sanchez-Pescador, R. and Urdea, M. S. (1984) Use of unpurified synthetic deoxynucleotide primers for rapid dideoxynucleotide chain termination sequencing. *DNA* **3**, 339–343.
15. Suggs, S. V., Hirose, T., Miyake, Y., Kawashima, E. H., and Johnson, M. J. (1981) Use of synthetic oligonucleotides for the isolation of specific cloned DNA sequences, in *Developmental Biology Using Purified Genes* (Brown, D. D., ed.), Academic, New York, pp. 683–693.
16. Mattila, P., Korpela, J., Tenkanen, T., and Pitkänen, K. (1991) Fidelity of DNA synthesis by the *Thermococcus litoralis* DNA polymerase—an extremely heat stable enzyme with proofreading activity. *Nucleic Acids Res.* **19**, 4967–4973.
17. Perrin, S. and Gilliland, G. (1990) Site-specific mutagenesis using asymmetric polymerase chain reaction and a single mutant primer. *Nucleic Acids Res.* **18**, 7433–7438.

CHAPTER 21

Site-Directed Mutagenesis Using a Rapid PCR-Based Method

Gina L. Costa, John C. Bauer,
Barbara McGowan, Mila Angert,
and Michael P. Weiner

1. Introduction

Site-directed mutagenesis is one of the fundamental tools available to probe the structure and function of proteins and cellular controlling mechanisms. Conventionally, site-directed mutagenesis methods can be reduced to two steps: strand separation and annealing of a mutagenesis deoxyoligonucleotide primer, and selection against the parental template. The strand separation step is necessary to allow effective competition between the naturally occurring complementing DNA and the much shorter mutagenesis primer. In non-polymerase chain reaction (PCR)-based methods, strand separation can be performed in vivo by the isolation of single-stranded vector through phage rescue or subcloning of a specific fragment on the single-stranded filamentous phage M13 *(1)*. Alternatively, with in vitro non-PCR-based methods, heat or physical separation of the two complementing strands can be used *(2)*. Most standard PCR-based mutagenesis methods use heat denaturation and often dilute template concentration in order to reduce the occurrence of reannealing the complementing DNA strands. PCR methods generally use a reduced template concentration to lower the nonmutagenized parental background *(3)*. Consequently, it is necessary to increase the cycle number for PCR to produce workable quantities of mutagenized DNA.

From: *Methods in Molecular Biology, Vol. 57: In Vitro Mutagenesis Protocols*
Edited by: M. K. Trower Humana Press Inc., Totowa, NJ

Parental selection in site-directed mutagenesis is often necessary to reduce the background of nonmutagenized template from overwhelming the reaction. Parental selection can be either in vivo-based as, for example, the incorporation of uridine in template DNA during growth in a suitable host *(4)*, or in vitro-based, as in an incorporation of phosphorothioates *(5,6)* or 5-methyl dCTP *(1)* during the first- or second-strand synthesis.

In the following site-directed method (*see* Fig. 1), we have modified and optimized specific steps in a PCR method *(7,8)*. These include:

1. Increasing the starting template concentration;
2. Reducing the number of cycles needed to generate the PCR fragment;
3. Use of *Taq* DNA polymerase and *Taq* Extender PCR additive *(9)* or *TaqPlus* DNA polymerase *(10)* to increase PCR robustness;
4. Incorporation of efficient parental selection *(11)*;
5. Polymerase polishing of the PCR-generated fragment to increase yield *(12)*; and
6. Intramolecular ligation to derive the desired end product.

The overall advantage to this method has been to reduce the possibility of second-site mutations and decrease the amount of time and effort needed to perform site-directed mutagenesis.

2. Materials

1. PCR primers (*see* Notes 1–3).
2. Plasmid template DNA (*see* Note 4).
3. 10X PCR mutagenesis buffer: 100 mM KCl, 100 mM (NH$_4$)$_2$SO$_4$, 200 mM Tris-HCl, pH 8.8, 20 mM MgCl$_2$, 1% Triton X-100, and 1 mg/mL BSA (*see* Note 5).
4. 25 mM dNTP mix: 6.25 mM each of dATP, dCTP, dGTP, and dTTP.
5. *Taq* DNA polymerase (5 U/µL) (Stratagene Cloning Systems, La Jolla, CA).
6. *Taq* Extender (5 U/µL) (Stratagene).
7. *TaqPlus* DNA polymerase (5 U/µL) (Stratagene).
8. Mineral oil.
9. *Dpn*I restriction enzyme (10 U/µL).
10. Cloned *Pfu* DNA polymerase (2.5 U/µL) (Stratagene).
11. 10 mM ATP mix (Stratagene).
12. T4 DNA ligase (4 U/µL) (Stratagene).
13. Falcon 2059 polypropylene tube (Becton-Dickenson Labware, Lincoln Park, NJ).
14. *Escherichia coli* competent cells.

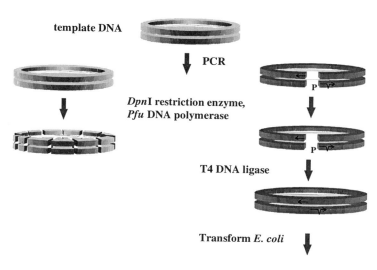

Fig. 1. Schematic of PCR mutagenesis. PCR mutagenesis is performed in four steps. In the first step, a reduced-cycle PCR is performed with a single primer set that incorporates the changes in one or both primer(s). *Taq* DNA polymerase and *Taq* Extender are used to increase the robustness and reliability of the reaction. Increased template concentration is used to offset the limited number of rounds of PCR. In the second step, the restriction enzyme *Dpn*I is used to digest any remaining parental DNA, and the *Pfu* DNA polymerase is used to end-polish and remove any *Taq*-generated extended nucleotide bases on the PCR fragment. In the third step, the reaction is diluted and T4 DNA ligase is added to intramolecularly ligate the ends of the PCR fragment. In the fourth and final step, the ligated solution is used to transform *E. coli* or other host strain.

3. Methods
3.1. PCR Mutagenesis Protocol

1. For the mutagenesis reaction, add the following reagents: 0.5 pmol of template DNA (0.5 pmol of template DNA = 0.33 μg/kb × size of the template [kb]); 2.5 μL 10X PCR mutagenesis buffer (*see* Note 5); 1 μL of dNTP mix; 15 pmol of each primer (15 pmol = 5 ng/base × size of the primer [bases]) (*see* Note 3); distilled, deionized water to 24 μL.
2. Next, add 1 μL *TaqPlus* DNA polymerase (or 0.5 μL of *Taq* DNA polymerase and 0.5 μL of *Taq* Extender) and overlay with mineral oil.
3. Cycle the reaction using the following suggested paramenters: one cycle of 4 min at 94°C, 2 min at 50°C, 2 min at 72°C; then 7–10 cycles of 1 min at 94°C, 2 min at 56°C, 2 min at 72°C; and finally, 5 min at 72°C.

4. Following the PCR, place the reaction on ice to cool to <37°C and add 1 µL of *Dpn*I restriction enzyme and 1 µL of cloned *Pfu* DNA polymerase directly into the aqueous solution, below the mineral oil overlay (*see* Note 6).
5. Incubate at 37°C for 30 min and then 72°C for an additional 30 min.
6. Next, add 100 µL of distilled, deionized water, 10 µL 10X PCR mutagenesis buffer, and 5 µL of 10 m*M* ATP.
7. Check a 10-µL aliquot of the reaction mixture by agarose gel analysis to confirm the presence of the desired PCR product (*see* Notes 7 and 8).
8. Remove a 10-µL aliquot of the reaction mixture to a new tube and add 1 µL of T4 DNA ligase (4 U). Incubate at 37°C for 60 min (*see* Note 9).

3.2. E. coli *Transformation Protocol*

1. Gently thaw *E. coli* competent cells on ice and aliquot 80 µL to a prechilled Falcon polypropylene tube. Add 2 µL of the ligase-treated DNA to the cells, swirl gently, and incubate for 30 min on ice.
2. Heat pulse for 45 s at 42°C and then place on ice for 2 min. The cells can now be plated directly onto the appropriate agar plates, or 1 mL of media added to the tube containing the transformed cells to allow for suitable outgrowth and recovery (*see* Note 10).

4. Notes

1. Mutagenesis primers are used to either add, delete, and/or substitute nucleotides in a given template sequence. The following considerations should be made for the design of the mutagenesis primers to be used for site-directed mutagenesis (also *see* Fig. 2 and the control example shown in Figs. 3 and 4, on pp. 244 and 245, respectively):
   a. The two primers must anneal to opposite strands of the plasmid.
   b. The primers should be capable of synthesizing a PCR product (*see* Note 5).
   c. One or both of the primers *must* be 5' phosphorylated. T4 polynucleotide kinase can be used for the 5' phosphorylation of an oligonucleotide primer (*13*).
   d. It is suggested that there be at least 15 bases (preferably 25–30 bases) of homology to the template at the 3' end of each primer.
   e. The distance between the primers is not crucial, but the primers cannot overlap. This feature of this PCR-based site-directed mutagenesis method makes it ideal for creating large loop-ins and deletions.
   f. Deletion mutants will result when either one or both primers misprime. It may be beneficial to change the conditions of the PCR or to modify the primer design (e.g., change the primer offset) to reduce the occurrence of mispriming.

Template DNA

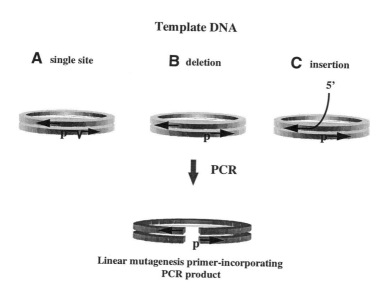

Fig. 2. Types of mutagenesis primers that can be used. Shown are several types of mutagenesis primers that can be used for PCR mutagenesis. These include primers that **(A)** lie adjacent to each other and can be used to create single-site changes, **(B)** are offset from each other and can be used to create deletions, and/or **(C)** contain extended lengths of noncomplementary regions for addition mutagenesis. Primer sets that employ a combination of these primer designs or the use of translationally silent mutations may also be used in this mutagenesis procedure *(15)*.

2. Primers may need to be HPLC or PAGE purified before using in the mutagenesis procedure, since unpurified primers used in the PCR may contain 5'-truncated oligonucleotides that are incorporated into the PCR product.
3. T4 DNA ligase will only efficiently ligate molecules containing 5'-termi-nal phosphates; therefore, one primer must be phosphorylated. Proper 5' phosphorylation can be achieved by the incorporation of a 5'-terminal phos-phate during synthesis of the oligonucleotides or by kinasing the oligo-nucleotide primer prior to use in the mutagenesis procedure.
4. Template DNA can be CsCl-purified or obtained from a miniplasmid preparation; both have been used successfully.
5. PCR templates vary in purity, length, GC content, and secondary struc-ture. For this reason, the PCR amplification step of the mutagenesis proce-dure should be conducted using a range of reaction buffers that differ in

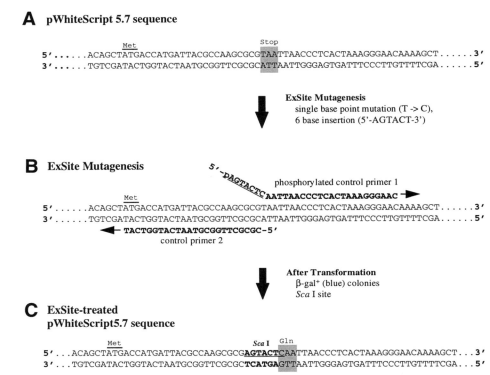

Fig. 3. Primer design of the mutagenesis control reaction. The mutagenesis
control oligonucleotide primers are used to simultaneously revert an ochre stop
codon (TAA) in the β-galactosidase gene encoded on the pWhitescript5.7 control template to a glutamine codon (Gln, CAA) and to insert six bases (corresponding to a *Sca*I restriction endonuclease site, 5'-AGTACT-3'). The
oligonucleotide control primer #2 does not overlap the phosphorylated oligonucleotide control primer #1. The oligonucleotide control primer set is used to
create full-length PCR product using *Taq* DNA polymerase and *Taq* Extender
PCR additive (or *TaqPlus* DNA polymerase; Stratagene). Following transformation, colonies can be screened for the β-galactosidase (β-gal+) (blue) phenotype and presence of an additional *Sca*I site.

buffering capacities (i.e., variation in salt concentration and pH) *(14)*. We
recommend the odd-numbered buffers from the Opti-Prime PCR Optimization kit (Stratagene). More specifically, Opti-Prime buffers #3, #7, and
#11 have been found to reproducibly PCR amplify the majority of double-
stranded templates. Reactions can be repeated with the optimized buffer
that yields the desired PCR product.

β-gal⁺ clones

control   #1   #2   #3   #4

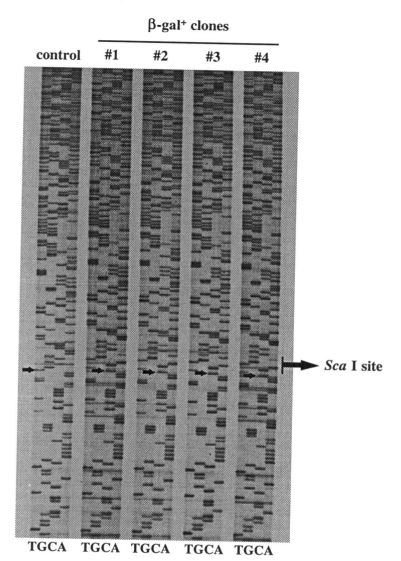

← *Sca* I site

TGCA   TGCA   TGCA   TGCA   TGCA

Fig. 4. Sequencing of wild-type and mutated plasmid DNA. The mutagenized region in the *lacZ* gene of the plasmid pWhiteScript5.7 was confirmed by dideoxy DNA sequence analysis using the M13(-20) oligonucleotide primer. Wild-type plasmid (control) and mutagenized plasmids (β-gal⁺ clones #1–4) from the PCR mutagenesis reaction were screened to confirm the reversion an ochre stop codon (TAA) in the control plasmid to a glutamine codon (CAA) and an insertion of a 6-base *Sca*I restriction endonuclease recognition site (5'-AGTACT-3').

6. Several good methods exist for selecting against parental DNA in site-directed mutagenesis procedures. In this rapid method the use of *Dpn*I restriction endonuclease was chosen because it can be used with almost all DNA obtained directly from *E. coli* without further modification *(11)*. *Dpn*I recognizes the methylated sequences (5'-G^{m6}ATC-3') that are modified by the *dam* gene of almost all common strains of *E. coli*. Unmethylated template DNA can be modified in vitro prior to step 1 using commercially available Dam protein. This step would be required for DNA obtained from a source other than a *dam*$^+$ *E. coli* (e.g., a yeast- or eukaryotic-sourced material).

The *Pfu* polishing step is necessary for the removal of bases extended onto the 3' ends of the PCR fragment by *Taq* DNA polymerase. Polishing has been shown to exhibit a sevenfold increase in mutagenesis efficiency *(12)*.

7. The following may explain the reasons for the absence or little PCR product as determined by agarose gel analysis:

   a. Template DNA is degraded. Check the integrity of the dsDNA. The template DNA should not be degraded. Both miniprep and cesium-banded DNA preparations are compatible with this mutagenesis procedure.

   b. PCR primers are incorrect. Review Figs. 1–3. Check for correct primer design and sequence.

   c. Reagent ratios are off. In order to provide for an efficient PCR-based site-directed mutagenesis method, it is necessary that the procedure be conducted utilizing an increased template concentration and a reduced cycling number. The suggested template:primer concentration ratios have been calculated to provide for optimal efficiencies in this PCR-based mutagenesis procedure. This ratio may need to be adjusted for efficient PCR with other templates or primers.

   d. PCR parameters require optimization. Pilot PCR amplification reactions may need to be conducted on each dsDNA template used in this mutagenesis procedure. Conditions such as buffer compatibility; primer design and concentration; and denaturing, annealing, and extension cycling parameters should be optimized to yield the desired PCR product prior to conducting mutagenesis procedures.

8. If multiple or spurious PCR products are generated during in vitro amplification, optimize reaction parameters using the "best" 10X reaction buffer. It may be advantageous to select a single 10X reaction buffer which yields the most robust desired PCR product. One can then modify the cycling parameters (e.g., times and temperatures of the denaturing, annealing, and extension cycles) in order to eliminate the spurious, secondary PCR products. A decrease in mutagenesis efficiency will result when undesired PCR products are present that are then subsequently ligated and transformed.

9. The reaction mixture is diluted prior to ligation to prevent the concatenation of highly concentrated DNA in solution. A dilution of 1:4 is recommended, but more or less may be optimal depending on the concentration of the starting material and efficiency of the PCR reaction. It should be noted that some manufacturers define a unit of T4 ligase differently. The four units recommended for this step is quantified on a blunt-ended linker molecule. This assay is representative of the actual reaction used for rapid PCR mutagenesis. If a new supplier (or a different lot from the same manufacturer) of ligase is used, it may be neccessary to test various concentrations in the reaction for optimal efficiency.
10. The quick transformation protocol described is useful for plasmid templates which contain a β-lactamase or chloramphenical selectable marker. For plasmids that use kanamycin (or neomycin) the post heat shock addition of a rich media and outgrowth period are required *(13)*.

Acknowledgments

The authors thank Dan McMullan, Loretta Callan, Matt Petre, and Cindy Murray for their discussions and contributions which aided in experimental design. G. L. Costa and M. P. Weiner also thank Sherrie Ramson and Mark Bergseid for the initial troubleshooting of this method.

References

1. Vandeyar, M., Weiner, M. P., Hutton, C., and Batt, C. (1988) A simple and rapid method for the selection of oligonucleotide-directed mutants. *Gene* **65,** 129–133.
2. Weiner, M. P., Felts, K. A., Simcox, T. G., and Braman, J. C. (1993) A method for the site-directed mono- and multi-mutagenesis of double-stranded DNA. *Gene* **126,** 35–41.
3. Picard, V., Erdsal-Badju, E., Lu, A., and Bock, S. C. (1994) A rapid and efficient one-tube PCR-based mutagenesis technique using *Pfu* DNA polymerase. *Nucleic Acids Res.* **22,** 2587–2591.
4. Kunkel, T. A. (1985) Rapid and efficient site-specific mutagenesis without phenotypic selection. *Proc. Natl. Acad. Sci. USA* **82,** 488–492.
5. Taylor, J. W. and Eckstein, F. (1985) The rapid generation of oligonucleotide-directed mutations at high frequency using phosphorothioate-modified DNA. *Nucleic Acids Res.* **13,** 8764–8785.
6. Sugimoto, M., Esaki, N., and Soda, K. (1989) A simple and efficient method for oligonucleotide-directed mutagenesis using plasmid DNA template and phosphorothioate-modified nucleotide. *Anal. Biochem.* **179,** 309–311.
7. Weiner, M. P. and Costa, G. L. (1994) Rapid PCR site-directed mutagenesis. *PCR Methods Appl.* **4,** S131–S136.
8. Weiner, M. P., Costa, G. L., Schoettlin, W., Cline, J., Mathur, E., and Bauer, J. C. (1994) Site-directed mutagenesis of double-stranded DNA by the polymerase chain reaction. *Gene* **151,** 119–123.

9. Nielson, K. B., Schoettlin, W., Bauer, J. C., and Mathur, E. (1994) *Taq* Extender™ PCR additive for improved length, yield and reliability of PCR products. *Strategies Mol. Biol.* **7,** 27.
10. Nielson, K., Scott, B., Bauer, J. C., and Kretz, K. (1994) *TaqPlus*™ DNA polymerase for more robust PCR. *Strategies Mol. Biol.* **7,** 64,65.
11. Nelson, M. and McClelland, M. (1992) The use of DNA methyltransferase/endonuclease enzyme combinations for megabase mapping of chromosomes. *Methods Enzymol.* **216,** 279–303.
12. Costa, G. L. and Weiner, M. P. (1994) Polishing with T4 or *Pfu* polymerase increases the efficiency and cloning of PCR fragments. *Nucleic Acids Res.* **22,** 2423.
13. Sambrook, J., Fritsch, E. F., and Maniatis, T. (eds.) (1989) *Molecular Cloning: A Laboratory Manual*, 2nd ed. Cold Spring Harbor Laboratory Press, Cold Spring Harbor, NY.
14. Schoettlin, W., Nielson, K. B. and Mathur, E. (1993) Optimization of PCR using the Opti-Prime kit. *Strategies Mol. Biol.* **6,** 43–44.
15. Weiner, M. P. and Scheraga, H. A. (1989) A set of Macintosh programs for the design of synthetic genes. *Comp. Appl. Biol. Sci. (CABIOS)* **5,** 191–198.

CHAPTER 22

A Simple Method
to Introduce Internal Deletions
or Mutations into Any Position
of a Target DNA Sequence

*Marjana Tomic-Canic, Françoise Bernerd,
and Miroslav Blumenberg*

1. Introduction

Site-directed mutagenesis is a powerful tool used in modern molecular biology for protein and genetic engineering. A number of simple and elegant protocols are available to introduce mutations into a target DNA sequence. However, there are only a few methods described for deletion mutagenesis *(1–4)*. In this chapter, we demonstrate a simple method for creating internal deletions into any desired position in a target DNA sequence. The procedure involves replacement of the DNA region to be deleted with a restriction site for an endonuclease. This also facilitates the insertion of other DNA sequences into the site or if desired restoration of the deleted fragment. Introduction of the new restriction site also provides a useful diagnostic tool for screening for positive clones following the transformation procedure.

The method we describe involves two basic molecular biology techniques: the polymerase chain reaction (PCR) and DNA cloning procedures. A diagram of the experimental design is presented in Fig. 1. The products of the first stage PCR reactions, split the template DNA into two halves, each containing a common internal restriction site defined by the inner primers (I-R and I-F). These products are then digested with

From: *Methods in Molecular Biology, Vol. 57: In Vitro Mutagenesis Protocols*
Edited by: M. K. Trower Humana Press Inc., Totowa, NJ

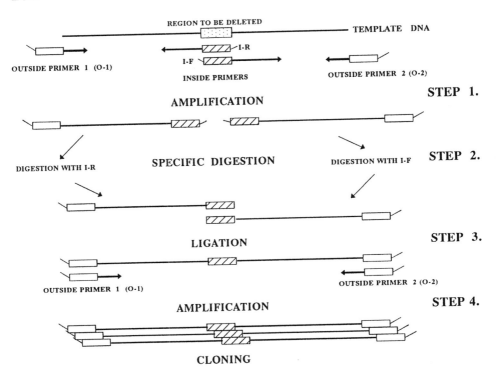

Fig. 1. Experimental design. The region to be deleted or mutagenized is represented by a dotted box. The black arrows on both the outside and inside primers represent annealing regions, whereas the slanted lines represent the additional three nucleotides that facilitate proper restriction digestion (*see* Note 1). The open and striped boxes on the outside and inside primers, respectively, represent the specific restriction enzyme recognition sites. Note that the inside primers specify an identical restriction sequence.

this restriction enzyme, and then the fragments are ligated together. This ligation reaction mix forms the template, with no further purification, for a second round of PCR using the outside primers (O1 and O2), which results in a single in vitro amplified product in high yields, that can be readily characterized to confirm that the desired DNA region has been deleted and replaced by the designed restriction site. This mutated product can then be easily cloned into a recipient vector, by digestion with the designed restriction endonuclease restriction sites incorporated by the flanking outer primers. We have used this method successfully to eliminate specific transcription sites selectively, including AP1, EGF-RE, K6-PAL and Site-A, from two different keratin promoters K6 and K5 *(5,6)*.

2. Materials

Solutions 1–6 are stored at –20°C, solution 13 is stored at 4°C, and all others at room temperature.

1. Synthesized single-stranded oligonucleotides.
2. *Taq* DNA polymerase (5 U/µL).
3. dNTP Stock 4 mM each: dATP, dCTP, dTTP, dGTP.
4. 10X PCR buffer: 100 mM Tris-HCl, pH 8.3, 500 mM KCl, 15 mM MgCl$_2$, 0.01% (w/v) gelatin.
5. Appropriate restriction enzymes and their corresponding buffers.
6. T4 DNA ligase (1 U/µL).
7. 10 mM ATP.
8. Agarose.
9. Ethidium bromide stock 10 mg/mL. Stored in a light-protected bottle.
10. 3M Sodium acetate, pH 4.8–5.2
11. 1X TBE buffer: 0.09M Tris-borate, 0.09M boric acid, 0.002M EDTA, pH 8.0.
12. TE buffer: 10 mM Tris-HCl, pH 7.5, 1 mM EDTA. Autoclave.
13. Phenol: double-distilled and saturated with TE buffer.
14. Chloroform, store in a light-protected bottle.
15. Ethanol: 100 and 80% (v/v) with distilled water.
16. PCR purification kit (optional, *see* Note 1).
17. Mineral oil.
18. Dialysis tubing for purification of DNA by electroelution.
19. Competent *Escherichia coli* cells.

3. Methods
3.1. First Stage PCR Reaction

1. Design four PCR primers, for two independent reactions, that will amplify the target template (excluding the region to be deleted) in two segments (*see* Figs. 2 and 3). In both cases incorporate restriction sites into the two outer primers that will be used for the final cloning into the desired vector. Include an identical restriction recognition sequence for both the inside primers. The sequences for the restriction sites should be placed at the 5' ends of all primers flanked by an additional three bases to ensure complete digestion by the endonucleases involved (*see* Note 2).
2. Use the following PCR reaction conditions (amount/tube) (*see* Note 3): 20 ng template DNA, 0.5 µM of each primer, 10 µL of 10X PCR buffer, 4 µL

5' TTT TCTAGA CAGCCCATGCTCTCC   3'   INSIDE PRIMER I-F

5' TTT TCTAGA TGAGCTTGCAGGTTG   3'   INSIDE PRIMER I-R

ORIGINAL TEMPLATE

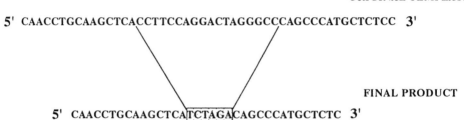

5' CAACCTGCAAGCTCACCTTCCAGGACTAGGGCCCAGCCCATGCTCTCC   3'

FINAL PRODUCT

5' CAACCTGCAAGCTCA TCTAGA CAGCCCATGCTCTC   3'

Fig. 2. An example of appropriately designed inside primers creating a deletion in the target DNA sequence. The dotted boxes represent the restriction site that is introduced into the target, replacing the deleted DNA segment.

5' TTT TCTAGA ACTAGGGCCCAGCCC   3'   INSIDE PRIMER I-F

5' TTT TCTAGA AGGTGAGCTTGCAGG   3'   INSIDE PRIMER I-R

ORIGINAL TEMPLATE

5' CAACCTGCAAGCTCACCTTCCAGGACTAGGGCCCAGCCCATGCTCTCC   3'

5' CAACCTGCAAGCTCACCT TCTAGA ACTAGGGCCCAGCCCATGCTCTCC   3'

FINAL PRODUCT

Fig. 3. An example of appropriately designed inside primers creating point mutations in the target DNA sequence. The dotted boxes represent the restriction site that is introduced into the target. Asterisks represent the introduced point mutations.

of dNTP mix, 0.5 µL of *Taq* DNA polymerase. Mix gently and bring the solution up to 100 µL with sterile, distilled water. Prepare three tubes for each reaction. Overlay the reactions with sufficient mineral oil to prevent evaporation. Initiate the following program for 30–40 cycles: denaturation, 1 min at 94°C; primer annealing, 1 min at 50°C; extension, 2 min at 74°C.

3. Analyze a small aliquot (10 µL) on an agarose gel to determine if each PCR reaction was successful (*see* Note 4). If products of the correct size are present, pool the reactions from each set of three tubes.

4. To purify the PCR products, use commercial columns (Wizard PCR Preps, Promega, Madison, WI) designed for this purpose (*see* Note 1). This will result in concentrated, clean DNA resuspended in a total volume of 50 µL.

3.2. PCR Product Digestion

The following standard procedure is performed on both of the first stage PCR products in parallel:

1. Place 20 µL of each PCR product into separate tubes and to each, add 2.5 µL of appropriate restriction buffer (10X) that is recommended with the endonuclease you decided to use, and 2.5 µL of endonuclease. Mix gently and leave the tubes at 37°C for a minimum of 1 h. Stop the reactions by adding 0.5*M* EDTA (pH 8.0) to a final concentration of 10 m*M*.

2. Load the digested first stage PCR products on a preparative agarose gel (*see* Note 4). Run the gel in 1X TBE buffer at 80 V (*see* Note 5) to separate the DNA fragments. Examine the gel on a long wavelength UV transilluminator and excise the bands using a clean scalpel.

3. DNA purification by electroelution (*see* Note 6). Enclose each of the excised agarose gel slices with 400–800 µL 0.5X TBE (*see* Note 7) in a clipped dialysis bag (avoid including air bubbles). Place the dialysis bags into the electrophoretic chamber filled with 0.5X TBE and pass the same electric current you normally use for agarose gel electrophoresis for 2 h (*see* Note 8). Without moving the bags, determine if DNA elution is complete (whether all the DNA migrated from the agarose slices into the solution) using a hand-held long wavelength UV lamp. If elution is complete, reverse the polarity for 1 min to detach the DNA from the walls of the bags. Open the dialysis bags and transfer all the buffer into fresh tubes; wash the bags with an additional 200 µL of 0.5X TBE buffer and combine with the samples in the tubes.

4. Purify the eluted DNA fragments using phenol–chloroform extraction (*see* Note 9). For each sample: Add an equal volume of phenol and mix by vortexing 10 s. Centrifuge 12,000*g* for 3 min. Remove the aqueous phase (top layer) and transfer to a fresh tube. Add an equal volume of chloro-

form, mix by vortexing 10 s, and spin for 3 min at 12,000g. Remove the top layer to a fresh tube and add 1/10 vol of 3M sodium acetate, pH 4.8–5.2, and 2 vol of 100% ethanol. Leave at –20°C for at least 10 min (*see* Note 10). Centrifuge for 15 min at 12,000g and aspirate the liquid carefully. At this point a small white pellet should be visible at the bottom of the tube (*see* Note 11). Add 500 μL of 80% ethanol and spin again for 5 min at 12,000g (*see* Note 12). Aspirate the supernatant and dry the sample in a vacuum centrifuge for 3–5 min, or air dry. A small white pellet should be visible. Resuspend the pellet in 25 μL of water or TE buffer.

3.3. DNA Ligation

To 0.5 μg DNA of each first stage PCR product, add 3 μL of 5X T4 ligase buffer and 1 μL T4 DNA ligase and bring to 15 μL with distilled water. Incubate for 1–4 h at either 16°C or at room temperature. Use this ligation mix directly in the second PCR reaction.

3.4. Second Stage PCR Reaction

1. PCR reaction conditions (amount per tube): 1 μL of ligation mixture, 0.5 mM of each of the outer primers, 10 μL of 10X PCR buffer, 4 μL of 4 mM dNTPs, and 0.5 μL of *Taq* polymerase. Mix gently using a pipetman (do not vortex) and bring the solution up to 100 μL with distilled water. Prepare three tubes for each PCR reaction. Overlay the reactions with sufficient mineral oil to prevent evaporation. Initiate the following program for 30–40 cycles: denaturation, 1 min at 94°C; primer annealing, 1 min at 50°C; extension, 2 min at 74°C.

2. Analyze a 10 μL aliquot of each reaction by agarose gel electrophoresis. A single PCR product, equal to the combined size of the first stage products, should have been generated. Pool and then purify the single DNA fragment as oulined in Section 3.1., step 4.

3. To the purified second stage PCR product, add 5 μL of appropriate 10X restriction buffer, 3 μL of each restriction enzyme to digest the 5' and 3' ends of the DNA fragment (as dictated by the sites incorporated into the PCR product during the amplification), and make up to 50 μL with distilled water. Mix gently and leave the tubes in the 37°C for a minimum of 1 h. Stop the reaction by adding 0.5M EDTA (pH 8.0) to a final concentration of 10 mM (*see* Note 13).

4. In parallel with the digestion of the second stage PCR product, cleavage of the recipient vector should be performed using identical restriction enzymes. Take 5 μg of clean, plasmid DNA and add 1/10 vol 10X restriction buffer, 3 μL of each restriction enzyme, and appropriate volume of distilled water. Mix gently and incubate as described.

5. Purify both PCR product and vector DNA by phenol–chloroform extraction followed by ethanol precipitation (as described in Section 3.2., step 4).
6. To 1 μg of the PCR product DNA and 300 ng of vector DNA, add 3 μL 5X T4 DNA ligase buffer, 1 μL of T4 DNA ligase, and distilled water to 15 μL (*see* Note 14). Mix gently and leave at either 16°C or at room temperature for 4 h. This ligation mixture can be directly used to transform competent *E. coli* cells by any standard protocol.

4. Notes

1. Purification of the PCR reaction product is a necessary step to remove excess primers, primer-dimers, and possibly nonspecific PCR products that can interfere with the following restriction digestion and ligations steps. Commercial columns are very convenient, but are costly. Alternatively, use phenol/chloroform extraction followed by ethanol precipitation as described in Section 3.2., step 4. The precipitated DNA should be resuspended in the 50 μL of distilled water or TE buffer.
2. There are a few important points one should keep in mind when designing the primers (*see* Figs. 2 and 3). The restriction site incorporated into both inner primers should be unique, i.e., present in neither the template DNA nor the recipient vector into which the mutant DNA will be cloned. Creation of such a site is useful for first determining that the second stage PCR product has incorporated the desired mutation(s) and second, it also serves as a convenient tool for rapidly screening plasmids following the cloning step. When designing the outside primers, it is better (if possible) to use two different unique restriction sites. This way, cloning of the final mutant DNA into the vector is directional, i.e., you do not have to worry about the orientation of the insert. It is particularly useful to choose two restriction enzymes that cut in the same buffer, saving both a purification and digestion step.
3. In the text we have described a basic PCR protocol that works well in our laboratory. For further information on this technique one may consult books such as *PCR Technology (7)*. In addition, there are many commercial PCR kits available that provide detailed instructions. For any PCR reaction being prepared you should ensure that the all the reagents are of the highest quality and that your template DNA is clean. We recommend the use of sterile pipet tips.
4. The percentage of the agarose required depends of the size of the DNA fragments you are expecting. However gels of 1–1.5% (w/v) agarose are convenient for the size of fragments generated by in vitro amplification.
5. The power of electrical current required depends on your gel apparatus, but generally it should be around 1.5 V/cm.

6. Isolation of the PCR products from the agarose gel is necessary, because the PCR reaction may contain nonspecific DNA products in addition to the desired fragment. We prefer to undertake this step by electroelution, since it is a fast procedure, providing an acceptable yield of DNA. However, commercial products based on DNA binding matrices may also be utilized, such as GlassMax (Life Technologies, Bethesda, MD) and GeneClean (Bio101, La Jolla, CA).
7. The volume of the buffer in the dialysis bag depends on both the thickness of the agarose slice and on the amount of the DNA present. Use approx 500 µL of buffer/g of agarose gel.
8. Care should be taken not to move the dialysis bags during electroelution, since the current should always be moving the DNA out of the agarose gel block.
9. This is the standard method for removing any remaining traces of agarose and proteins from the DNA. Although the PCR product DNA is usually clean, it sometimes happens that during the phenol extraction the upper (aqueous) phase is cloudy. That does not affect later stages of the procedure.
10. This is convenient step to stop at if required, since the DNA may be stored in ethanol at −20°C overnight
11. Sometimes it is very difficult to see the pellet and rather than white, it looks "transparent." Do not get discouraged, the DNA is there!
12. The 80% ethanol wash step improves DNA solubility after precipitation.
13. If restriction enzymes that cut outside primers are not active in the same restriction buffer, two separate digestion reaction should be performed. First, digest with one enzyme, purify the DNA by phenol–chloroform extraction and ethanol precipitation as described in Section 3.2., step 4), and then proceed with the second digestion.
14. If the size of the insert is significantly smaller than the vector, than the ratio between the PCR product and vector DNA concentrations should be 3:1 in the ligation reaction. If, however, they are of similar size modify the ratio to 1:1.

Acknowledgments

We especially thank I. M. Freedberg for generous support of our research, as well as careful reading of the manuscript. We also thank E. Collado-Nunez for the synthetic oligonucleotides and J. Avins for secretarial help. Our research is supported by National Institutes of Health grants AR30682, AR40522, AR41850, and the NYU Skin Disease Research Center Grant AR39749. M. Blumenberg is a recipient of the Irma T. Hirschl Career Scientist Award and M. Tomic-Canic is a recipient of the Ken Burdick Memorial Fellowship Award granted through the Dermatology Foundation.

References

1. Legerski, R. J., Hodnett, J. L., and Gray, H. B., Jr. (1978) Extracellular nucleases of pseudomonas BAL 31. III. Use of the double-strand deoxyribonuclease activity as the basis of a convenient method for the mapping of fragments of DNA produced by cleavage with restriction enzymes. *Nucleic Acid Res.* **5,** 1445–1464.
2. Sakonju S., Bogenhagen, D. F., and Brown, D. D. (1980) A control region in the center of the 5S RNA gene directs specific initiation of transcription: I. The 5' border of the region. *Cell* **19,** 13–25
3. Sambrook, J., Fritsch, E. F., and Maniatis, T. (1989) *Molecular Cloning: A Laboratory Manual.* Cold Spring Harbor Laboratory Press, Cold Spring Harbor, NY.
4. King, P. and Goodbourn, S. (1992) A method for sequence-specific deletion mutagenesis. *Nucleic Acid Res.* **20,** 1039–1044.
5. Ohtsuki, M., Tomic-Canic, M., Freedberg, I. M., and Blumenberg, M. (1992) Nuclear proteins involved in transcription of the human K5 keratin gene. *J. Invest. Dermatol.* **99,** 206–215.
6. Bernerd, F., Magnaldo, T., Freedberg, I. M., and Blumenberg, M. (1993) Expression of the carcinoma-associated keratin K6 and the role of AP-1 proto-oncoproteins. *Gene Expression* **3,** 187–199.
7. Erlich, M. (ed.) (1989) *PCR Technology: Principles and Applications for DNA Amplification,* Stockton Press, New York.

CHAPTER 23

A Simple Method for Site-Specific Mutagenesis that Leaves the Rest of the Template Unaltered

Marjana Tomic-Canic, Ivana Sunjevaric, and Miroslav Blumenberg

1. Introduction

Site-directed mutagenesis is an important component of modern molecular biology. The use of this technique became necessary both in our studies of promoter function and in the analysis of protein structure–function relationships. Although several polymerase chain reaction (PCR)-based methods of site-specific mutagenesis have been described *(1–4)*, we have developed a simple procedure that can introduce either a single or a small cluster of mutations into any DNA segment in the range 0.3–3 kb. Importantly, using this technique, only the designed changes are incorporated into the target sequence, all other positions remain unaltered.

This method, described herein, is based on two very simple and widely used molecular biology techniques: PCR and restriction digestion with Type II restriction endonucleases that cut double-stranded DNA at a short distance from their recognition sites. The experimental design is presented in Fig 1. The procedure involves PCR between two pairs of primers, denoted outside and inside in Fig. 1. The inside primers incorporate both the desired mutation(s) and restriction recognition sequences for a Type II enzyme. A list of such enzymes is presented in Table 1. Following in vitro amplification, the two PCR products are digested with the

From: *Methods in Molecular Biology, Vol. 57: In Vitro Mutagenesis Protocols*
Edited by: M. K. Trower Humana Press Inc., Totowa, NJ

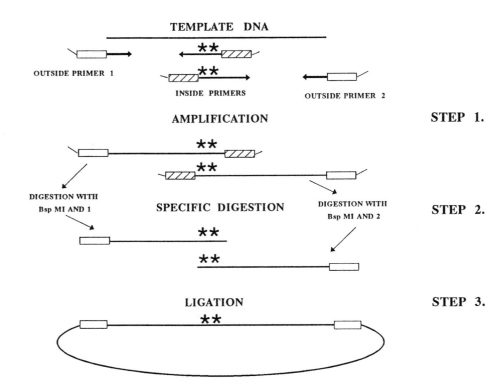

Fig. 1. Experimental design. Point mutations to be introduced are represented by the asterisks. On the outside primers the black arrows represent annealing regions, the open boxes represent the restriction sites, and the slanted lines represent the additional three nucleotides that allow proper digestion (*see* Note 1). On the inside primers the black arrows represent the annealing region, the striped boxes represent the specific Type II enzyme restriction site (*see* Note 2) and the slanted lines represent the additional three nucleotides segments that allow proper digestion.

designated type II enzyme, thereby removing the associated recognition sequences from their ends. Subsequent ligation and cloning steps recreate the original template except for the designed mutations (*see* Fig. 2, for an example). We have used *Bsp*MI in our protocol because its restriction site is close to its recognition sequence and therefore the length of the inside primers used in the PCR reaction can be kept short. An additional advantage is that the 4 base staggered restriction

Table 1
List of Type II Restriction Enzymes that are Self-Eliminating
and that Cleave the DNA at a Distance from Their Recognition Sequences

*Bbs*I	5'... GAAGAC(N)$_2$.... 3' 3'... CTTCTG(N)$_6$.... 5'	*Ear*I	5'... CTCTTC(N)$_1$ ... 3' 3'... GAGAAG(N)$_4$ ... 5'
*Bbv*I	5'... GCAGC(N)$_8$ ... 3' 3'... CGTCG(N)$_{12}$ ... 5'	*Fok*I	5'... GGATG(N)$_9$ ... 3' 3'... CCTAC(N)$_{13}$ ... 5'
*Bpm*I	5'... CTGGAC(N)$_{16}$ ... 3' 3'... GACCTC(N)$_{14}$ ... 5'	*Hga*I	5'... GACGC(N)$_5$ ... 3' 3'... CTGCG(N)$_{10}$ ... 5'
*Bsa*I	5'... GGTCTC(N)$_1$ ... 3' 3'... CCAGAG(N)$_5$ ... 5'	*Hph*I	5'... GGTGA(N)$_8$ ... 3' 3'... CCACT(N)$_7$ ... 5'
*Bsg*I	5'... GTGCAG(N)$_{16}$ ... 3' 3'... CACGTC(N)$_{14}$ ... 5'	*Mbo*II	5'... GAAGA(N)$_8$ ... 3' 3'... CTTCT(N)$_7$ ... 5'
*Bsm*AI	5'... GTCTC(N)$_1$ ... 3' 3'... CAGGG(N)$_{14}$ ... 5'	*Mnl*I	5'... CCTC(N)$_7$ ... 3' 3'... GCAGAAG(N)$_4$ ... 5'
*Bsm*FI	5'... GTCCC(N)$_{10}$ ... 3' 3'... CAGGG(N)$_{14}$ ...5'	*Sap*I	5'... GCTCTTC(N)$_1$ ... 3' 3'... CGAGAAG(N)$_4$ ... 5'
*Bsp*MI	5'... ACCTGC(N)$_4$ ... 3' 3'... TGGACG(N)$_8$ ... 5'	*Sfa*NI	5'... GCATC(N)$_5$ ... 3' 3'... CGTAG(N)$_9$ ... 5'

site of *Bsp*MI also promotes ligation of the two PCR products by T4 DNA ligase.

We have successfully used this approach to identify retinoic acid and thyroid hormone nuclear receptor binding sites in the promoter of the K14 keratin gene *(5,6)*.

2. Materials

Solutions 1–6 are stored at –20°C, solution 11 at 4°C, all others at room temperature.

1. 0.5 m*M* Synthesized single-stranded primer stocks.
2. 5 U/µL *Taq* polymerase.
3. 10X PCR buffer: 100 m*M* Tris-HCl, pH 8.3, 500 m*M* KCl, 15 m*M* MgCl$_2$, 0.1% (w/v) gelatin.
4. dNTP stock: 4 m*M* each of dATP, dTTP, dGTP, dCTP.
5. Appropriate restriction enzymes, including *Bsp*MI and their corresponding buffers.
6. 1 U/µL T4 DNA ligase.
7. Agarose.

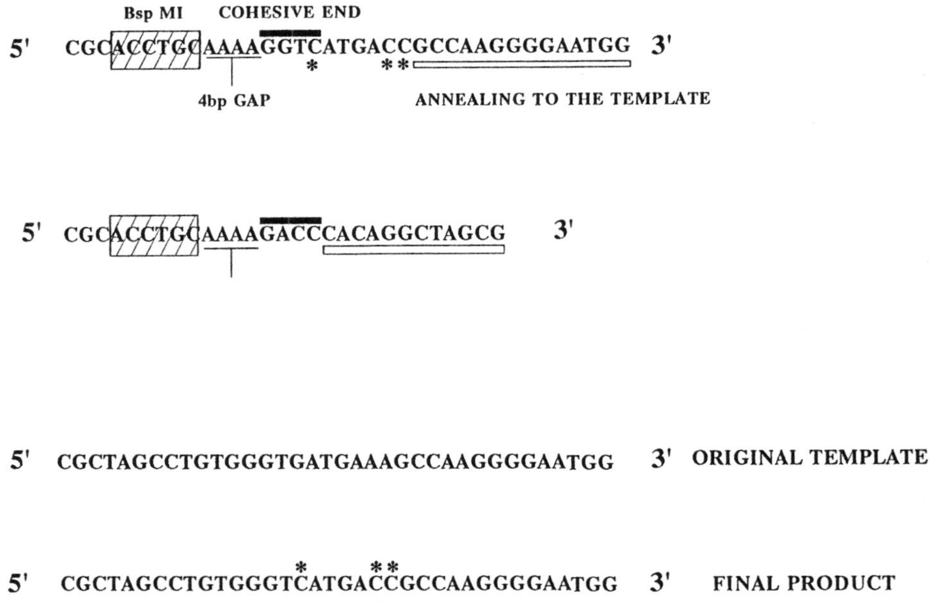

Bsp MI   COHESIVE END

5' CGCACCTGCAAAAGGTCATGACCGCCAAGGGGAATGG 3'
                    *   **
4bp GAP   ANNEALING TO THE TEMPLATE

5' CGCACCTGCAAAAGACCCACAGGCTAGCG 3'

5' CGCTAGCCTGTGGGTGATGAAAGCCAAGGGGAATGG 3' ORIGINAL TEMPLATE

5' CGCTAGCCTGTGGGTCATGACCGCCAAGGGGAATGG 3' FINAL PRODUCT

Fig. 2. An example of appropriately designed inside primers creating point
mutations. Point mutations are represented by asterisks. The striped boxes represent the restriction site for *Bsp*MI. They are followed by a four nucleotide
gap. The black, thick lines represent cohesive ends and open, thick lines represent the annealing region of the primers. Below are the sequences for the original template, followed by the sequence of the final product with the designed
point mutations.

8. 1X TBE buffer: 0.09M Tris-borate, 0.09M boric acid, 2 mM EDTA,
   pH 8.0.
9. 10 mg/mL Ethidium bromide stock. Store in a light-protected bottle.
10. TE buffer: 10 mM Tris-HCl, pH 7.5, 1 mM EDTA. Autoclave.
11. 0.5M EDTA, pH 8.0
12. Phenol: double-distilled and saturated with TE buffer.
13. Chloroform, store in a light-protected bottle.
14. Ethanol: 100 and 80% (v/v) with distilled water.
15. 3M Sodium acetate, pH 4.8–5.2.
16. Wizard PCR preps kit (Promega, Madison, WI) for PCR product purifica-
    tion (optional).
17. T4 DNA ligase and 5X reaction buffer.
18. Competent *Escherichia coli* cells.

3. Methods
3.1. PCR Reactions

Correct primer design is essential to the procedure and should be carefully undertaken. A total of four primers is required for two independent PCR reactions that will amplify the target template DNA in two segments (*see* Fig. 1). The two outside primers should incorporate convenient restriction sites at their 5' ends for final cloning into the desired vector (*see* Note 1).

The two inside primers should be designed such that each has an identical recognition sequence for *Bsp*MI (or if desired other Type II site), followed by 4 bases (the number of bases is dependent on the restriction enzyme used) that are complementary to each other. These sequences should be incorporated into the 5' ends of each primer and lie close to the site(s) of mutation. Mismatches can be introduced in one or both of the inside primers. For further guidance on the design of these primers it is advisable to consult Fig. 2.

Both the outside and inside primers should incorporate a minimum of 15 bases of sequence complementary to the template at their 3' ends to ensure specific annealing to the target DNA during the PCR reaction (*see* Note 2). Furthermore, the restriction endonuclease recognition sequences in all four primers must be flanked (at their 5' ends) by an additional 3-base tail to ensure complete digestion by the enzymes involved.

1. PCR reaction conditions are as follows (amount/tube): 20 ng template DNA, 0.5 μ*M* of each primer pair (outside and inside primer combination); 10 μL 10X PCR buffer, 4 μL stock dNTPs, and 0.5 μL of *Taq* polymerase. Mix gently (do not vortex) and make up to 100 μL with sterile, distilled water. Prepare three tubes for each PCR reaction. Overlay each reaction mix with sufficient mineral oil to prevent evaporation. Use the following program for 30–40 cycles: denaturation, 1 min at 94°C; annealing, 1 min at 50°C; and extension, 2 min at 74°C (*see* Note 3).
2. Analyze a small aliquot (10 μL) from each tube on an agarose gel to determine reaction specificity. If products of the correct size are present, pool the reactions from each set of three tubes.
3. Purify the PCR products using the Wizard PCR prep columns following their detailed protocol (*see* Note 4). This will result in concentrated, clean DNAs, each in a total volume of 50 μL.

3.2. PCR Product Digestion

The following procedure is independently performed on both purified PCR products. First, the amplified DNA segments are restricted, in separate tubes, with *Bsp*MI enzyme. Following purification, the DNA is then cut with the enzymes specified by the outside primers to allow cloning into a recipient plasmid vector digested with identical enzymes.

1. Place the purified PCR products into separate tubes (20 µL each), and to each add 2.5 µL of 10X *Bsp*MI restriction buffer, and 2.5 µL of *Bsp*MI restriction enzyme. Mix gently and incubate at 37°C for a minimum of 1 h (*see* Note 5). Stop the reaction by adding 0.5*M* EDTA, pH 8.0 to a final concentration of 10 m*M* (*see* Note 6).

Purify the DNA from both reactions using phenol-chloroform extraction/ethanol precipitation. For each sample:

2. Add an equal volume of phenol and mix by vortexing for 10 s. Centrifuge at 12,000*g* for 3 min. Remove the aqueous phase (top layer) and transfer into a fresh tube (*see* Note 7).
3. Add an equal volume of chloroform, mix by vortexing for 10 s, and spin for 3 min at 12,000*g* (*see* Note 8). Remove the top layer to a fresh tube.
4. Add 1/10 total volume of 3*M* sodium acetate, pH 4.8–5.2, and two volumes of 100% ethanol. Mix and then leave at –20°C for at least 10 min (*see* Note 9).
5. Centrifuge for 15 min at 12,000*g* and carefully aspirate the liquid. At this point a small white pellet should be visible at the bottom of the tube (*see* Note 10).
6. Add 500 µL of 80% ethanol and spin again for 5 min at 12,000*g* (*see* Note 11). Aspirate the supernatant and dry the sample either in a vacuum centrifuge for 3–5 min or air-dry. A small white pellet should be visible. Resuspend the pellet into 25 µL of either water or TE buffer.
7. To each tube, add 2.5 µL of the appropriate 10X restriction buffer that is recommended with the enzyme specified by the particular outside primer, and 2.5 µL of its associated restriction enzyme. Mix gently and leave the tubes at 37°C for minimum of 1 h (*see* Note 5). Stop the reactions by adding 0.5*M* EDTA, pH 8.0 to a final concentration of 10 m*M*.
8. In parallel with the digestion of the amplified PCR products, cleavage of the recipient plasmid vector should be undertaken with identical restriction enzymes (again as specified by the outside primers). Take 5 µg of plasmid DNA and add 1/10 of the volume of appropriate 10X restriction buffer, 3 µL of each restriction enzyme (*see* Note 12), and appropriate volume of

distilled water. Mix gently and leave the tubes at 37°C for a minimum of 1 h (*see* Note 5). As before, stop the reaction by adding 0.5*M* EDTA, pH 8.0 to a final concentration of 10 m*M*.

9. Repeat the purification of both the PCR products and plasmid vector DNA using phenol/chloroform extraction, followed by ethanol precipitation as described in steps 2–6.

3.3. DNA Ligation

Mix 0.5 µg of each digested and purified PCR product, with 100 ng of vector DNA, 3 µL of 5X T4 ligase buffer, and 1 µL of T4 DNA ligase. Make up to 15 µL with distilled water. Incubate for 1–4 h at either 16°C or room temperature. This ligation mixture can be directly used to transform competent *E. coli* cells using standard protocols.

4. Notes

1. When designing the outside primers, it is preferable to use two different unique restriction sites. This way, cloning of the mutant DNA into the vector will be directional (i.e., you do not have to worry about the orientation of the insert). Furthermore, the use of different restriction sites will prevent the two PCR products ligating to each other at their "wrong" ends. Since the procedure requires restoration of the original template sequence (apart from the designed mutations), this can only be achieved through ligation of the amplified DNA segments at their *Bsp*MI sites. It is particularly useful to choose two enzymes that cut in the same buffer, thereby saving a purification and additional digestion step.

2. *Bsp*MI cuts with a 4 base, 3' overhang. It is of great importance that the PCR product's cohesive ends generated on digestion are complementary to both the template and to each other, because after restriction, the full length template is restored by their ligation.

3. The described conditions work in most cases, but if the template is unusual in size or sequence, resulting in either no product formation or nonspecific products, they may be modified. There are many commercially available PCR optimization kits (Boerhinger Mannheim [Mannheim, Germany], Invitrogen [San Diego, CA], and Stratagene [La Jolla, CA]; all provide such products for instance) and we strongly recommend following the protocols provided by these manufacturers. In addition, for any PCR reaction being prepared, you should ensure that all the reagents are of the highest quality and that your DNA template is clean. We recommend the use of sterile pipet tips.

4. Alternatively, you can purify the PCR products using phenol/chloroform extraction followed by ethanol precipitation as described in detail in Section 3.2., steps 2–6.

5. Although the majority of enzymes cut most efficiently at 37°C, there are some that have a different optimum temperature. Ensure that the digestion reaction is being incubated at the optimum temperature for the restriction enzyme.

6. Alternatively, some enzymes may be heat inactivated by incubating the digestion mixture at 65°C for 5–10 min. Information on whether a particular enzyme is heat labile is usually found in the manufacturer's catalog.

7. The purpose of phenol extraction is to remove proteins from the DNA sample. Sometimes even after centrifugation, the top layer is very cloudy. If this occurs, repeat the phenol extraction before continuing with the next step.

8. Chloroform extraction is a necessary step after phenol extraction and its purpose is to remove the remains of the phenol from your DNA sample. One extraction is usually sufficient.

9. This is a convenient stop-point in the protocol. You may leave the precipitated DNA samples in ethanol at –20°C for as long as you wish.

10. The size of the pellet is dependent on the amount of the DNA that you have and therefore when small amounts are involved, it may be very difficult to see.

11. The 80% ethanol wash step improves the solubility of the DNA following precipitation.

12. If the restriction enzymes that cut the outside primers are not active in the same buffer, two separate digestion reactions should be performed. First digest with one enzyme, purify the DNA by phenol–chloroform extraction, and ethanol precipitation (*see* Section 3.2, steps 2–6), and then proceed with the second digestion.

Acknowledgments

We especially thank I. M. Freedberg for generous support of our research as well as careful reading of the manuscript. We also thank E. Collado-Nunez for the synthetic oligonucleotides and J. Avins for secretarial help.

Our research is supported by National Institutes of Health Grants AR30682, AR40522, AR41850, and the NYU Skin Disease Research Center Grant AR39749. M. Blumenberg is a recipient of Irma T. Hirschl Career Scientist Award and M. Tomic-Canic is a recipient of Ken Burdick Memorial Fellowship Award granted through The Dermatology Foundation.

References

1. Lanhdt, O., Grunert, H.-P., and Hahn, U. (1990) A general method for rapid site-directed mutagenesis using the polymerase chain reaction. *Gene* **96,** 125–128.
2. Stemmer, W. P. C. and Morris, S. K. (1992) Enzymatic inverse PCR: a restriction site independent, single fragment method for high-efficiency, site-directed mutagenesis. *Biotechniques* **13,** 215–220.
3. Kupiers, O. P., Boot, H. J., and de Vos, W. M. (1991) Improved site-directed mutagenesis method using PCR. *Nucleic Acids Res.* **19,** 4558.
4. Sharrocks, A. D. and Shaw, P. E. (1992) Improved primer design for PCR-based, site-directed mutagenesis. *Nucleic Acids Res.* **20,** 1147.
5. Tomic, M., Sunjevaric, I., Savtchenko, E. S., and Blumenberg, M. (1990) A rapid and simple method for introducing specific mutations into any position of DNA leaving all other positions unaltered. *Nucleic Acids Res.* **18,** 1656.
6. Tomic-Canic, M., Sunjevaric, I., Freedberg, I. M., and Blumenberg, M. (1992) Identification of the retinoic acid and thyroid hormone receptor-responsive element in the human K14 keratin gene. *J. Invest. Dermatol.* **99,** 842–847.

CHAPTER 24

Multiple Site-Directed Mutagenesis

Kolari S. Bhat

1. Introduction

Site-directed mutagenesis techniques allow selective engineering of gene sequences. In in vitro site-directed mutagenesis, base alterations are introduced into a target sequence by incorporating DNA base changes within a primer utilized in the DNA synthesis step. Several site-directed mutagenesis procedures based on this general principle have been described *(1,2)*. However, application of these methodologies for multiple site-directed mutagenesis requires several cloning steps. I have developed a polymerase chain reaction (PCR)-based multiple site-directed mutagenesis procedure *(3)*. This technique utilizes a combination of DNA amplification and chain extension to alter specific bases, starting from one end of a target DNA molecule and progressing to the other end. This multiple site-directed mutagenesis procedure is outlined in Fig. 1. Each mutagenesis cycle involves three steps: PCR, restriction digestion, and DNA chain extension. The PCR step introduces base changes into the DNA and then amplifies the mutated fragment. Restriction digestion, followed by gel electrophoresis is then used to select for this mutagenized DNA fragment. Finally, the chain extension reaction step extends the mutagenized DNA fragment along the target DNA, generating template for the next mutagenic primer to bind. This mutagenesis cycle is repeated until all the desired site-specific mutations are completed in the target DNA sequence.

I describe the multiple site-directed mutagenesis procedure as applied to the removal of all *Sau*3AI (GATC) and *Tsp*509I (AATT)

From: *Methods in Molecular Biology, Vol. 57: In Vitro Mutagenesis Protocols*
Edited by: M. K. Trower Humana Press Inc., Totowa, NJ

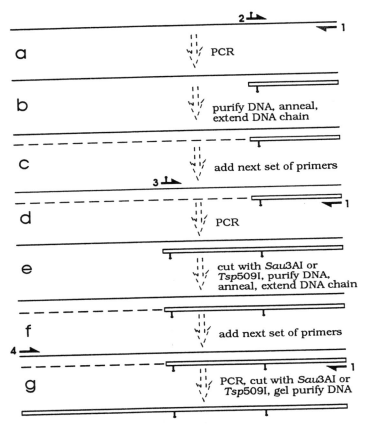

Fig. 1. Outline of the multiple site-directed mutagenesis procedure. This figure illustrates mutagenesis steps (a–g) to create two separate base changes in a target DNA fragment. The DNA template is represented as a thin line, whereas the mutagenized DNA is shown as the open box. The arrows in the primers point to the 3' ends. The primers are numbered 1–4. From ref. *3* with permission.

sites from the kanamycin resistance gene cartridge of plasmid pBRkan1 *(3)*. This general procedure, however, can be applied to create multiple site-directed mutations at all positions along any DNA molecule *(see* Note 1).

2. Materials

Solutions are stored at room temperature unless stated otherwise.

2.1. Preparation
of Plasmid (pBRkan1) DNA Template

1. Plasmid: Plasmid pBRkan1 *(3)* in *Escherichia coli* DH5αMCR.
2. LB medium: To make 1 L, dissolve 10 g bactotryptone, 5 g yeast extract, and 5 g NaCl in about 800 mL distilled water. Adjust the pH to 7.4 with 1*N* NaOH. Adjust the volume to 1 L with distilled water and autoclave. Store away from direct light.
3. Cell suspension buffer: Make a solution containing 50 m*M* Tris-HCl, pH 8.0 and 10 m*M* EDTA and autoclave. Cool, add DNase free-RNaseA to 100 μg/mL concentration. Store at 4°C.
4. Lysis buffer: 0.2*N* NaOH, 1% SDS. It is desirable to make this buffer fresh from stock solutions of 1*N* NaOH and 10% SDS.
5. 3*M* Potassium acetate buffer, pH 5.5. Adjust the pH with glacial acetic acid. Filter through a 0.2-μm filter and autoclave.
6. NaCl/PEG: Dissolve 13 g polyethylene glycol 6000 and 4.68 g NaCl in a total volume of 100 mL distilled water. Filter sterilize through a 0.2-μm filter. Store at 4°C.
7. TE (low EDTA): 10 m*M* Tris-HCl, pH 8.0, 0.2-m*M* EDTA. Autoclave.
8. 4*M* NaCl: Dissolve 23.38 g NaCl in a total volume of 100 mL distilled water, filter through a 0.2-μm nitrocellulose filter, and autoclave.
9. Kanamycin (100X stock): Prepare a 3.5 mg/mL solution of kanamycin sulfate in distilled water. Filter sterilize and store in small aliquots at –20°C.
10. Phenol (distilled): Saturate with glass distilled water and store at 4°C. Before use, take a phenol aliquot and equilibrate with 100 m*M* Tris-HCl, pH 8.0.
11. Chloroform.
12. Isopropanol.
13. 70% Ethanol.

2.2. Mutagenesis Reaction and Cloning

1. *Taq* DNA polymerase: *AmpliTaq* polymerase (5 U/μL) (Perkin-Elmer, Cetus, Norwalk, CT). Store at –20°C.
2. 10X *Taq* polymerase buffer: 0.1*M* Tris-HCl, pH 8.3, 0.5*M* KCl, 15 m*M* MgCl$_2$, and 0.1% gelatin. Store at –20°C.
3. dNTP stock: 2 m*M* each of dATP, dCTP, dGTP, and dTTP. Store in aliquots at –20°C.
4. Oligonucleotide primers: 100 μ*M* stock in distilled water. Store at –20°C (*see* Notes 2–4).
5. Wizard DNA purification kit (Promega, Madison, WI). Any other DNA purification reagents based on the general procedure of Vogelstein and Gillespie *(4)* are also suitable.

6. Agarose: Low-melting temperature agarose.
7. TAE electrophoresis buffer (10X stock): 400 m*M* Tris-acetate and 20 m*M* EDTA, pH 8.3.
8. Competent cells: Frozen competent cells of *E. coli* such as strain DH5αMCR (Life Technologies, Bethesda, MD) prepared according to Hanahan *(5)*. Store these cells in 200 μL aliquots at –80°C.
9. LB agar plates containing 35 μg/mL kanamycin. Store at 4°C.
10. Restriction endonucleases: *Sau*3AI, *Tsp*509I, *Aat*II, and *Bsp*HI with their reaction buffers (New England Biolabs, Beverly, MA).
11. T4 DNA ligase and 10X reaction buffer (New England Biolabs).

3. Methods
3.1. Preparation of Template DNA

The mutagenesis protocol does not require the target DNA to be cloned into a specialized vector. Any homogeneous DNA fragment cloned into plasmid or ssDNA vectors or obtained by PCR amplification may be used in the protocol (*see* Note 5). In the procedure described, the first step requires preparing plasmid DNA of pBRkan1. This vector contains a kanamycin resistance gene within a 1-kb region flanked by restriction endonuclease sites *Aat*II and *Bsp*HI. Many published plasmid protocols generally yield adequate quality template DNA. A modified alkaline lysis plasmid purification protocol may be utilized as follows:

1. Streak a kanamycin-containing LB plate with a frozen stock of pBRkan1 clone and grow overnight at 37°C.
2. Pick a large colony and inoculate 5 mL of LB medium containing 35 μg/mL kanamycin. Grow with vigorous aeration at 37°C for 12–16 h or overnight.
3. Transfer 3 mL of the overnight culture into two 1.5-mL microcentrifuge tubes and centrifuge at 10,000*g* for 2 min. Remove the supernatant completely with a pipet tip.
4. Gently resuspend and combine the pellets in 150 μL of cell suspension buffer. At this stage, the cells should be completely suspended. Cells may be suspended by repeated pipeting. Leave the suspension at room temperature for 10 min.
5. Add 150 μL of SDS/NaOH solution. Mix by inversion and leave at room temperature for 5 min.
6. Add 150 μL of potassium acetate buffer and mix by inversion. Incubate the mixture on ice for at least 20 min. Centrifuge the mixture at 12,000*g* for 20 min. Carefully transfer the supernatant to a new tube.

7. Add 400 µL of Tris-HCl equilibrated phenol and vigorously vortex for 1 min. Separate the phases by centrifugation at 12,000*g* for 2 min. Carefully transfer the upper aqueous phase to a new tube.

8. Add 200 µL each of phenol and chloroform. Vigorously vortex for 1 min. Separate the phases by centrifugation at 12,000*g* for 2 min. Carefully transfer the aqueous phase to a new tube.

9. Add 0.75 volume of isopropanol and mix. Leave at room temperature for 20 min or longer. Collect the precipitate by centrifugation at 2000*g* for 15 min. Remove all the supernatant. Wash the pellet with 70% ethanol and air dry. Resuspend the pellet in 50 µL TE buffer.

10. Add 50 µL of NaCl/PEG solution, mix, and incubate in ice for 1 h. Centrifuge at 12,000*g* for 15 min at 4°C. Carefully remove all supernatant. Wash with 70% ethanol and air dry. Finally, redissolve the pellet in 150 µL TE buffer.

11. Estimate the DNA concentration by measuring the absorbance at 260 nm (1 OD U = 50 µg/mL of DNA). The yield is usually approx 12–15 µg. Store the DNA at –20°C.

3.2. PCR-Mediated Site-Directed Mutagenesis Reaction and Cloning

Each of the mutagenesis cycles consists of three steps:

1. The amplification reaction that introduces the desired site-directed mutation and amplifies the DNA region between the mutation site and one end of the DNA molecule.

2. Restriction digestion reaction that removes unaltered DNA molecules by cleavage with endonucleases (*Sau*3AI or *Tsp*509I in this example). A subsequent agarose gel electrophoresis run removes unincorporated oligonucleotide primers and restriction digested unaltered DNA fragments.

3. A DNA chain extension step, in which the mutated DNA is annealed to the target DNA and extended by DNA polymerase. After this extension reaction, the native plasmid DNA need not be separated from the reaction mixture. Instead, the next round of mutagenesis is initiated by the amplification reaction, using the contents of the same tube.

Note that the final round of amplification before the product will be cloned may require the use of an "end-primer" pair into which convenient restriction endonuclease sites are incorporated. These restriction enzyme recognition sequences should be compatible with the cloning vector to be used (*see* Note 4). Experimental details of the mutagenesis cycle are as follows:

1. Mix 50 ng pBRkan1 plasmid DNA, 15 μL 10X *Taq* polymerase buffer, 15 μL dNTP stock, 1.5 μL of each PCR primers (primer 1 and 2 for the first mutagenesis cycle, *see* Fig. 1), and 1.0 μL (5 U) of *Taq* DNA polymerase enzyme. Adjust the final reaction volume to 150 μL with distilled water. Perform the amplification reaction in a thermal cycler at the following cycle settings: 94°C, 1 min; 45°C, 1 min; and 72°C, 1 min for 3 cycles followed by 94°C, 1 min; 50°C, 1 min; and 72°C, 1 min for 9 more cycles (*see* Note 6).

2. Purify the PCR product by Wizard DNA purification system (*see* Note 7) and digest the DNA with *Sau*3AI or *Tsp*509I restriction endonuclease (depending on the mutation required) in a 100 μL reaction volume. Separate the DNA on a 1.5% low melting temperature agarose gel (*see* Note 8). After staining with ethidium bromide and visualizing the DNA bands, excise the DNA band of interest and again purify the DNA by the Wizard DNA purification system. Quantitate the purified DNA spectrophotometrically (*see* Section 3.1., step 11).

3. For the chain extension reaction, mix 30 ng of plasmid DNA and 60 ng of the gel-purified PCR reaction product in a 25-μL final volume. Heat the mixture to 95°C for 5 min in a water bath. Add 15 μL of 10X *Taq* DNA polymerase reaction buffer. Allow the mixture in the water bath to cool slowly to 45°C over a 1-h period. Add 15 μL dNTP stock, 2 μL *Taq* polymerase, and 90 μL distilled water. Incubate the mixture at 60°C for 2 min followed by 72°C for 5 min.

4. Add 1.5 μL of each of the next primer set (primer 1 and 3 for mutagenesis cycle 2, *see* Fig. 1). Perform the amplification cycles according to the PCR conditions described in step 1 (*see* Note 9).

5. Repeat this mutagenesis cycle until all the desired mutations are completed. After the last mutagenesis cycle, digest the reaction product with *Aat*II and *Bsp*HI. Gel purify the final product as in step 2 and determine the DNA concentration.

6. Prepare a linearized vector fragment of pBRkan1 by completely digesting 1 μg of the plasmid DNA with *Aat*II and *Bsp*HI. From this digest, isolate the 1.4-kb vector fragment by agarose gel electrophoresis followed by purification using the Wizard DNA purification system as outlined in step 2. Quantitate the isolated DNA fragment.

7. For the DNA ligation step, combine 60 ng of the vector fragment from step 6 with 40 ng of mutagenized DNA product of step 5. Add 1 μL T4 DNA ligase and 2 μL 10X ligase buffer. Adjust the final volume to 20 μL and incubate at 16°C for 4–16 h.

8. Transform 1–2 μL of the ligated DNA into a competent *E. coli* strain and plate out on a selective media (*see* Note 10).

The transformation should yield about 1–6 × 10^3 colonies. Typically, >80% of the colonies should contain the multimutagenized DNA sequence (*see* Note 11).

4. Notes

1. The multiple site-directed mutagenesis procedure is also applicable for more generalized base changes at any position in a DNA molecule without depending on restriction endonuclease sites. For such universal multiple site-directed mutagenesis, a uracil-containing DNA template should be utilized. Single- or double-stranded uracil-containing DNA templates can be generated in vivo by utilizing *dut⁻, ung⁻* strains of *E. coli (6)*. Alternatively, uracil-incorporated DNA templates can be synthesized in vitro by PCR in which UTP is substituted for dTTP. In multiple site-directed mutagenesis reactions using uracil-containing DNA templates, after DNA chain extension reaction, the uracil-containing template is removed by a combination of UDP-glycosylase reaction and a 5-min heat treatment at 90°C. Thus, the chain extension, template DNA cleavage, and subsequent PCR-mediated mutagenesis step are all carried out in a single tube.

2. The success of the mutagenesis procedure largely depends on careful choice of the mutagenic primer. The primer should have at least eight bases of complimentarity at its ends. The primer can be 18–50 bases in length and up to four base changes may be introduced into the oligonucleotide sequence. When selecting a primer for mutagenesis, avoid regions of direct and inverted repeats. In addition, avoid more than four continuous G and C residues within the primer sequence.

3. The mutagenesis protocol does not require phosphorylation of the oligonucleotide primers. The oligonucleotide primer quality is critical to the success of this procedure. Oligonucleotides less than 25 bases appear to perform well with no purification. However, it is recommended that oligonucleotides over 25 bases are purified following their synthesis. Hydrophobic C-18 column (oligo-purification cartridge) is adequate for this purpose.

4. Restriction endonuclease recognition sites may be incorporated at the 5' end of each end-primer for convenient cloning, depending on the vector the mutagenized PCR product is to be subcloned into. These restriction enzyme sites should be flanked by at least four additional bases to ensure efficient digestion of the resulting PCR product.

5. The mutagenesis procedure works best with target DNAs under 1 kb size. DNAs over 1 kb tend to lower the DNA yield during the mutagenesis cycle. In addition, longer DNA templates reduce the chain extension efficiency. When working with a target DNA of over 1 kb, it is recommended to carry out mutagenesis steps on smaller fragments of the target sequence.

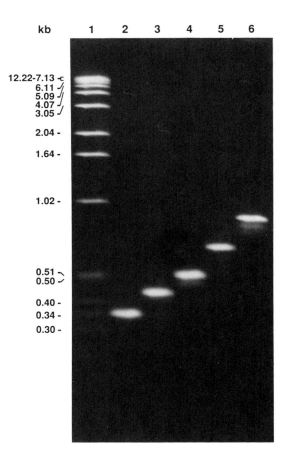

Fig. 2. Agarose gel analysis of multiple mutagenesis intermediates. The figure shows DNA intermediates during the mutagenesis of the kanamycin resistance gene of pBRkan1. Lane 1, DNA standard marker 1-kb ladder (Life Technologies) with sizes indicated on the left side. Lanes: 2, 1st PCR product; 3, 2nd PCR product; 4, 3rd PCR product; 5, 4th PCR product; 6, 5th PCR product. The DNA samples were separated on a 1.5% agarose gel. From ref. *3* with permission.

6. Limiting the amplification reaction to under 15 cycles appears to eliminate undesirable mutations. Other thermostable polymerases (*Pfu, Vent*, etc.) with lower error rate may also be used. However, these polymerases require careful optimization of Mg^{2+} concentration in the reaction buffer.
7. When an amplification reaction yields insufficient DNA product, the product should be increased by scaling up the reaction rather than increasing the number of PCR cycles.

8. The agarose gel electrophoresis separation is utilized to remove primers and unaltered DNA, after restriction digestion. Size comparison of DNA samples from different mutagenesis cycles by gel electrophoresis can also be used to monitor the progress of multiple site-directed mutagenesis stages (*see* Fig. 2).

9. The protocol should generate excess amplified DNA at every mutagenesis cycle. This excess DNA can be utilized to repeat an unsuccessful mutagenesis cycle. Failure of a mutagenesis cycle is generally owing to inefficient extension by the DNA polymerase from the primer. In such a case the primer region should be checked carefully for potential secondary structure formations. In addition, the PCR reaction conditions may also be modified to amplify difficult template regions.

10. Lack of colonies after transformation may be due to low competency of *E. coli* cells or inadequate ligation. The transformation efficiency of competent cells should be measured by transforming a control plasmid DNA. Inadequate ligation is usually owing to incomplete restriction digestion. Many restriction endonucleases require at least four extra bases beyond their recognition sites for optimum cleavage (*see* Note 4).

11. The mutations can be tested by resistance of the DNA to restriction digestion. However, accuracy of these mutations should be confirmed by DNA sequencing.

References

1. Kunkel, T. A. (1985) Rapid and efficient site-specific mutagenesis without phenotypic selection. *Proc. Natl. Acad. Sci. USA* **82**, 488–492.
2. Vandeyar, M. A., Weiner, M. P., Hutton, C. J., and Batt, C. A. (1988) A simple and rapid method for the selection of oligonucleotide-directed mutants. *Gene* **65**, 129–133.
3. Bhat, K. S. (1993) Generation of a plasmid vector for deletion cloning by rapid multiple site-directed mutagenesis. *Gene* **134**, 83–87.
4. Vogelstein, B. and Gillepsie, D. (1979) Preparative and analytical purification of DNA from agarose. *Proc. Natl. Acad. Sci. USA* **76**, 615–619.
5. Hanahan, D. (1985) Techniques for transformation of *E. coli*, in *DNA Cloning: A Practical Approach*, vol. 1 (Glover, G. M., ed.), IRL, Oxford, UK, pp. 109–135.
6. Trower, M. K. (1994) Site-directed mutagenesis using a uracil-containing phagemid template. *Methods Mol. Biol.* **31**, 67–77.

CHAPTER 25

Construction of Linker-Scanning Mutations by Oligonucleotide Ligation

Grace M. Hobson, Patricia P. Harlow, and Pamela A. Benfield

1. Introduction

The purpose of linker-scanning mutagenesis is to create a series of mutant molecules in which individual sections are sequentially replaced with the same "neutral" mutant sequence (*see* Fig. 1). Typically the technique has been applied to DNA and has most commonly been used to determine the *cis*-regulatory roles of upstream flanking regions of genes. The technique has several advantages over more random mutational analysis:

1. The approach is systematic and implies no previous prejudice about the location of functional elements;
2. The same mutated segment is substituted in each mutant, so that potential contributions to activity from the mutated segment are minimized when comparing mutants; and
3. Most importantly, the spacing and torsional orientation of remaining functional elements remains unchanged in the mutants.

Linker-scanning mutagenesis was first promoted by McKnight and his colleagues *(1)*, and the name arises from the fact that they used a replacement segment containing an endonuclease restriction site generated by the addition of synthetic linker DNA to appropriate DNA fragments generated by deletion. As a result, the replaced segment DNA was small (approx 10 bp) and contained a restriction site that could then be further

From: *Methods in Molecular Biology, Vol. 57: In Vitro Mutagenesis Protocols*
Edited by: M. K. Trower Humana Press Inc., Totowa, NJ

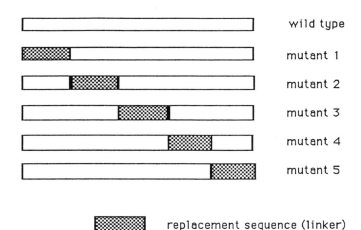

Fig. 1. A schematic representation of a series of linker-scanning mutants in a biopolymer such as DNA or protein. The open boxes represent the wild-type sequence and the hatched boxes represent a replacement mutant segment.

used to generate mutations (e.g., internal deletions). For analysis of gene regulatory function the technique is usually used to examine relatively short stretches of DNA (200–300 bp) in more detail, having established the location of potential regulatory sites by more gross deletion experiments. Technically, however, the principle can be applied to analysis of other biopolymers, e.g., proteins. Alanine scanning mutagenesis *(2)* represents an extension of linker scan technology to analysis of functionally important residues in proteins.

This chapter describes a modification of the linker-scanning method described by Karlsson et al. *(3)*. A series of synthetic oligonucleotides is produced to cover both strands of the DNA sequence under investigation. Each oligonucleotide is designed to span partially the two adjacent complementary strands as outlined in the sample scheme in Fig. 2. The entire set of oligonucleotides anneal together to assemble a complete DNA region. Sufficient oligonucleotides to create a totally wild-type sequence are synthesized, but by exchanging pairs of wild-type for mutant oligonucleotides, changes can be introduced at any position in the DNA region. By ensuring that the terminal oligonucleotides possess the cohesive ends of restriction enzyme sites, the synthetic region is then used to replace a corresponding restriction enzyme fragment in the piece of DNA under investigation. Although obviously the efficiency of the

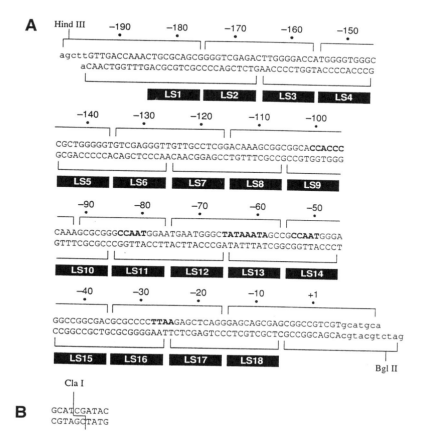

Fig. 2. Sample strategy *(4)* for construction of linker scan (LS) mutant promoter fragments for the rat brain creatine kinase *(ckb)* promoter. **(A)** Sequence of the wild-type *ckb* promoter DNA insert showing the location of overlapping oligonucleotides used for its construction. Black boxes labeled LS1–LS18 indicate the positions of the linkers in the LS mutants. Lower case letters indicate non-*ckb* sequences. *Hind*III and *Bgl*II overlaps used to insert synthetic promoter regions into the vector are indicated. **(B)** The sequence of the *Cla*I linker showing the *Cla*I restriction site. The sequences of mutant oligonucleotides used to construct the LS mutants can be deduced by replacing the wild-type sequences shown in A with the *Cla*I linker for each LS mutant.

method will decrease as the length of the segment to be constructed increases, we have used this method successfully to prepare linker-scanning mutations through a 200-bp section of the brain creatine kinase *(ckb)* promoter *(4)*.

2. Materials

1. Synthetic oligonucleotides: These may be generated using a variety of commercially available synthesis machines using the β-cyanoethyl phosphoramite chemistry with a dimethoxytrityl blocking group (*see* Note 1). Oligonucleotides (not gel purified before use) were resuspended to a concentration of 1 mg/mL. The design of oligonucleotides is discussed in Notes 2–5.
2. 10X Kinase buffer: $0.5M$ Tris-HCl, pH 7.5, $0.1M$ MgCl$_2$, 50 mM DTT, 1 mM spermidine, 1 mM EDTA. Store at –20°C.
3. ATP: 42 mM adenosine triphosphate (ATP) solution. Store at –20°C.
4. T4 Polynucleotide kinase: Store as 20 U/μL stock at –20°C.
5. $10M$ Ammonium acetate.
6. Ethanol: 100 and 70% (v/v) solutions.
7. TE: 10 mM Tris-HCl, pH 8.0, 1 mM EDTA.
8. 100 mM MgCl$_2$.
9. $3M$ Na acetate.
10. 10X ligase buffer: $0.5M$ Tris-HCl, pH 7.5, $0.1M$ MgCl$_2$, 100 mM DTT, 10 mM ATP. Store at –20°C.
11. T4 DNA ligase: Store as 6 U/μL stock at –20°C.
12. Appropriate restriction endonucleases and their buffers.
13. Agarose: Low melting point agarose. Use a grade appropriate for cloning, e.g., Seaplaque GTG agarose (FMC).
14. TBE gel running buffer: 89 mM Tris, 89 mM borate, 2.5 mM EDTA, pH 8.3.

3. Methods

1. Kinase all oligonucleotides, except the terminal ones (*see* Note 6), separately as follows. Mix 40 μL of oligonucleotide, 6 μL of 10X kinase buffer, 1.5 μL of 42 mM ATP, 10 μL of dH$_2$O, and 1 μL of T4 polynucleotide kinase in a microfuge tube (*see* Note 7).
2. Incubate at 37°C for 1 h, then heat to 65°C for 15 min to stop the reaction. At this point oligonucleotides may be stored at –20°C.
3. Mix appropriate oligonucleotides together. Use 3.3 μL of the two unphosphorylated terminal oligonucleotides and 5 μL of each kinased internal oligonucleotide stock. For mutants leave out the appropriate wild-type pair and substitute with the corresponding mutant pair.
4. Heat to 95°C and slowly cool to room temperature in a water bath. This is usually best performed in a 1-L beaker. Boil 300 mL of water in the beaker; remove from heat. Float tubes containing the hybridization reactions in the water bath and allow to cool to room temperature.

5. Add 1/5 vol of 10M ammonium acetate to each tube and ethanol precipitate by adding 2 vol of 100% ethanol. Cool in dry ice/ethanol for 5–10 min. Pellet by spinning for 15 min in a microfuge. Wash the pellet with 70% ethanol and respin. Remove the supernatant and dry pellet. Resuspend in 200 μL TE.

6. Add 25 μL of 100 mM MgCl$_2$ and 25 μL of 3M Na acetate. Ethanol precipitate as described in step 5. Resuspend in 42.5 μL of H$_2$O.

7. Add 5 μL of 10X ligase buffer and 2.5 μL of T4 DNA ligase. Incubate at 14°C overnight. Ligated oligonucleotides may be stored at 4°C (*see* Note 8).

8. Double digest 1 μg of vector DNA with appropriate restriction enzymes as directed by the supplier. Electrophorese on a 0.6% low melting temperature agarose gel in TBE running buffer. Visualize DNA by staining with ethidium bromide. Excise the vector band and melt in 4 vol of 10 mM Tris-HCl, pH 8.0. This results in a total volume of approx 300 μL (*see* Note 9).

9. Set up the following ligations: 16 μL of vector DNA, 1 μL of oligonucleotide insert, 2 μL of 10X ligase buffer, and 1 μL of T4 DNA ligase (*see* Note 10). Incubate overnight at 14°C.

10. Transform into a suitable *E. coli* host strain (*see* Note 11). Pick colonies and determine which colonies contain appropriately sized inserts by restriction and sequence (*see* Note 12).

4. Notes

1. Oligonucleotides synthesized using the methyl phosphite protecting group contain up to 30% methylated thymidine residues: These lead to mutations if read as cytidine *(5)*.

2. We have found it useful to design the terminal oligonucleotides so that the overhang constitutes a restriction site. Preferably these restriction sites should be different to allow insertion of the final synthetic fragment into an appropriately doubly digested vector. The remaining oligonucleotides should be made in two forms, one that allows generation of the wild-type sequence and one that allows replacement of each segment with a section of DNA that contains the linker restriction site of choice. Oligonucleotides should be designed to minimize any potential redundancy in the overlap regions. In this way the correct annealing scheme should be greatly favored and unwanted deletions or mutations can be avoided.

3. It is preferable to pick unique and different restriction sites for the terminal oligonucleotides and for the linker. In choosing these sites it is advisable to consider further manipulations that might be desired and avoid restriction sites that might appear elsewhere in the DNA constructs. Try to avoid any sites that might contain sequences of potential functional relevance, since the aim is to make the linker as "neutral" as possible.

4. Oligonucleotides do not have to be the same size. We have used oligo-nucleotides between 16 and 27 bases in length successfully. This allows some flexibility in the design scheme—for example, to avoid redundant overlaps and repeated sequences.
5. Try to avoid oligonucleotides with internal repeats that might allow hair-pin bend formation.
6. Terminal oligonucleotides are not kinased to avoid multimerization of the synthetic fragment.
7. This procedure produces a generous amount of kinased oligonucleotides. Considerably less material could be kinased for the mutant sequences that are only used in a limited number of ligations compared with the wild-type sequences.
8. Presence of the appropriately sized band could now be checked by agarose gel electrophoresis and gel purified for subsequent ligation into the vector. We have always seen multiple bands and even a smear interrupted by discrete bands when checking the ligation reaction by electrophoresis. It is probable that most of the material smaller than the appropriate insert size does not have the appropriate restriction site ends for liga-tion into the vector. Although in some cases we have gel purified the insert, we have found this to be unnecessary. In general, we do not check ligation mixtures by electrophoresis or gel purify the inserts; nevertheless, we have had a high success rate in isolating appropriate clones after ligation and transformation.
9. Alternatively, the restriction enzyme can be inactivated following restriction digestion by heating to 65°C for 10 min (for heat sensitive enzymes). The vector can then be used without gel purification if the restriction enzyme digestion was efficient.
10. Different vector insert ratios can be tried if problems are encountered.
11. Usually we use pUC based vectors as recipients for our linker scanned segments and transform into *E. coli* [DH5] by electroporation *(6)* to achieve high transformation efficiencies.
12. Plasmid DNA has been prepared from drug resistant colonies by the boil-ing preparation described by *(7)*. Plasmid DNA containing appropriately sized inserts has been sequenced using the USB Sequenase kit using the conditions suggested by the manufacturer.

References

1. McKnight, S. L. and Kingsbury, R. (1982) Transcriptional control signals of a eukaryotic protein-coding gene. *Science* **217,** 316–324.
2. Cunningham, B. C. and Wells, J. A. (1989) High-resolution epitope mapping of hGH-receptor interactions by alanine-scanning mutagenesis. *Science* **244,** 1081–1085.

3. Karlsson, O., Edlund, T., Moss, J. B., Rutter, W. J., and Walker, M. D. (1987) A mutational analysis of the insulin gene control region: expression in beta cells is dependent on two related sequences within the enhancer. *Proc. Natl. Acad. Sci. USA* **84,** 8819–8823.
4. Hobson, G. M., Molloy, G. R., and Benfield, P. A. (1990) Identification of cis-acting regulatory elements in the promoter region of the rat brain creatine kinase gene. *Mol. Cell. Biol.* **10,** 6533–6543.
5. Bell, L. D., Smith, J. C., Derbyshire, R., Finlay, M., Johnson, I., Gilbert, R., Slocombe, P., Cook, E., Richards, H., Clissold, P., Meredith, D., Powell-Jones, C. H., Dawson, K. M., Carter, B. L., and McCullagh, K. G. (1988) Chemical synthesis, cloning and expression in mammalian cells of a gene coding for human tissue-type plasminogen activator. *Gene* **63,** 155–163.
6. Dawes, W. J., Miller, J. F., and Ragsdale, C. W. (1988) High efficiency transformation of *E. coli* by high voltage electroporation. *Nucleic Acids Res.* **16,** 6127–6145.
7. Sambrook, J., Fritsch, E. F., and Maniatis, T. (1989) In vitro amplification of DNA by the polymerase chain reaction, in *Molecular Cloning: A Laboratory Manual,* 2nd ed., Chapter 14. Cold Spring Harbor Laboratory, Cold Spring Harbor, NY, pp. 14.1–14.35.

CHAPTER 26

Construction of Linker-Scanning Mutations Using PCR

Patricia P. Harlow, Grace M. Hobson, and Pamela A. Benfield

1. Introduction

In Chapter 25 we described linker scanning mutagenesis by oligo-nucleotide ligation. In this chapter we describe a more recent and versatile procedure that makes use of amplification by the polymerase chain reaction (PCR). For a description of the traditional method of generating linker scanning mutants by combination of deletion fragments, *see* ref. *1*.

Use of PCR provides an economical approach to linker scanning since fewer oligonucleotides are required to generate a set of mutants. Three general methods have been described for mutagenesis: the overlapping, asymmetric, and circular methods. The overlapping method *(2,3)* involves four oligonucleotides and three PCR reactions to create point, substitution, insertion, or deletion mutations at any point within a DNA fragment. Asymmetric methods *(4–6)* reduce the number of oligonucleotides to three and the number of PCR reactions to two for each mutation, but require purification of the PCR fragment from the first PCR reaction before proceeding to the second PCR reaction. Both the overlapping and asymmetric methods limit the amount of DNA sequencing required, but both require unique restriction sites appropriately placed near the ends of the fragment to be mutagenized. These methods have also been applied to the mutagenesis of proteins *(4–9)*. The circular method *(10,11)* reduces the number of PCR reactions and obviates the

From: *Methods in Molecular Biology, Vol. 57: In Vitro Mutagenesis Protocols*
Edited by: M. K. Trower Humana Press Inc., Totowa, NJ

requirement for appropriately placed restriction sites. However, if appropriate restriction sites are not available, the circular method increases the amount of DNA sequencing to be performed. Recently, Jayaraman et al. *(12)* combined the oligonucleotide ligation and a PCR method to synthesize DNA encoding horseradish peroxidase.

To create 18 linker-scan mutations in a 200-bp promoter, the oligonucleotide ligation method (*see* Chapter 25) requires 56 oligonucleotides (36 mutant and 20 wild-type). The PCR methods require fewer: 38 for the overlapping method, 20 for the asymmetric method, and 36 for the circular method. Although the asymmetric PCR method minimizes both the number of oligonucleotides and the amount of DNA sequencing required to create a series of linker-scan mutations, it requires purification of the fragment produced in the first PCR reaction.

We have successfully used the overlapping method without any intervening purification of PCR fragments to create mutations in the *ckb* promoter, and it is this method we describe in this chapter. The method can be adapted to the asymmetric PCR method by carrying out only one of the initial PCR reactions using a mutant and one common oligonucleotide. The resulting fragment, however, must be purified before proceeding to the second PCR reaction (Fig. 1).

2. Materials

1. Synthetic oligonucleotides: These may be generated using a variety of commercially available synthesis machines using the β-cyanoethyl phosphoramite chemistry with a dimethoxytrityl blocking group (*see* Note 1). Oligonucleotides (not gel purified before use) were resuspended to a concentration of 1 mg/mL. The oligonucleotides used in this protocol are named in accordance with Fig. 1. For a discussion of oligonucleotide design, *see* Note 2.
2. Template DNA: The template DNA is generally plasmid DNA that contains the region to be mutagenized (*see* Note 3).
3. 10X PCR reaction buffer: 500 mM KCl, 15 mM MgCl$_2$, 100 mM Tris-HCl, pH 8.3, 0.1% gelatin (*see* Note 4).
4. 2 mM dNTP mix: 2 mM of each dNTP, neutralized to pH 7.0. Store in aliquots at –20°C.
5. Mineral oil.
6. *Taq* DNA polymerase: DNA *Thermus aquaticus* DNA polymerase or AmpliTaq™ (Perkin Elmer Cetus, Norwalk, CT). Store according to manufacturer's instructions.

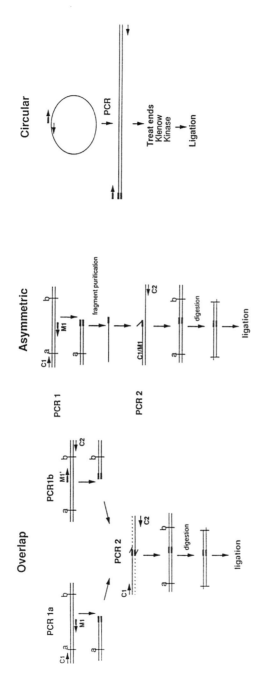

Fig. 1. Site-directed mutagenesis by PCR. In the overlapping and asymmetric methods the common oligonucleotides are C1 and C2, whereas the mutant oligonucleotides are M1 and M1'. The unique restriction sites are labeled a and b. In the asymmetric method the fragment produced from the first PCR reaction is labeled C1/M1. In the circular method only one oligonucleotide is required to be a mutant (M1); the other oligonucleotide may be a wild-type or mutant oligonucleotide.

7. Chloroform.
8. Appropriate gels, either agarose or acrylamide, and DNA size markers for checking reaction products and possibly purifying appropriate sized fragments.
9. Appropriate restriction endonucleases and their buffers for digesting the PCR fragments and the recipient vector.
10. Phenol/chloroform: A 1:1 (v/v) mix of Tris-HCl, pH 7.4 buffered phenol and chloroform.
11. 10X ligase buffer: $0.5M$ Tris-HCl, pH 7.5, $0.1M$ MgCl$_2$, 100 mM DTT, 10 mM ATP. Store at $-20°$C.
12. T4 DNA ligase: Store as 6 U/μL stock at $-20°$C.
13. Vector DNA: Appropriately digested plasmid DNA, e.g., pUC. Phenol extracted, ethanol precipitated, and resuspended at 3 ng/μL. Store at $-20°$C.

3. Methods
3.1. PCR Reaction 1

For each mutation set up two PCR reactions, 1a and 1b, in appropriately sized microfuge tubes.

1. In tube 1a place 2 μL of 10 μM (20 pmol) common oligonucleotide 1 (C1); 2 μL of 10 μM (20 pmol) mutant oligonucleotide 1 (M1); 5 μL of 10X PCR reaction buffer; 2.5 μL of 2 mM dNTP mix; 0.5–1 ng (0.15–0.3 fmol) of template DNA; and sterile water to 50 μL (*see* Notes 4 and 5).
2. In tube 1b place 2 μL of 10 μM (20 pmol) common oligonucleotide 2 (C2); 2 μL of 10 μM (20 pmol) complementary mutant oligonucleotide (M1'); 5 μL of 10X PCR reaction buffer; 2.5 μL of 2 mM dNTP mix; 0.5–1.0 ng of template DNA, and sterile water to 50 μL.
3. Overlay each reaction with a drop (about 50 μL) of mineral oil. Heat the reaction to 95°C for 5 min. Allow the reaction to cool to 70°C (*see* Note 6), then add below the oil layer 0.5–1.0 U of *Taq* polymerase that has been diluted into 1X PCR reaction buffer, and mix with the pipet tip.
4. Perform a PCR reaction in a programmable thermal cycler of 25–35 cycles of denaturation at 94°C for 30 s; annealing at an appropriate temperature for 1 min; extension at 72°C for 30 s; or an appropriate time for the length of fragment expected (*see* Note 7).
5. Extract the two reactions with chloroform to remove the mineral oil (*see* Note 8).

Remove an aliquot (1/10) from each reaction and electrophorese on an appropriate gel (agarose or acrylamide) to determine whether a single PCR fragment of the appropriate size has been produced. If there is only a single fragment, proceed to PCR reaction 2 (Section 3.2.). If there are multiple fragments, decide on the basis of number and intensity whether it would be advantageous to purify the appropriate sized fragment, repeat the reaction using different conditions, or proceed (*see* Note 9). If no PCR fragment has been produced, then repeat the PCR reaction using different conditions (*see* Note 4).

3.2. PCR Reaction 2

1. In an appropriately sized microfuge tube place: 0.5–5.0 μL of PCR reaction 1a (*see* Note 10); 0.5–5.0 μL of PCR reaction 1b; 2 μL of 10 μM (20 pmol) common oligonucleotide 1 (C1); 2 μL of 10 μM (20 pmol) common oligonucleotide 2 (C2); 5 μL of 10X PCR reaction buffer; 2.5 μL of 2 mM dNTP mix; and sterile water to 50 μL.
2. Overlay with mineral oil and heat to 95°C for 5 min. Allow the reaction to cool to 70°C and add below the mineral oil 0.5–1.0 U of *Taq* polymerase diluted in 1X reaction buffer.
3. Perform a PCR reaction in a programmable thermal cycler of 25–35 cycles of denaturation at 94°C for 30 s; annealing at an appropriate temperature for 1 min; extension at 72°C for 30 s.
4. Extract the reaction at least once with chloroform to remove the mineral oil.

Remove an aliquot (1/10), and electrophorese the sample on an appropriate gel (agarose or acrylamide) to determine whether a single PCR fragment of the appropriate size has been produced. If there is a single fragment, proceed to digest the fragment with appropriate restriction endonucleases. The choice of restriction endonuclease will determine whether the fragment can be digested without an intervening ethanol precipitation step (*see* Note 11). If multiple fragments are produced, decide whether it would be advantageous to purify the appropriate sized fragment, repeat the reaction using different conditions, or proceed directly.

3.3. Restriction Endonuclease Digestion and Ligation

1. Add the appropriate restriction endonucleases and digest for 2 h. Remove an aliquot (1/10), and electrophorese on an appropriate gel to determine if the expected sized fragments are present (*see* Note 12).
2. Extract the digested fragments with phenol/chloroform and then chloroform (*see* Note 13). Precipitate the fragments with ethanol. Estimate the concentration of the fragment by electrophoresis of an aliquot on an appropriate gel in comparison to a known amount of marker DNAs.

3. Add 1 μL of the digested fragments to 16 μL (50 ng) of an appropriatel; digested vector, 2 μL of 10X ligase buffer, and 1 μL of T4 DNA ligase Incubate overnight at 14°C (*see* Note 14).
4. Transform the ligated DNA into an appropriate *E. coli* host (*see* Note 15)
5. Screen the mutant clones either by restriction digestion of miniprep DN/ (*see* Note 16) or by hybridization with the mutant oligonucleotide (*se* Note 17).
6. Sequence the mutant clones using the common oligonucleotides, C1 and C2 to confirm that only the expected mutation was generated (*see* Note 18).

4. Notes

1. Oligonucleotides synthesized using the methyl phosphite protectin; group contain up to 30% methylated thymidine residues that can caus mutations if read as cytidine. Generally the oligonucleotides do no need to be purified by acrylamide electrophoresis, although batches o nucleotides with a high proportion of short products may produc lower amounts of PCR reaction products or require alteration of PCF conditions (e.g., temperature).
2. The design of the oligonucleotides to be chemically synthesized is critical The number of changes from the wild-type template affect the length o oligonucleotide required. When making a cluster of changes from the wild type sequence, as is the case when making linker-scan mutations, th changes should be confined to the 5' end of the oligonucleotide. The lengtl and sequence of the 3' portion of the oligonucleotide that hybridizes to th template should be such that the melting temperature, T_m, of hybridizatio: to the template is within a reasonable annealing temperature range (40–60°C). The T_m is estimated from the equation: $T_m = 4(G + C) + 2(A + T)$ Since the template DNA for PCR 2 is the annealed product of the PCF fragments from reactions 1a and 1b, it is critical when designing the mutan oligonucleotides, M1' and its complement (*see* Fig. 1), to have overlappinᵍ sequences with a reasonable T_m (40–60°C). The common oligonucleotide C1 and C2 (*see* Fig. 1) should be chosen so that their T_m is similar to th mutant oligonucleotides. It helps for subsequent cloning of the fragment t incorporate into C1 or C2 at least one restriction enzyme site that cleave: to produce a 5' or 3' overhang.
3. We have successfully utilized miniprep DNA prepared by the alkaline lysi: or boiling preparation procedures as template DNA. The plasmid DN^ may be either circular or linearized at a unique restriction site located awa: from the region to be mutagenized. If the DNA is linearized, it need not b: purified from the restriction digestion reaction when the concentration i: high (>1 ng/μL). Because PCR can amplify very small amounts of tem-

plate DNA, precautions against contamination are sometimes required. In the method described here, relatively large amounts of template DNA are used. Therefore, extraordinary precautions against contamination are not required. However, reasonable care to prevent contamination should be exercised (*see* ref. *13*).

4. As in any PCR reaction, the $MgCl_2$ concentration may need to be adjusted for a particular set of oligonucleotides *(14)*. The concentration used here has been used successfully for many oligonucleotide pairs. However, if no PCR fragment is observed, optimization of the $MgCl_2$ concentration is suggested.

5. Since the amount of template DNA can influence the frequency of unexpected mutations, Ho et al. *(3)* recommended a high initial template concentration. However, a high concentration may necessitate that the PCR fragments from PCR 1a and 1b be purified. We have found that a lower initial template concentration (0.5–1.0 ng) allowed us to recover mutant clones without having to purify the fragments from PCR 1.

6. After the initial denaturation of the DNA, maintenance of the reaction above the annealing temperature prevents spurious hybridization of the oligonucleotides that can result in the production of multiple PCR fragments.

7. The exact annealing temperature used for PCR will depend on the oligonucleotides chosen. Since *Taq* DNA polymerase extends nucleotides at the rate of 60 nucleotides/s *(15)* at 70°C, a 30-s extension time is sufficient to prepare PCR fragments of 1 kb or less. A longer extension time is necessary to prepare larger fragments. In order to reduce extraneous mutations, the number of cycles should be kept as low as possible. Usually 25–35 cycles are sufficient to produce a detectable amount of fragment starting with 1 ng of initial template.

8. The chloroform extraction step can be eliminated if an aliquot is carefully removed from the oil layer. This is sometimes easier if the reaction mix is dispensed onto a piece of parafilm.

9. Even if multiple bands result from the PCR reactions, we may proceed to PCR 2 if the expected sized band represents at least 30–50% of the ethidium bromide stained fragments. In some cases, however, we have purified the PCR fragments from PCR 1, especially when generating point mutations.

10. To dilute the wild-type template and eliminate purification of PCR fragments 1a and 1b, only 0.5–5.0 µL of PCR reactions 1a and 1b should be used.

11. We have successfully digested the PCR fragments from reaction 2 with *Hin*dIII/*Bgl*II without an intervening ethanol precipitation step by adjusting the pH, NaCl, and $MgCl_2$ concentrations before adding the enzymes. Some restriction endonucleases have different requirements and an intervening ethanol precipitation step may be necessary.

12. Although we have noted multiple bands for some PCR reactions, digestion with restriction endonucleases results primarily in the expected sized fragment.
13. A phenol extraction is used to inactivate the restriction endonucleases. If the restriction endonuclease utilized can be inactivated by heating to 70°C, the phenol/chloroform extractions can be eliminated.
14. Different vector insert ratios can be tried if problems are encountered. Vector to insert ratios of 1:1 to 1:3 are usually effective.
15. Usually we use pUC based vectors as recipients for our linker-scanned segments and transform them into *E. coli* [DH5] by electroporation to achieve high transformation efficiencies *(16)*.
16. Plasmid DNA may be prepared from drug resistant colonies by the boiling preparation described in ref. *13*.
17. If linker-scan mutations are generated by replacement with a unique restriction site, mutants may be screened by restriction digestion of miniprep DNA from a limited number of clones, however, when generating point mutations it may be necessary to screen many more clones by hybridization with a labeled mutant oligonucleotide.
18. Sequencing of potential positive mutants is essential before functional studies are initiated. We sequence using the USB Sequenase kit using the conditions suggested by the manufacturer. Oligonucleotides used in mutant preparation can often be used as sequencing primers. Not only is it necessary to confirm that the expected mutation was generated, but it is also necessary to rule out spurious mutations in the region of interest. *Taq* DNA polymerase has a poor fidelity, so unexpected mutations can occur generally at a rate of approx 1/10,000 bases per cycle *(17)*. We have also noted unexpected mutations, which apparently were present in the initial mutant oligonucleotides. Additionally, *Taq* DNA polymerase can add an additional nucleotide, generally an adenine residue, to the 3' end of a fragment *(18)*. Kuipers et al. *(19)* suggested that this potential error may be eliminated by appropriately choosing the first 5' nucleotide of the mutant oligonucleotide to follow a thymidine residue in the same strand of the template. Use of other thermostable polymerases (e.g., vent, *Pfu* polymerase) may overcome some of these problems.

References

1. McKnight, S. L. and Kingsbury, R. (1982) Transcriptional control signals of a eukaryotic protein-coding gene. *Science* **217,** 316–324.
2. Higuchi, R., Krummel, B., and Saiki, R. K. (1988) A general method of in vitro preparation and specific mutagenesis of DNA fragments: study of protein and DNA interactions. *Nucleic Acids Res.* **16,** 7351–7367.

3. Ho, S. N., Hunt, H. D., Horton, R. M., Pullen, J. K., and Pease, L. R. (1989) Site-directed mutagenesis by overlap extension using the polymerase chain reaction. *Gene* **77,** 51–59.
4. Sarkar, G. and Sommer, S. S. (1990) The "megaprimer" method of site-directed mutagenesis. *Biotechniques* **8,** 404–407.
5. Nelson, R. M. and Long, G. L. (1989) A general method of site-directed mutagenesis using a modification of the *Thermus aquaticus* polymerase chain reaction. *Anal. Biochem.* **180,** 147–151.
6. Perrin, S. and Gilliland, G. (1990) Site-specific mutagenesis using asymmetric polymerase chain reaction and a single mutant primer. *Nucleic Acids Res.* **18,** 7433–7438.
7. Horton, R. M., Cai, Z., Ho, S. N., and Pease, L. R. (1990) Gene splicing by overlap extension: tailor–made genes using the polymerase chain reaction. *Biotechniques* **8,** 528–535.
8. Horton, R. M., Hunt, H. D., Ho, S. N., Pullen, J. K., and Pease, L. R. (1989) Engineering hybrid genes without the use of restriction enzymes: gene splicing by overlap extension. *Gene* **77,** 61–68.
9. Vallette, F., Mege, E., Reiss, A., and Adesnik, M. (1989) Construction of mutant and chimeric genes using the polymerase chain reaction. *Nucleic Acids Res.* **17,** 723–733.
10. Hemsley, A., Arnheim, N., Toney, M. D., Cortopassi, G., and Galas, D. J. (1989) A simple method for site-directed mutagenesis using the polymerase chain reaction. *Nucleic Acid Res.* **16,** 6545–6551.
11. Jones, D. H. and Howard, B. H. (1990) A rapid method for site-specific mutagenesis and directional subcloning by using the polymerase chain reaction to generate recombinant circles. *Biotechniques* **8,** 178–183.
12. Jayaraman, K., Fingar, S. A., Shah, J., and Fyles, J. (1991) Polymerase chain reaction-mediated gene synthesis: synthesis of a gene coding for isozyme c of horseradish peroxidase. *Proc. Natl. Acad. Sci. USA* **88,** 4084–4088.
13. Sambrook, J., Fritsch E. F., and Maniatis T. (1989) In vitro amplification of DNA by the polymerase chain reaction, in *Molecular Cloning: A Laboratory Manual,* 2nd ed., Chapter 14, Cold Spring Harbor Laboratory, Cold Spring Harbor, NY, pp. 14.1–14.35.
14. Saiki, R. K. (1989). The design and optimization of the PCR, in *PCR Technology: Principles and Applications for DNA Amplification* (Erlich, H. A., ed.), Stockton, New York, pp. 7–16.
15. Gelfand, D. H. (1989) *Taq* DNA polymerase, in *PCR Technology: Principles and Applications for DNA Amplification* (Erlich, H. A., ed.), Stockton, New York, pp. 7–122.
16. Dawes, W. J., Miller J. F., and Ragsdale, C. W. (1988) High efficiency transformation of *E. coli* by high voltage electroporation. *Nucleic Acids Res.* **16,** 6127–6145.
17. Tindall, K. R. and Kunkel, T. A. (1988) Fidelity of DNA synthesis by the *Thermus aquaticus* DNA polymerase. *Biochemistry* **24,** 6008–6013.
18. Clark, J. M. (1988) Novel non-templated nucleotide addition reactions catalyzed by prokaryotic and eukaryotic DNA polymerases. *Nucleic Acids Res.* **16,** 9677–9686.
19. Kuipers, O. P., Boot, H. J., and de Vos, W. M. (1991) Improved site-directed mutagenesis method using PCR. *Nucleic Acids Res.* **19,** 4558.

CHAPTER 27

Use of Codon Cassette Mutagenesis for Saturation Mutagenesis

Deena M. Kegler-Ebo,
Glenda W. Polack, and Daniel DiMaio

1. Introduction

Cassette mutagenesis methods that introduce site-specific sequence changes into a target gene are powerful tools for the manipulation of proteins to analyze their structure and function *(1–3)*. Typically, a small target region is excised by cleavage at two constructed or naturally occurring restriction enzyme sites that flank this region, and the excised portion is replaced with oligonucleotides containing the desired mutation. In general, this method is used to mutagenize regions bracketed by closely spaced cleavage sites for restriction endonucleases that do not cleave elsewhere in the target plasmid. Use of cassette and other site-directed mutagenesis methods for saturation of one or more positions in a protein with all possible amino acid substitutions requires the costly synthesis of many customized oligonucleotides both to generate the necessary cleavage sites and to introduce each desired amino acid change. Much of the cost of oligonucleotide synthesis can be avoided by using degenerate oligonucleotides that have the potential to create several different mutations *(4,5)*. However, the use of degenerate oligonucleotides often requires substantial screening efforts because of the difficulty in identifying the final few nucleotide changes required to complete the set of desired mutants.

The method described here, Codon Cassette Mutagenesis *(6)*, utilizes a set of 11 universal oligodeoxyribonucleotide cassettes to generate mutations.

From: *Methods in Molecular Biology, Vol. 57: In Vitro Mutagenesis Protocols*
Edited by: M. K. Trower Humana Press Inc., Totowa, NJ

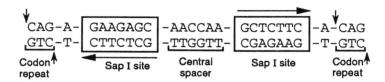

Fig. 1. Structure of a representative mutagenic codon cassette. The two copies of the recognition sequence for *Sap*I are enclosed in the boxes, with the horizontal arrows pointing toward the sites of cleavage that are indicated by the vertical arrows. The direct terminal repeats that correspond to the codon eventually introduced are indicated, as is a central spacer segment between the divergent *Sap*I recognition sites. The cassette shown here would introduce a CAG codon (glutamine) if inserted in the orientation shown and a CUG codon (leucine) if inserted in the other orientation. Reprinted from ref. *6* by permission of Oxford University Press.

The major advantage of this method is that this single set of mutagenic codon cassettes can be used to substitute or insert codons encoding all possible amino acids at any predetermined position in any gene. Thus, the expense of customized oligonucleotide synthesis is greatly reduced. Each mutagenic codon cassette (Fig. 1) contains two recognition sequences for *Sap*I, a restriction endonuclease that cleaves outside of its recognition sequence. The *Sap*I recognition sequences are arranged in opposite orientations (i.e., with their cleavage sites at opposite ends of the cassette) and are separated by a central spacer region. At each end of the cassette is a 3-bp direct repeat, positioned such that the sites of *Sap*I cleavage bracket each repeat, generating three base cohesive single-strand ends. The codon ultimately introduced by each cassette corresponds to this terminal repeat. Therefore, the identity of the codon cassette used in each mutagenesis reaction determines the mutations that are generated.

The use of mutagenic codon cassettes to create codon substitutions involves the steps illustrated in Fig. 2. First, a linear target molecule devoid of *Sap*I cleavage sites must be constructed that contains a double-strand blunt end at the site of mutagenesis. If the double-strand break is located between adjacent codons in the wild-type sequence, codon cassette mutagenesis will introduce single codon insertions. Single codon substitutions will be obtained if, as shown in the figure, the double-strand breaks are positioned immediately upstream and downstream of the

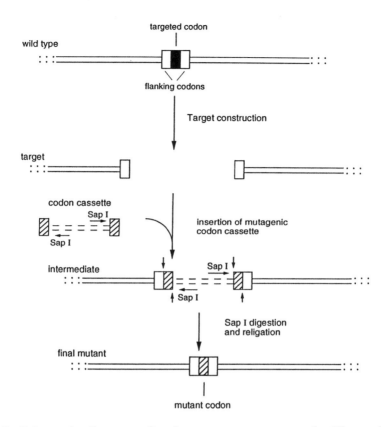

Fig. 2. Schematic diagram of codon cassette mutagenesis. The codon targeted for mutagenesis is represented by the solid box, and the codons immediately adjacent to the targeted codon are represented by the open boxes. The direct repeat at the ends of the mutagenic codon cassette and the final mutant codon are represented by the cross-hatched boxes. The *Sap*I recognition sequences and sites of *Sap*I cleavage are indicated by horizontal arrows and short vertical arrows, respectively.

codon selected for replacement (i.e., the targeted codon is deleted from the linear target molecule). Mutagenic codon cassettes are inserted into the target molecule by ligation at the site of the blunt ends to generate an intermediate molecule (*see* Note 1). The intermediate molecule containing the inserted cassette is then resolved by *Sap*I cleavage (which excises all of the cassette except for three base cohesive ends derived from the direct repeat) followed by intramolecular ligation of these single-strand tails. These manipulations in effect transfer a single copy of the thee base direct repeat from the cassette into the target molecule, thereby generating the final mutation. We discuss in this chapter how to use the codon cassette mutagenesis methodology to substitute or insert codons. We include a discussion of the construction of suitable target molecules, the insertion and resolution of the codon cassettes, and screening to identify intermediate molecules and final mutants.

2. Materials

Enzymes (which were obtained from New England Biolabs, Beverly, MA, unless stated otherwise), reaction buffers, oligonucleotides, and Sequenase kit are stored at –20°C. Other materials are stored at room temperature unless stated otherwise.

2.1. Reagents
for Target Construction and Mutagenesis

1. Universal codon cassettes of the general structure shown in Fig. 1 were obtained from New England Biolabs, and diluted to 10 ng/µL in TE.
2. T4 DNA ligase (400 U/µL).
3. 10X Ligase reaction buffer: 500 mM Tris-HCl, pH 7.8, 100 mM MgCl$_2$, 100 mM dithiothreitol, 10 mM ATP, 250 µg/mL bovine serum albumin.
4. *Sap*I restriction endonuclease (1 U/µL).
5. 10X *Sap*I reaction buffer: 500 mM K acetate, 200 mM Tris-acetate, 100 mM magnesium acetate, 10 mM dithiothreitol, pH 7.9.
6. Klenow fragment of DNA polymerase I (5 U/µL).
7. 10X Klenow reaction buffer: 100 mM Tris-HCl, pH 7.5, 50 mM MgCl$_2$, 75 mM dithiothreitol.
8. TE: 10 mM Tris-HCl, pH 8.0, 1 mM EDTA.
9. 10X dNTP mix for Klenow reaction: 500 µM each in TE (store at –20°C).

2.2. Colony Hybridization

1. Denaturation buffer: 0.5M NaOH, 1.5M NaCl.
2. Neutralization buffer: 1.0M Tris-HCl, pH 7.5, 1.5M NaCl.
3. 20X SSC: 173.5 g of NaCl, 88.2 g sodium citrate, 800 mL H$_2$O; adjust pH to 7.0 with 10N NaOH, and adjust volume to 1 L. (This stock solution is diluted with H$_2$O to generate 6X SSC and 2X SSC.)
4. 10% SDS stock: 100 g SDS, 900 mL of H$_2$O; adjust pH to 7.2 with HCl and adjust volume to 1 L.
5. Denhardt's reagent 50X stock: 5 g Ficoll (type 400, Pharmacia, Uppsala, Sweden), 5 g polyvinylpyrrolidone PVP-360 (Sigma, St. Louis, MO), 5 g bovine serum albumin (Fraction V, Sigma), H$_2$O to 500 mL (aliquot and store at –20°C).

6. Prehybridization buffer: 6X SSC, 5X Denhardt's Reagent, 0.5% SDS, 100 mg/mL denatured salmon sperm DNA (or calf thymus DNA), 50% deionized formamide.
7. Hybridization wash solution: 6X SSC, 0.1% SDS.
8. T4 Polynucleotide kinase (10 U/μL).
9. 10X Kinase buffer: 700 mM Tris-HCl, pH 7.6, 100 mM MgCl$_2$, 50 mM dithiothreitol.
10. Single-strand deoxyribonucleotide SAPP-5'-AGAAGAGCAACCAAGC-3' (500 μg/mL in TE), which hybridizes to all codon cassettes.
11. Nitrocellulose membrane, 82-mm circles (Schleicher and Schuell, Keene, NH).
12. [γ^{32}P]-ATP, 10 mCi/mL, 6000 Ci/mmol (Amersham, Arlington Heights, IL) (store at –20°C).

2.3. Other Reagents

1. Sequenase Version 2.0 DNA Sequencing Kit (US Biochemical, Cleveland, OH).
2. Phenol/chloroform/isoamyl alcohol: 25:24:1 mixture of TE-saturated phenol, chloroform, and isoamyl alcohol (store at 4°C).
3. 3M Na acetate, pH 5.2.
4. Ethanol (100 and 70%, store at –20°C).
5. Speedprep buffer: 50 mM Tris-HCl, pH 8.0, 4% Triton X-100, 2.5M LiCl, 62.5 mM EDTA.
6. tRNA: 10 mg/mL yeast tRNA (Sigma) (store at –20°C).
7. 3-mm Chromatography paper, 46 × 57 cm sheets (Whatman, Maidstone, UK).
8. RNase A, from bovine pancreas (Boehinger Mannheim Biochemicals, Mannheim, Germany).
9. 1M NaOH.
10. 3.75M ammonium acetate, pH 5.0.

3. Methods
3.1. Target Construction

To use codon cassette mutagenesis, a target molecule must first be constructed that is devoid of endogenous *Sap*I cleavage sites and contains a double-strand blunt break at the site of mutagenesis (*see* Note 2). The following steps are involved in constructing target molecules:

1. Remove endogenous *Sap*I sites from vector or target gene (if necessary).
2. Construct a pretarget molecule that contains restriction endonuclease cleavage sites that can be used to generate blunt ends at the appropriate position for codon substitution or insertion.
3. Digest the pretarget molecule (and fill in ends if necessary) to generate the desired target with the appropriate blunt ends.

The presence of *Sap*I recognition sequences within the target molecule is not compatible with the use of the codon cassette methodology. Although the *Sap*I recognition sequence is 7-bp long and occurs relatively rarely in DNA, such sequences may be present in the gene or plasmid vector selected for mutagenesis, so these sites must be removed by subcloning or standard mutagenesis procedures (*see* Note 3) *(7–10)*.

After removal of any endogenous *Sap*I sites, a blunt end target must be constructed at the site of mutagenesis. First, a strategy to generate the correct blunt ends in the target gene must be designed, then a pretarget molecule is constructed that contains restriction sites that allow generation of these ends. Cleavage by restriction endonucleases that generate blunt ends (as shown in Fig. 3A,B) is the simplest method to generate the target, but this approach cannot be used at all positions (*see* Note 4). A general method of constructing targets involves the use of *Sap*I to generate the appropriate blunt end sites (Fig. 3C). To generate a target for codon substitution by using this method, the targeted codon is replaced with a segment of DNA containing *Sap*I cleavage sites, arranged so that *Sap*I cleavage and subsequent filling in of the resulting recessed ends removes the *Sap*I sites and generates blunt ends at the appropriate position for cassette insertion. Since the *Sap*I sites are removed and the wild-type codons flanking the site of mutagenesis are regenerated on either side of the blunt end site, this approach can be used at any amino acid sequence. Furthermore, since the vector and gene by necessity contain no other *Sap*I sites, this method can be used in any targeted gene.

Once the strategy of generating the necessary blunt ends is designed, sequences that allow the execution of this strategy must be incorporated into the gene of interest. If the codon of interest is contained on a small segment of DNA bounded by sites for restriction endonucleases that do not cut elsewhere in the plasmid, this segment can be excised from the gene and replaced with synthetic oligonucleotides containing the desired sequences. If the codon of interest is not contained on such a segment, overlap (or recombinant) PCR mutagenesis can be used to insert the necessary sequence alterations into any segment of DNA (*see* Note 5) *(11,12)*.

3.1.1. Preparation of Blunt End Target Molecule by Using Sap*I and Klenow Polymerase*

1. In a microcentrifuge tube, mix 2 μL of 10X *Sap*I reaction buffer, 5 μL (5 μg) pretarget molecule, 8 μL water, and 5 μL *Sap*I. Incubate at 37°C for 4 h.

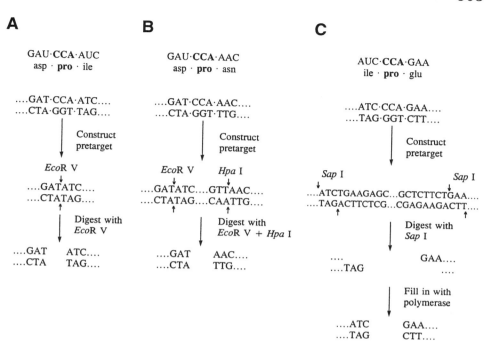

Fig. 3. Generation of blunt end target molecules for codon substitution. The top line in each panel shows the wild-type sequence of the codon targeted for mutagenesis (in bold face) and the two flanking codons, together with the amino acids they encode. The second line shows the corresponding wild-type DNA sequence. The third line shows the DNA sequence of a constructed pretarget molecule containing restriction endonuclease recognition sites that allow the generation of the necessary blunt ends. The fourth line shows the ends generated by digestion with the indicated restriction endonucleases. In the case of (A) and (B), this is the final target molecule. The fifth line in (C) shows the final target molecule after filling-in the *Sap*I ends with Klenow polymerase. (A) Generation of blunt ends by digestion with a single restriction endonuclease that leaves a blunt end. Note that the 5' half of the *Eco*RV site, GAT, and the 3' half of the *Eco*RV site, ATC, correspond to the codons encoding the flanking amino acids, aspartic acid and isoleucine, respectively. (B) Generation of blunt ends by digestion with two different restriction endonucleases that leave blunt ends. Note that the 5' half of the *Eco*RV site, GAT, and the 3' half of the *Hpa*I site, AAC, correspond to codons encoding the flanking amino acids, aspartic acid and asparagine, respectively. (C) Generation of blunt ends by digestion with *Sap*I that leaves a three-base single-strand extension followed by filling in with the Klenow fragment of DNA polymerase I. Note that the triplets generated in this example, ATC and GAA, correspond to codons encoding the flanking amino acids, isoleucine and glutamic acid, respectively.

2. Check an aliquot by agarose gel electrophoresis with an uncut standard to confirm that digestion is complete.

3. Add 30 µL TE, extract DNA by vortex mixing with 50 µL phenol/chloroform/isoamyl alcohol, and centrifuge. Transfer upper layer to new tube, add 5 µL Na acetate, vortex mix, add 100 µL ethanol, vortex mix, incubate at –20°C for 2 h or on dry ice/ethanol for 15 min, precipitate by centrifugation, rinse with 70% ethanol, dry, and dissolve in 20 µL TE.

4. To 16 µL (4 g) of ethanol-precipitated *Sap*I-digested DNA, add 2 µL 10X Klenow reaction buffer, 1 µL 10X deoxyribonucleoside triphosphate mix, and 1 µL Klenow polymerase. Incubate at 22°C for 15 min.

5. Add TE and extract DNA with phenol/chloroform/isoamyl alcohol and ethanol precipitate as described in step 3. Dissolve in 20 µL TE.

3.2. Use of Codon Cassettes to Generate Codon Substitutions and Insertions

Ligation of mutagenic codon cassettes at a target site and their subsequent resolution result in the codon substitution or insertion. Each cassette has the potential to introduce two different codons, depending on the orientation in which the cassette is inserted, and codons encoding all 20 amino acids are represented in the set of 11 mutagenic cassettes (*see* Note 6).

3.2.1. Cassette Insertion and Resolution

Once the target molecule with the appropriate blunt ends is prepared, 11 ligation reactions are set up, one for each mutagenic cassette (*see* Note 7). In many cases, insertion of the codon cassette is very efficient, and isolates with inserted cassettes can be identified readily by restriction analysis and sequencing of DNA prepared from individual bacterial colonies (*see* Note 8). Since there are only two predicted outcomes of each ligation reaction (i.e., the cassette inserted in the two orientations), screening a handful of isolates generated from each reaction is usually sufficient to identify intermediate molecules with cassettes in the two orientations. Once an isolate is identified with the correct sequence, it is resolved to yield the final mutation. Resolution entails linearization of each intermediate plasmid with *Sap*I and recircularization of the molecule via the cohesive ends that correspond to the introduced codon (*see* Note 9). Intramolecular recircularization of the *Sap*I-digested intermediate molecule is very efficient, and since there is only one desired outcome of each resolution reaction, minimal screening is required to identify the final mutation (*see* Notes 10 and 11).

Saturation Mutagenesis 305

3.2.1.1. INSERTION OF CODON CASSETTES

1. Ligate blunt end target molecule and codon cassette at a molar ratio of approx 1:25. For each cassette, set up a separate reaction containing 1 µL 10X ligase buffer, 1 µL (200 ng) blunt end target molecule, 2.5 µL double-stranded codon cassette, 4.5 µL water, and 1 µL T4 DNA ligase. Incubate overnight at 16°C.
2. To each reaction add 40 µL TE and 2 µL of tRNA carrier, and extract with phenol/chloroform and ethanol precipitate as described in step 3 in Section 3.1.1. Dissolve pellet in 10 µL TE.
3. Transform competent *Escherichia coli* separately with 2.5 µL of solution from each reaction. (Typically, we use strains HB101 or DH5α.)
4. To identify plasmids with inserted cassettes, screen colonies by colony hybridization (*see* Section 3.2.2.) or prepare DNA from individual bacterial colonies (*see* Section 3.2.1.2.) for analysis by *Sap*I digestion (*see* Note 12) or DNA sequencing.

3.2.1.2. PREPARATION OF MINIPREP DNA FROM INDIVIDUAL BACTERIAL COLONIES *(13)*

1. Pick a colony into 3 mL growth medium supplemented with the appropriate antibiotic and grow overnight at 37°C with agitation.
2. Transfer 1.5 mL of overnight culture to microcentrifuge tube and pellet cells with a 30 s spin in microfuge (*see* Note 13).
3. Aspirate media, disperse pellet, and lyse cells by vortexing in 150 µL of Speedprep buffer. (Pellets should be completely dispersed for best results.) Leave at room temperature for 5 min.
4. Add 150 µL phenol/chloroform/isoamyl alcohol, vortex mix 10 s, spin 2 min to separate layers.
5. Transfer upper layer to a new microcentrifuge tube, add 300 µL 100% ethanol to precipitate DNA, and vortex well.
6. Microfuge at 13,000*g* for 5 min at room temperature.
7. Wash pellet with cold 70% ethanol, and dry.
8. Dissolve in 20 µL TE, pH 8.0, containing 100 µg/mL RNase A. Leave at room temperature for 5 min. DNA solution can be stored at −20°C.

3.2.1.3. DNA SEQUENCING FROM MINIPREP DNA

1. Denature DNA by adding 4 µL 1*M* NaOH to 16 µL miniprep DNA. Incubate for 10 min at room temperature.
2. Add 2.5 µL NH₄ acetate and vortex mix. To precipitate DNA, add 100 µL ice-cold 100% ethanol and chill for 20 min at −70°C, or for at least 2 h at −20°C.
3. Pellet in microcentrifuge, discard supernatant, wash with cold 70% ethanol, and dry pellet.

4. Dissolve pellet in 7 µL water, and proceed with primer annealing and sequencing as outlined in Sequenase Version 2.0 manual *(14)*. We use 3 pmol primer for each annealing reaction.

3.2.1.4. RESOLUTION OF INTERMEDIATE MOLECULES TO GENERATE FINAL MUTATIONS

1. Set up a separate reaction to resolve each intermediate molecule. Mix 2 µL 10X *Sap*I reaction buffer, 5 µL miniprep DNA of the intermediate molecule, 11 µL water, 2 µL *Sap*I. Incubate at 37°C for at least 4 h.
2. Check an aliquot by gel electrophoresis with an uncut standard to confirm that digestion is complete.
3. To circularize digested intermediate molecule, add 5 µL 10X ligase buffer, 10 µL *Sap*I-digested intermediate DNA, 34 µL water, 1 µL T4 DNA ligase. Incubate at room temperature for at least 1 h (*see* Note 14).
4. Add 2 µL tRNA, extract with phenol/chloroform/isoamyl alcohol and ethanol precipitate. Dissolve pellet in 10 LTE.
5. Transform competent *E. coli* separately with 2-4 µL of DNA solution from each reaction.
6. To detect transformants lacking cassettes, screen colonies by colony hybridization (*see* next section) or analyze miniprep DNA by *Sap*I digestion (*see* Note 15).
7. Carry out DNA sequence analysis on isolates without the cassette to confirm codon substitution or insertion.

3.2.2. Screening Transformants by Colony Hybridization

If cassette insertion or resolution is not readily detected by random screening of a few colonies by restriction endonuclease digestion or sequencing, colony hybridization can be used to screen for the presence of the codon cassette and for its resolution (*see* Note 16). The same oligonucleotide, SAPP, which is complementary to a portion of all codon cassettes, is used as a probe in each case. Colonies hybridizing to the probe when intermediate molecules are screened possess cassettes and are further processed. After *Sap*I digestion of intermediate molecules and religation, the same probe can also be used to identify colonies that no longer hybridize and from which the cassette has been removed. These are the mutants that possess a codon change. Both intermediate molecules and final mutants are verified by DNA sequence analysis.

1. Use toothpicks to lift colonies from agar plate containing the transformants. Prepare a master plate and a duplicate plate for hybridization by stabbing agar using a grid to orient isolates (*see* Note 17).

Remember to include positive and negative controls (colonies harboring plasmids with and without an inserted cassette, respectively). Grow at 37°C overnight.

2. Place nitrocellulose membrane onto the hybridization plate for 5 min and lift filter to obtain imprint of bacteria.

3. Place filter, bacteria side up, on a series of stacks of 3-mm paper soaked in the following solutions at room temperature: 10% SDS for 5 min, denaturation buffer for 5 min, neutralization buffer for 10 min, and 2X SSC for 5 min. Air dry nitrocellulose (*see* Note 18).

4. Fix DNA to the membrane by baking *in vacuo* at 80°C for 2 h or by UV crosslinking (*see* Note 19).

5. To phosphorylate the oligonucleotide probe, mix 1 µL oligonucleotide-SAPP, 2 µL 10X kinase buffer, 5 µL [γ^{32}P]-ATP, 11 µL water, 1 µL T4 polynucleotide kinase. Incubate for 45 min at 37°C.

6. Add 30 µL TE, extract with phenol/chloroform/isoamyl alcohol, and spin upper layer though a Sephadex G50 spin column. Count 1 µL of the flowthough (which contains labeled probe) with scintillation fluid. Properly dispose of used spin column in radioactive waste.

7. Prehybridize filter in 5–10 mL prehybridization buffer for 30 min to 2 h at 37°C.

8. Hybridize overnight at 37°C in 5–10 mL of prehybridization buffer supplemented with 2,500,000 cpm of probe. Wash in 200-mL hybridization wash solution once at room temperature for 5 min, and twice at 37°C for 30 min each. Air dry, cover filter with Saran wrap, and expose to film.

9. Recover positive or negative colonies, as appropriate, from the master plate and grow bacteria for preparation of DNA for further analysis.

4. Notes

1. Because codon cassettes have blunt ends, they can be inserted into any blunt end site.

2. Target construction requires the only custom designed oligonucleotides used in codon cassette mutagenesis. In our experience, the effort and expense of target construction are rapidly offset by the savings obtained by using the universal mutagenic cassettes for saturation mutagenesis.

3. Several strategies can be used to eliminate endogenous *Sap*I sites. Most simply, the target gene can be recloned into a vector that lacks *Sap*I sites, or a small segment of DNA containing the *Sap*I site can be excised from a nonessential portion of the vector or target gene. Alternatively, a small segment of DNA devoid of *Sap*I sites but containing the codon to be mutagenized can be cloned into a vector without *Sap*I sites. After codon cassette mutagenesis is carried out, the mutant fragment can be recloned

into the full-length gene for analysis. Although this approach requires additional cloning steps for each mutant, it may be appropriate if the target gene contains multiple *Sap*I sites. If the target gene only contains one or a few *Sap*I sites, the site(s) can be eliminated by standard site-directed point mutagenesis procedures *(7–10)*. Because of the degenerate nature of the genetic code, it is possible to inactivate any *Sap*I site without altering the amino acid sequence of a protein encoded by that segment of DNA.

4. In order to use this approach, the recognition sequence of the restriction endonuclease(s) used must be compatible with the sequence of the codons flanking the site of mutagenesis. Currently described endonucleases can accommodate codons encoding approximately one-half of all possible amino acids in these flanking positions (*see* Table 1 of ref. *6*). As restriction endonucleases with novel specificities are discovered, this approach will become appropriate at more positions. Because the enzymes used to generate blunt ends must not cut elsewhere in the plasmid, it may be necessary to remove additional cleavage sites as described in Note 3 for endogenous *Sap*I sites.

5. In overlap PCR mutagenesis (described in detail in Chapters 15–17), two separate PCR reactions are first carried out to generate two DNA segments with a small region of overlap containing the desired sequence change (in this case, restriction endonuclease cleavage sites that allow generation of blunt ends). The 5' DNA segment is generated by PCR with a 5' flanking primer (which can be quite distant from the targeted codon) and an internal primer (which contains the sequence change). The 3' DNA segment is generated by PCR with a 3' flanking primer and the other internal primer, which is complementary to the first internal primer. A third PCR reaction is then carried out by using the two overlapping segments as templates and the two flanking primers. This will amplify the entire region between the two flanking primers while incorporating the desired sequence change from the region of overlap. Standard subcloning procedures are then used to insert the amplified region into the target gene.

6. The 11 mutagenic cassettes are listed in Table 2 of ref. *6*. These codon cassettes can be purchased from New England Biolabs under the trade name code 20 cassette mutagenesis kit.

7. The ligation and transformation reactions can be carried out for all 11 cassettes in parallel to reduce the amount of effort required in this step. In addition, prior to bacterial transformation, in some cases it is possible to digest the ligation reaction with the restriction endonuclease used to generate the blunt end during target construction. This will eliminate plasmids without an inserted cassette, thereby reducing the effort required to identify the correct intermediate molecules. *Sap*I digestion cannot be used in this enrichment step since the desired cassette contains *Sap*I sites.

8. This analysis proceeds rapidly if it is carried out on miniprep DNA, which must be very clean in order for it to be suitable for sequencing. We have adapted the protocol of Goode and Feinstein *(13)*, but other methods are also suitable. DNA sequence analysis at this stage will confirm the insertion of a single cassette, determine the orientation of the cassette, and document the absence of unanticipated deletions at the junctions between the cassette and the target molecule (which we have observed on rare occasions).

9. *Sap*I redigestion following ligation can be used to eliminate intermediate molecules from which the cassette was not excised. Such molecules can arise either because of incomplete *Sap*I digestion, or because of reinsertion of the excised cassette into the digested intermediate molecule.

10. By using this approach, we have successfully used all 11 codon cassettes and obtained all predicted codon substitutions.

11. An alternative approach for mutant isolation eliminates the need for analyzing or sequencing the intermediate molecules. In this approach, several colonies are pooled following ligation of the cassette and bacterial transformation. DNA is prepared from the pooled colonies, digested with *Sap*I, religated, and used to transform bacteria. DNA is then prepared from individual colonies and screened by sequencing to identify the two possible mutations generated by each cassette. This approach may afford considerable savings of time and effort, but it requires that most members of the pool contain inserted cassettes and that the two orientations are about equally represented.

12. Intermediate molecules containing an inserted cassette will be linearized by *Sap*I digestion. However, if *Sap*I digestion and filling in is used to generate the target molecule, *Sap*I digestion should not be used to screen for inserted cassettes.

13. It is also possible to scale up this procedure, if necessary, to obtain more DNA.

14. This reaction dilutes the DNA to favor intramolecular ligation.

15. The final mutants are now resistant to *Sap*I digestion.

16. We are also attempting to improve the design of the codon cassettes by incorporating a *lac* operator sequence, which should allow the ready identification of intermediate and resolved plasmids on indicator plates.

17. Since the same oligonucleotide probe is used to screen for both cassette insertion and resolution, colonies derived from multiple different insertion and resolution reactions can be screened on a single plate.

18. If the nitrocellulose becomes yellow or brittle, it was not adequately neutralized. A second neutralization step can be performed before 2X SSC treatment.

19. We use a Stratagene [La Jolla, CA] UV crosslinker 1800 on the auto-crosslink setting.

Acknowledgments

This procedure was developed with the support of an NIH grant (CA37157). The authors thank C. Docktor-Wolfe for assistance during the initial development of Codon Cassette Mutagenesis, New England Biolabs for the gift of *Sap*I and oligonucleotides, and J. Zulkeski for secretarial help.

References

1. Matteucci, M. D. and Heyneker, H. L. (1983) Targeted random mutagenesis: the use of ambiguously synthesized oligonucleotides to mutagenize sequences immediately 5' of an ATG initiation codon. *Nucleic Acids Res.* **11**, 3113–3121.
2. Wells, J. A., Vasser, M., and Powers, D. B. (1985) Cassette mutagenesis: an efficient method for generation of multiple mutations at defined sites. *Gene* **34**, 315–323.
3. Stone, J. C., Vass, W. C., Willumsen, B. M., and Lowy, D. R. (1988) p21-*ras* effector domain mutants constructed by "cassette" mutagenesis. *Mol. Cell. Biol.* **8**, 3565–3569.
4. Hill, D. E., Oliphant, A. R., and Struhl, K. (1987) Mutagenesis with degenerate oligonucleotides: an efficient method for saturating a defined DNA region with base pair substitutions. *Methods Enzymol.* **155**, 558–568.
5. Horwitz, B. H. and DiMaio, D. (1990) Saturation mutagenesis using mixed oligonucleotides and M13 templates containing uracil. *Methods Enzymol.* **185**, 599–611.
6. Kegler-Ebo, D. M., Docktor, C. M., and DiMaio, D. (1994) Codon cassette mutagenesis: a general method to insert or replace individual codons by using universal mutagenic cassettes. *Nucleic Acids Res.* **22**, 1593–1599.
7. Zoller, M. J. and Smith, M. (1982) Oligonucleotide-directed mutagenesis of DNA fragments cloned into M13 vectors. *Methods Enzymol.* **100**, 468–500.
8. Itakura, K., Rossi, J. J., and Wallace, R. B. (1984) Synthesis and use of synthetic oligonucleotides. *Ann. Rev. Biochem.* **53**, 323–356.
9. Botstein, D. and Shortle, D. (1985) Strategies and applications of in vitro mutagenesis. *Science* **229**, 1193–1201.
10. Kunkel, T. (1985) Rapid and efficient site-specific mutagenesis without phenotypic selection. *Proc. Natl. Acad. Sci. USA* **82**, 488–492.
11. Higuchi, R., Krummel, B., and Saiki, R. K. (1988) A general method of in vitro preparation and specific mutagenesis of DNA fragments: study of protein and DNA interactions. *Nucleic Acids Res.* **16**, 7351–7367.
12. Ho, S. N., Hunt, H. D., Horton, R. M., Pullen, J. K., and Pease, L. R. (1989) Site-directed mutagenesis by overlap extension using the polymerase chain reaction. *Gene* **77**, 51–59.
13. Goode, B. L. and Feinstein, S. C. (1992) "Speedprep" purification of template for double-stranded DNA sequencing. *Biotechniques* **12**, 373–374.
14. United States Biochemical (1994) Step-By-Step Protocols for DNA Sequencing with Sequenase Version 2.0 T7 DNA Polymerase (8th ed.).

CHAPTER 28

Saturation Mutagenesis by Mutagenic Oligonucleotide-Directed PCR Amplification (Mod-PCR)

Lillian W. Chiang

1. Introduction

Saturation mutagenesis is one approach for determining the contributions of individual base pairs or amino acids to the structure and function of defined DNA sequence elements or proteins, respectively (1). If a simple phenotypic screen is available, saturation mutagenesis can be used to determine the relative importance of regions (larger than single basepairs or amino acids) by dividing a large element into smaller regions and independently saturating each small region with random point mutations. The number and degree of phenotypic changes exhibited by each regionally distinct population of mutants indicate the importance of each region to the activity of the whole element (2).

For both analyses, the mutagenesis method for generating random base substitutions must allow for the isolation of populations of DNA molecules that are randomly and efficiently mutagenized in the targeted region and wild-type (WT) in the remaining nontargeted bases. This chapter describes mutagenic oligonucleotide-directed PCR amplification (Mod-PCR) wherein, base substitution mutations within the targeted region are incorporated during synthesis of a degenerate oligonucleotide to be used as a primer for PCR, and, PCR amplification with the degenerate primer and an opposing WT primer leads to incorporation of the mutant primer and restoration of the remaining WT bases of the element (Fig. 1). Cloning of the PCR products containing random mutations is

From: *Methods in Molecular Biology, Vol. 57: In Vitro Mutagenesis Protocols*
Edited by: M. K. Trower Humana Press Inc., Totowa, NJ

311

DNA SEQUENCE ELEMENT:

activator footprint

< AGCCGTT GCCGGTTATT AAGG CCGACACT GCCACCTGATT TTTTAGACTTGC CATCAGA >

-35 region   *-10 region*

Degenerate oligonucleotide synthesis (15% misincorporation, 10-base target)

DEGENERATE OLIGONUCLEOTIDE:

AATGGATCCAGCCGTT gccggttatt AAGG

BamHI

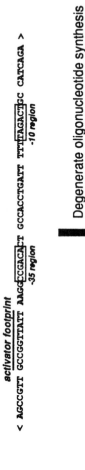

PCR amplification to incorporate mutations and produce double-stranded products.

EcoRI

opposing wildtype primer

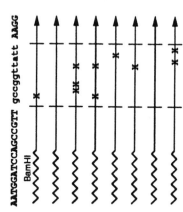
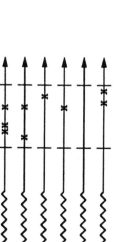

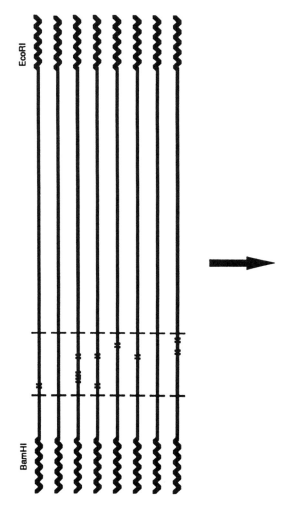

CLONE MUTANT POPULATION FOR SEQUENCING AND PHENOTYPIC ASSAYS

Fig. 1. Saturation mutagenesis of a DNA sequence element by Mod-PCR. The WT sequence of a hypothetical DNA sequence element is shown. The goal is to saturate the activator footprint (a 10-base target region) with base-substitution mutations. In the first step, a degenerate oligonucleotide encompassing the targeted region is synthesized on an automated DNA synthesizer (primers are drawn to correspond to the sequence with an arrowhead designating the 3'-end). When a nucleotide targeted for mutagenesis is reached (indicated by lowercase), the WT nucleotide is doped with 5% of each of the non-WT nucleotides (an X indicates a non-WT base incorporated during synthesis). In the second step, the remaining WT bases in the DNA sequence element are restored by PCR amplification using a WT primer for the opposing end. Restriction sites such as *EcoRI* and *BamHI* (indicated by jagged lines) engineered into the 5'-ends of the primers allow subsequent cloning of the mutant population for sequencing and phenotypic assays.

achieved by engineering restriction sites into the 5' ends of the PCR primers. Because the random mutagenesis is limited to the primer region, Mod-PCR is efficient for saturation mutagenesis of a 1–30-base region, depending on the primer length. Mod-PCR can be used with an overlap PCR strategy to extend the mutagenized region beyond 30 bases.

2. Materials

Solutions are stored at room temperature and enzymes are stored in a nonfrost-free −20°C freezer unless stated otherwise.

2.1. Degenerate Oligonucleotide Synthesis

1. Applied Biosystems DNA synthesizer model 380B.
2. β-Cyanoethyl phosphoramidites: Dilute from 1.0 g stocks (Applied Biosystems, Foster City, CA; A, #400326; G, #400327; C, #400328; and T, #400329) to 0.1M in acetonitrile under dry nitrogen gas to prevent reagent decomposition.
3. A/G/C/T cyanoethyl phosphoramidite (Applied Biosystems #400334).
4. 30% Ammonium hydroxide.
5. Ether: Saturate with H_2O just prior to use.

2.2. PCR Amplification, DNA Recovery, and Cloning

1. AmpliTaq polymerase (Perkin-Elmer Cetus, Norwalk, CT; 5 U/µL).
2. 10X amplification buffer: 100 mM Tris-HCl, pH 8.3, 500 mM KCl, 0.01% (w/v) gelatin. Store at −20°C.
3. 50 mM $MgCl_2$: Store at 4°C, not at −20°C, to prevent precipitation.
4. 10 mM dNTP stock: Dilute in H_2O from 100 mM stocks (Pharmacia, Uppsala, Sweden; pH 7.5, stored at −70°C) of dATP, dCTP, dGTP, and dTTP. Store 10 mM stock at −20°C for up to 1 mo.
5. WT primers at 20 µM in H_2O. Store at −20°C. For primer design, *see* Note 1.
6. WT PCR template can be a plasmid clone, genomic DNA, or cDNA, depending on the available source. The template preparation should be of sufficient quantity and quality to allow for efficient PCR amplification.
7. PCR grade mineral oil.
8. Chloroform: $CHCl_3$ is mixed at a 24:1 ratio by volume with isoamyl alcohol.
9. Phenol-chloroform: Phenol should be double-distilled and saturated with Tris-HCl, pH 8.0, then combined in equal ratio with chloroform solution (prepared as described in item 8). Store at −20°C. Thaw a stock that may be kept at 4°C until oxidation is observed by the appearance of pink color.
10. 1 mg/mL Bovine serum albumin (BSA): Diluted in H_2O from 10 mg/mL stock (New England Biolabs, Beverly, MA). Store at −20°C.
11. NuSieve agarose (FMC Bioproducts, Rockland, ME).

12. T4 DNA ligase (New England Biolabs; 400 U/µL).
13. 10X ligation buffer: 660 mM Tris-HCl, pH 7.5, 50 mM MgCl$_2$, 50 mM dithiothreitol, 10 mM ATP. Store at –20°C for up to 1 mo.
14. Cloning vector: Digested with appropriate restriction endonucleases (*Eco*RI and *Bam*HI are used for the example in this chapter), treated with calf intestine alkaline phosphatase (Boehringer Mannheim, Mannheim, Germany; stored at 4°C) to prevent religation of vector without insert during cloning, and gel purified.
15. 10X *Eco*RI/*Bam*HI restriction buffer: 1.5% Triton X-100, 1M NaCl, 500 mM Tris-HCl, pH 7.5, 100 mM β-mercaptoethanol, 50 mM MgCl$_2$.
16. Restriction enzymes *Eco*RI and *Bam*HI (New England Biolabs).

3. Methods

3.1. Degenerate Oligonucleotide Synthesis

Mutagenesis is achieved by synthesizing a degenerate primer for each target region. Alternatively, degenerate oligomers may be purchased from a custom synthesis facility. The strategy for introducing degeneracy to oligomers synthesized on an Applied Biosystems DNA synthesizer using the phosphoramidite method *(3,4)* is described below:

1. During synthesis of the WT portion of the degenerate oligomer (for primer design, *see* Note 2), during which the appropriate WT nucleotide is added to the synthesis chamber from one bottle (A, G, C, or T).
2. When a nucleotide targeted for mutagenesis is reached, the machine is programmed to add simultaneously equal volumes from two different bottles: one containing the WT nucleotide; the other containing an equimolar mixture of all four nucleotides. Thus, the resulting nucleotide mixture in the synthesis chamber contains mostly the WT nucleotide at that position, and a small amount of the three non-WT nucleotides depending on the dilution factor of the equimolar mixture (Fig. 2, *see* Note 3).
3. After synthesis is complete, a pool of oligonucleotides is obtained with random base substitutions in the targeted region at a misincorporation rate dependent on the dilution factor described step 2 (Fig. 2; *see* Notes 3 and 4).

Once the primers have been synthesized carry out the following:

4. Detach and remove the oligonucleotide protecting groups in 30% ammonium hydroxide by incubation at 55°C overnight.
5. Dry the primers down under vacuum and resuspend in 200 µL of H$_2$O.
6. Extract each primer three times with an equal volume of ether, ethanol precipitate, and resuspend in 100 µL of H$_2$O.

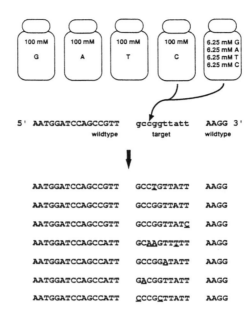

Fig. 2. Degenerate oligonucleotide synthesis. Symbols within bottles indicate concentrations of specific nucleotide presursors used for synthesis. In the nucleotide sequence, a, g, c, and t indicate positions targeted for misincorporation; for these positions, nucleotide precursors from two bottles are added simultaneously. In the resulting products A, G, C, and T indicate the nucleotide present; underlined nucleotides within the target region differ from the WT sequence.

3.2. PCR Amplification, DNA recovery, and Cloning

The random mutations generated by degenerate oligonucleotide synthesis are incorporated by using the degenerate primer in a PCR amplification reaction with the WT primer for the opposing end (Fig. 1). After restriction endonuclease digestion, the PCR products can be cloned into an appropriate vector for phenotypic assay and sequence analysis. A detailed protocol for PCR amplification, DNA recovery, and cloning is described herein. This chapter provides some commentary where appropriate concerning PCR and cloning optimization; a more detailed discussion can be obtained from a variety of PCR or cloning manuals *(5)*.

1. Carry out PCR amplifications in 100-μL reaction volumes containing 1X amplification buffer, 1.5–10 mM MgCl$_2$ optimized for specificity and

recovery of amplified product, 200 μM of each dNTP, 1 μM of the degenerate primer, 1 μM of the WT primer, 2.5 U of AmpliTaq polymerase, and 1 ng of denatured template (*see* Note 5). Overlay with 50 μL of mineral oil, and subject the reactions to 35 cycles of PCR: 1 min at 94°C to denature, 30 s at 45–55°C to anneal, and 2 min at 72°C to extend.

2. Extract the amplification products once with chloroform to remove the mineral oil, and then subject a 5-μL aliquot to minigel agarose electrophoresis to monitor the amount of product recovered.

3. Extract the remaining PCR product (~95 μL after minigel analysis) once with an equal volume of phenol-chloroform and then ethanol precipitate. Resuspend the pellet directly in 10 μL of 1X *Eco*RI/*Bam*HI restriction buffer containing 5 U of *Bam*HI and 2 U of *Eco*RI, and 0.1 mg/mL BSA. Carry out the digestions for 2 h at 37°C or overnight at room temperature.

4. Gel purify the products from a 4% NuSieve agarose gel and carry out ligations in the melted agarose according to the FMC Bioproducts protocols. Briefly, cut desired fragments from the gel after visualization by ethidium bromide staining, taking care to minimize exposure to short wavelength UV. Melt gel fragments at 65–68°C for 15 min, dilute at least threefold with warm (37–65°C) H$_2$O, and keep molten at 37°C. Add an appropriate amount of fragment (*see* Note 6) in a 10 μL volume to a 40 μL ligation reaction containing 0.5 μg vector, 1X ligase buffer, 0.05 mg/mL BSA, and 1 μL T4 DNA ligase. Leave on benchtop (room temperature) overnight to ligate.

5. Transform 8 μL of the ligation reaction into an appropriate competent *Escherichia coli* host strain and plate onto selective media (*see* Note 7).

Following transformation, colonies should be purified and cultured for plasmid preparation. Each clone needs to be sequenced to determine the individual base substitution mutations obtained. The distribution of mutant classes (0, 1, 2, or more substitutions per clone) is predicted by the binomial theorem and is dependent on the misincorporation rate during degenerate oligonucleotide synthesis. However, the observed distribution is influenced by other factors such as the differential hybridization efficiency of primers with variable numbers of mismatches during PCR (*see* Notes 8–10). After sequencing 374 clones generated with six different degenerate oligonucleotides synthesized at a misincorporation rate of 0.15, Chiang and Howe *(2)* observed that 20–66% of the sequenced clones contained mutations (34–80% of the clones contained no substitutions and were WT) (*see* Note 10).

4. Notes

1. Oligomers to be used as primers for PCR and DNA sequence analysis are designed to satisfy, as well as possible, the following criteria: 17–20 nucleotides (nt) homology to the template, a T_m of 52–56°C (by an estimate of 2°C for each A – T basepair and 4°C for G – C), an overall G + C content of 40–50%, pyrimidine tracts ≤6 nt, G-tracts ≤4 nt, purine tracts ≤ 4 nt, and an apparent lack of secondary structure. Restriction endonuclease sites (such as *Eco*RI and *Bam*HI), and 2–4 extra 5' nucleotides were designed into the primer 5'-ends to allow for and ensure complete restriction endonuclease cutting. Primer pairs for PCR should have <2 bp complementarity at the 3' ends to minimize primer-dimer formation.

2. In addition to the criteria described in Note 1, the degenerate primers should be designed with at least four WT nucleotides (nonmutagenized positions) on the 3' end to ensure efficient priming during the PCR step.

3. A sample calculation of misincorporation rate is given. If the equimolar A/G/C/T mix is diluted to 0.025M, each nucleotide is present at 6.25 mM or 1/16th of the 0.1M WT bottles (Fig. 2). The resulting nucleotide mixture in the synthesis chamber would contain 5% each of the three non-WT nucleotides and 85% WT, resulting in a misincorporation rate of 0.15/ nucleotide. If the region targeted for misincorporation were 10 bases, this would result in an average of 1.5 misincorporations (non-WT nucleotides) per oligomer, a level that maximizes the proportion of one- and two-base substitutions in the resulting pool of degenerate oligomers.

4. The five-bottle method described in this chapter (a total of five bottles containing nucleotide precursors for A, G, C, T, and A/G/C/T are required) minimizes nonrandom substitution that can result with the alternate method of preparing separately spiked A, G, C, and T mixes in addition to the WT bottles (eight bottles total). Chiang, Kovari, and Howe demonstrated that the mutagenesis is sufficiently random *(6)*. The distribution of base changes recovered in one experiment are shown in Fig. 3.

5. For PCR, 100 ng of a linearized plasmid is alkali denatured in a 10-µL vol of 0.2M NaOH for 15 min at room temperature, followed by 10-fold dilution into H$_2$O. One nanogram of denatured template is used immediately in each PCR amplification reaction. Alkali denaturation of the template may not be necessary for efficient PCR amplification. Alternatively, a 5-min incubation at 94°C prior to PCR thermal cycling may be sufficient to ensure complete denaturation of the template before the first annealing cycle. In addition, any of a variety of techniques such as Hot Start PCR may be used to maximize the yield of product.

6. A fragment:vector ratio of 1:1 to 3:1 works well for most ligations.

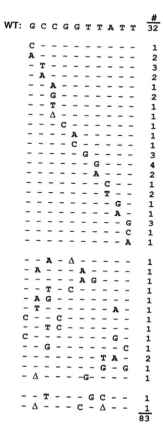

Fig. 3. Distribution of base changes recovered by Mod-PCR. A 10-base region in the *lys* promoter of bacteriophage Mu was mutagenized by Mod-PCR *(2,6)*. The WT DNA sequence of the region targeted for mutagenesis is shown at the top. The number of times a specific sequence was found is indicated on the right. For the mutants, only the mutant nucleotides are indicated; Δ represents a deleted nucleotide; the G in the last double mutant represents an inserted G.

7. A lack of any colonies present on the plate after transformation is usually attributable to low competency of the host strain. Obtaining clones at one order of magnitude dilution below that observed for intact control plasmid is an indication of a very successful ligation. For example, if ~200 colonies plate at a 10^{-1} dilution of the transformation mix for the intact plasmid, then ~200 colonies should appear for the undiluted transformation mix of the ligation reaction. Efficient mutagenesis by Mod-PCR requires efficient clon-

ing of the PCR product (i.e., ≥1000 transformants/ligation reaction). Another good control is to ligate vector without the PCR fragment added; the appearance of very few or zero colonies indicates complete restriction endonuclease digestion and thorough alkaline phosphatase treatment of the vector.

8. Parameters affecting annealing conditions during PCR, such as temperature, $MgCl_2$ concentration, and primer length/sequence are predicted to affect the distribution of mutant classes recovered. Each pool of degenerate primers generated is expected to consist of a binomial distribution of 0, 1, 2, and more base substitutions per oligomer depending on the misincorporation rate and target length. Annealing conditions are expected to have differential effects on the number of mismatches tolerated during hybridization of each mutant primer to the WT template for extension by *Taq* polymerase. Some have observed a bias against multiple mismatches *(2,6)*, others have not (Irina Artsimovitch and Martha M. Howe, personal communication, January 16, 1995).

9. The cloning step also contributes to variability in the distribution of mutant classes recovered. Since the degenerate primers consist of a heterogeneous population of primer sequences, some proportion of the PCR amplification product consists of heteroduplexes. This proportion approaches 100% if the PCR amplification plateaus and opposite-strand product out competes primers for hybridization to template. The DNA repair systems of the host strain will determine which strand of the heteroduplex is repaired.

10. The easiest way to alter the observed distribution of mutant classes is to change the misincorporation rate during degenerate oligonucleotide synthesis. For good Mod-PCR results, some time should be spent in optimizing PCR and cloning conditions. However, a considerable amount of time can be saved if multiple degenerate oligonucleotides (two or three) are synthesized using increasing misincorporation rates. Once mutants are obtained, a representative sampling (10–20) generated from each different primer can be sequenced to determine if an acceptable rate of mutagenesis was achieved. Alternatively, a colony hybridization assay *(7)* with a WT primer as probe can be used to detect and eliminate WT clones from further analysis.

Acknowledgments

I thank Martha M. Howe for providing support and advice while I was developing these techniques during my tenure in her laboratory, and David Albagli, Irina Artsimovitch, and Mallika Srinivasan for critical reading of the manuscript.

References

1. Bowie, J. U. and Sauer, R. T. (1989) Identifying determinants of folding and activity for a protein of unknown structure. *Proc. Natl. Acad. Sci. USA* **86,** 2152–2156.
2. Chiang, L. W. and Howe, M. M. (1993) Mutational analysis of a *C*-dependent late promoter of bacteriophage Mu. *Genetics* **135,** 619–629.
3. Matteucci, M. D. and Caruthers, M. H. (1981) Synthesis of deoxynucleotides on a polymer support. *J. Am. Chem. Soc.* **103,** 3185–3191.
4. Beaucage, S. L. and Caruthers, M. H. (1981) Deoxynucleoside phosphoramidites— a new class of intermediates for deoxypolynucleotide synthesis. *Tetrahedron Lett.* **22,** 1859–1862.
5. Cohen, D. M. (1991) Enzymatic amplification of DNA by PCR: standard procedures and optimization, in *Current Protocols in Molecular Biology* (Ausubel, F. M., Brent, R., Kingston, R. E., Moore, D. D., Seidman, J. G., Smith, J. A., and Struhl, K., eds.), Wiley, NY, pp. 15.1.1–15.1.7.
6. Chiang, L. W., Kovari, I., and Howe, M. M. (1993) Mutagenic oligonucleotide-directed PCR amplification (Mod-PCR): an efficient method for generating random base substitution mutations in a DNA sequence element. *PCR Methods Appl.* **2,** 210–217.
7. Duby, A., Jacobs, K. A., and Celeste, A. (1988) Using synthetic oligonucleotides as probes, in *Current Protocols in Molecular Biology* (Ausubel, F. M., Brent, R., Kingston, R. E., Moore, D. D., Seidman, J. G., Smith, J. A., and Struhl, K., eds.), Wiley, NY, pp. 6.4.1–6.4.10.

CHAPTER 29

Random Mutagenesis
of Short Target DNA Sequences via PCR
with Degenerate Oligonucleotides

Frank Kirchhoff
and Ronald C. Desrosiers

1. Introduction

Polymerase chain reaction (PCR) is a powerful technique for the amplification of specific DNA sequences, for the generation of chimeric molecules, and for site-directed mutagenesis. It allows the rapid generation of relatively large quantities of mutated DNA. Drawbacks are the costs of synthesizing oligonucleotide primers and the high error rates of thermostable polymerases relative to other DNA polymerases. In cases where extensive collections of mutations in defined target sequences are desired, it is often more efficient and cost effective to synthesize degenerate oligonucleotides in a single step. One elegant method to create primer libraries with the potential of all possible point mutations is to dope each of the four nucleoside phosphoamides with small amounts of the other three *(1)*. Alternatively, primers can also be generated by allowing misincorporation only at selected sites *(2)*. The frequencies and types of mutations in the degenerate oligonucleotides can be easily varied by the selection of doping nucleotide percentages at each step of the synthesis. In the early protocols, the complementary mutagenic oligonucleotides bore cohesive ends *(3)*, or contained flanking restriction sites *(4)*, to allow cloning. These approaches did not have general utility because of the need for conveniently located restriction sites at the

From: *Methods in Molecular Biology, Vol. 57: In Vitro Mutagenesis Protocols*
Edited by: M. K. Trower Humana Press Inc., Totowa, NJ

ends of the target sequence. In this chapter, we present a method that uses complex oligonucleotide mixtures to generate numerous changes in short target DNA sequences by PCR via splicing by overlap extension (SOE-PCR) *(5,6)*. The use of SOE-PCR makes it possible to use restriction sites distant from the target sequence for easy cloning, and also to minimize the size of the mutagenized PCR fragment compared to other PCR-based strategies in which complete plasmids are generated *(7–9)*. However, it is also possible to use recombinant PCR (R-PCR), in which the entire plasmid is amplified during PCR and recovered by homologous recombination after transformation of *Escherichia coli (9)*. It has recently been described that using alkaline denatured plasmid template results in both reduced background of wild-type clones and higher efficiencies of amplification *(10)*. SOE- and R-PCR with degenerate oligonucleotides provide rapid, simple, and effective means to generate a large number of mutant clones in defined target sequences.

2. Materials

Solutions are stored at room temperature unless stated otherwise.

2.1. Oligonucleotide Synthesis and PCR

1. Laboratory equipment:
   a. An automated DNA synthesizer plus the reagents and solvents for DNA synthesis. Degenerate oligonucleotides are also available from commercial suppliers.
   b. A thermocycler for PCR.
   c. Equipment and reagents for agarose gel electophoresis.
2. Ammonium hydroxide solution (25% [v/v]).
3. Oligonucleotide purification cartridges and reagents (Applied Biosystems, Foster City, CA).
4. 10 mM dNTPs (store at −20°C).
5. 10X PCR-buffer: 100 mM Tris-HCl, pH 8.3, 500 mM KCl (store at −20°C).
6. 25 mM MgCl$_2$ (store at −20°C).
7. *Taq* DNA Polymerase (5 U/µL) (store at −20°C).

Alternatively, other thermostable DNA polymerases can be used:

8. Mineral oil.
9. Reagents to purify DNA fragments from agarose gels (e.g., GeneClean or Mermaid kits, Bio 101 [La Jolla, CA]).

2.2. Cloning and Sequencing

1. Appropriate enzymes for restriction endonuclease digestion (store at –20°C).
2. T4 DNA ligase and ligation buffer (store at –20°C).
3. A suitable vector.
4. Competent *E. coli* (store at –80°C). Can be purchased from commercial suppliers (e.g., Stratagene [La Jolla, CA]).
5. Reagents and buffers for transformation and propagation of *E. coli*. Either as recommended by the suppliers of competent *E. coli*, or following the various standard protocols.
6. Equipment and reagents for DNA sequence analysis (store as suggested by the manufacturer).

3. Methods
3.1. Oligonucleotide Design and Synthesis

The two inner mutagenic oligonucleotides are designed so that they span the entire target sequence (*see* Note 1). The 3' ends of these primers should extend 3–5 nucleotides into the region outside the area to be mutagenized to obtain mutations over the entire target sequence with a comparable efficiency. Mismatches close to the 3' ends of the mutagenic primers result in inefficient amplification. Therefore, these positions are less frequently mutagenized in the final PCR product.

Depending on the GC-content and mismatch frequencies, the 5' ends should overlap by at least 15–20 nucleotides (*see* Note 2). Based on the specific experiment, the lengths, positions, as well as the mutation frequencies of the respective oligonucleotides will vary (*see* Note 3).

The outer primers are used to generate amplification products containing convenient restriction sites for cloning. The oligonucleotides themselves can contain unique restriction sites, or alternatively, convenient restriction sites may be present within the amplified fragment (*see* Note 4).

If random point mutations over the whole oligonucleotide sequence are desired, dope the nucleoside phoshoamidite solutions with the chosen amount of the others prior to synthesis of the inner primerset (Fig. 1A) (*see* Note 5). The frequency of change for each position can be briefly calculated on the basis of the amounts of the precursors present in the solution. For example, we obtained approximately a 4.5% mutation rate by doping each vial of phosphoamidites with 1.5% (v/v) of the other three (*see* Note 6). The mutation frequencies can easily be changed by altering the concentrations of the respective phosphoamidite mixes.

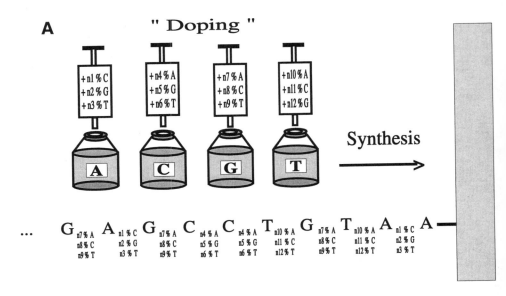

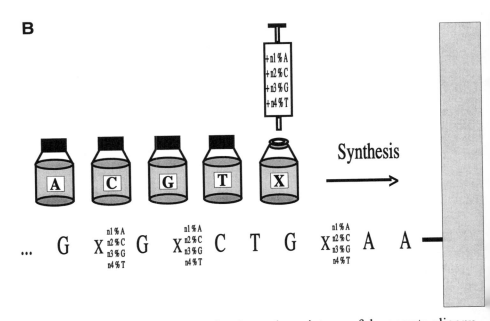

Fig. 1. Strategies for the synthesis of complex mixtures of degenerate oligonucleotides. **(A)** Each vial of phosphoamidites may be doped with various percentages
(n1–n12) of the other three to obtain mutagenic changes throughout the entire synthesis. **(B)** Incorporation of changes at certain positions using the X position.

Moreover, changes can be introduced just at certain nucleotide positions, e.g., by doping just the A-amidite, or changes to a certain nucleotide can be introduced at all positions, e.g., by just adding the A-amidite solution to the other three (*see* Note 7).

Changes can also be introduced at particular positions by using the X-position of the synthesizer. Prior to synthesis the appropriate amounts of nucleoside phoshoamidites to be used are poured in the X-flask (*see* Fig. 1B). For most synthesizers the program can be interrupted at certain steps and the X-flask can be replaced if different combinations of A/C/ G/T phosphoamidites are desired (*see* Note 8).

1. Synthesize the oligonucleotides. Prior to synthesis make sure that the reagents are fresh (*see* Note 9). It is useful to flush the reagent lines prior to synthesis to remove old, homogenous phoshoamidite solutions (*see* Note 10).
2. Cleave the protected oligonucleotides from the columns by standard treatment with ammonium hydroxide following synthesis and purify the primers on oligonucleotide purification cartridges (Applied Biosystems) according to the protocols of the manufacturer. Adjust the oligonucleotide concentrations after purification (e.g., to 100 pmol/2.5 µL in water).

3.2. PCR Conditions

An outline of the procedure is given in Fig. 2. We describe a basic protocol that worked in our hands for most applications and should be used before attempting variations. However, in some experiments the annealing temperature, the pH of the buffer, the dNTP concentrations and/or the Mg^{2+} concentration need to be adjusted to obtain a satisfactory amount of specific product (*see* Notes 11 and 12).

1. Prepare two separate standard PCR reactions to generate two PCR products that contain mutations in the region of overlap as follows (*see* Note 13). Add 10 µL PCR buffer, 3 µL of each dNTP, 10 µL 25 m*M* MgCl$_2$, 2.5 U *Taq* DNA polymerase, 10–50 ng of template DNA, and 25–100 pmol of each primer (*see* Note 14) to a 0.5-mL Eppendorf tube and adjust the total reaction volume to 100 µL with distilled water. Overlay the reaction mix with mineral oil to prevent evaporation.
2. Transfer the tubes to a thermal cycler and initiate the cycling program (25 cycles, 1 min at 94°C, 1 min at 45°C, 1 min at 72°C) (*see* Note 15). After the final cycle an additional step at 68–72°C for 5 min should be performed to ensure complete extension. To optimize the a replication fidelity, the initial annealing temperatures should be as high as possible, while still allowing efficient amplification with the degenerate primers.

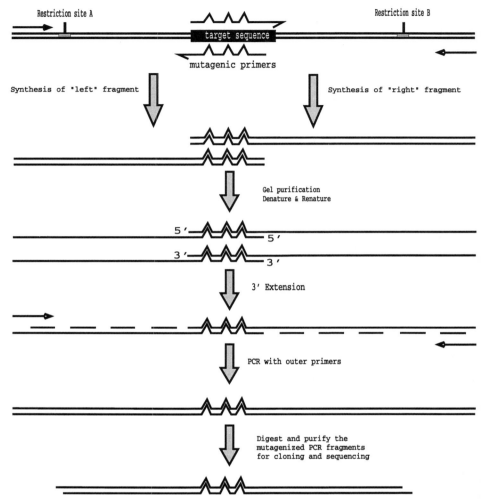

Fig. 2. Strategy for random mutagenesis of defined target sequences by SOE-PCR. The right and left halves are first amplified separately with overlapping "inside" primers containing mismatches. Subsequently, the two separate PCR products are combined and full-length products are obtained by 3' extension and amplification with the outer set of primers. Finally the mutagenized PCR products are digested with appropriate restriction enzymes, cloned, and sequenced.

3. Run 20 µL PCR product on a 1% agarose gel to determine the yield of the PCR reaction. Excise the correct sized band and purify the DNA by standard methods to remove excess primers and wild-type sequences (*see* Note 16).

4. Analyze an aliquot (20–50%) of the purified fragments by electrophoresis in an agarose gel to estimate the amount of DNA obtained (*see* Note 17).
5. Combine the purified primary PCR products in approximately equimolar amounts. Setup the secondary PCR reaction as described (*see* Section 3.2., step 1); add only the outer primers (*see* Fig. 2) and about 0.1–0.5 pmol of the mixed left and right half fragments to the reaction mix. Transfer to a thermocycler and start cycling as described (*see* Section 3.2., step 2 and Note 18). Under PCR conditions, heteroduplex molecules will form that can be extended at their 3' ends and amplified with the outer set of primers to generate a double-stranded fragment with random changes in the target sequence.

3.3. Cloning and DNA Sequencing

Cloning strategies and research applications vary with the individual experiments. Therefore, we give only a brief outline of the basic procedure which may need to be modified to fit the different applications.

1. Run 20 µL of the second PCR reaction on an agarose gel.
2. If only the correct-sized product is visible under UV light, digest an aliquot of the secondary PCR product with the appropriate restriction enzyme(s) and ligate it to a cleaved and dephosphorylated vector. If additional bands are visible, excise the signal of interest and purify the DNA prior to cutting (*see* Note 16).
3. Transform an aliquot of the ligation reaction into a suitable competent strain of *E. coli*.
4. Depending on the subsequent application, the target sequences of randomly picked individual clones can be determined by dideoxynucleotide sequencing, or mixed plasmid populations can be used for selection experiments prior to sequence analysis. Clones selected for further analysis should be sequenced across the entire PCR-derived portion (*see* Note 19).

4. Notes

1. The length of the target region which can be mutagenized in one step depends on the efficiency of the oligonucleotide synthesis. Some automated DNA synthesizers can produce degenerate oligonucleotides >100 nucleotides in length. Moreover, larger target regions can be mutagenized by using several sets of mutagenic primers corresponding to different segments of the target sequence *(1,2)*. Also, the oligonucleotides do not need to overlap completely. Therefore, two degenerate 40-mers with a 15-bp overlap region allow mutagenesis over 65 bp of target sequence. Note that

the frequency of changes is higher in the overlapping region because both strands contain mutations.

2. The primary PCR products must overlap enough to allow efficient binding. As with the PCR primers, the length of the overlap, necessary to achieve this, depends on the PCR conditions, GC content, and the degeneracy of the oligonucleotides used.

3. As indicated in Fig. 1, the frequencies and types of mutations can be easily varied during synthesis. The major limitation is simply that a substantial percentage of the degenerate primers must still bind to its target sequence to allow efficient amplification. Although low annealing temperatures and high MgCl$_2$ concentrations during cycling will favor nonspecific amplification, it is usually not useful to incorporate more than 1 change per 10 bases.

4. If the restriction sites used for cloning are inside the amplified fragment, it is easy to visualize the efficiency of the restriction digests by gel electrophoresis. If the restriction sites are the outer primers, be sure to add a few bases to the 5' ends of the outer primers to allow efficient restriction endonuclease digestion.

5. We mixed the predisolved phosphoamidite solutions prior to synthesis *(1)*. Others prepared their doped amidite pots by mixing preweighted aliquots of the individual nucleoside phosphoramidites *(11)*.

6. We and others *(1,2,9)* observed somewhat lower than expected mutation frequencies. Inefficient PCR amplification with mismatched primers and inefficient survival of mismatched sequences in *E. coli* may contribute to lower than expected frequencies of mutation. These discrepancies will increase, the more degenerate the mutagenic oligonucleotides are, and finally lead to inefficient amplification.

7. A method in which A residues in particular were mutagenized has been described *(2)*. In this paper they also controlled the number of changes per oligonucleotide by adjusting the proportion of A versus C/G/T in the X reservoir.

8. Some synthesizers allow programmed mixing, or have up to eight positions for phoshoamidite solutions. This makes it even more convenient to alter the misincorporation rate at each individual coupling step.

9. It is important to use fresh reagents particularly for the mixed phosphoamidite solutions to minimize any bias in nucleotide addition. G residues in particular are added relatively poorly if the reagents are not fresh.

10. Residual homogenous phosphoamidite solutions will reduce the misincorporation rate for the first of each G/A/T and C nucleotide added to the column if the reagent lines are not flushed prior to synthesis.

11. An applicable annealing temperature is usually 5°C below the T_m of the primers used for amplification. The T_m (°C) value can very roughly be calculated by the formula:

(number of G + C residues) × 4 + (number of A + T residues) × 2

Stringent annealing temperatures will help to increase specificity. However, with mixtures of degenerate oligonucleotides, selection of too high annealing temperatures is problematic; only well-matched primers will allow amplification under these conditions, resulting in reduced mutation frequencies and product yield. Therefore, depending on the frequency of mismatches present in the primers, lower annealing temperatures have to be used. The *Taq* DNA polymerase is active over a broad range of temperatures and will allow primer extension.

12. It can be highly advantageous to optimize the PCR. PCR optimization kits from various suppliers might be useful for some applications. *Taq* DNA polymerase concentrations of 0.5–5 U/100 µL reaction may give satisfactory results. dNTP concentrations between 20 and 200 µ*M* are recommended; low concentrations increase specificity and fidelity. Higher concentrations have to be used to amplify long DNA fragments. All four dNTPs have to be used at equivalent amounts. The Mg^{2+} concentration affects the product specifity and optimization over the range of 0.5–6 m*M* magnesium might be benefical. EDTA or other chelators can disturb the apparent optimum.

13. Alternatively, R-PCR with the degenerate primers can be used to amplify the whole plasmid. This method has the advantage that no enzymatic reaction other than PCR is required, and only two sets of oligonucleotides and a single step of PCR are necessary prior to cloning in *E. coli*. However, inefficient amplification of full-length plasmid may result in inefficient retrieval of mutant clones. Moreover, background levels of unmutated template plasmids can be relatively high. Du et al. *(10)* recently described R-PCR with alkaline-denatured plasmid template. This procedure resulted in reduced background and better yields of PCR products. As with SOE-PCR, sequencing is required to authenticate DNA fragments to be used.

14. For degenerate primers, degeneracy at the 3' ends is not useful because these primers are inefficiently extended. Complementarity at the 3' ends promotes the formation of primer-dimers and reduces the yield of the desired product. The primers should not contain palindromic sequences. Furthermore, more than two Cs or Gs at the 3' ends should be avoided to prevent mispriming at G + C-rich sequences. The use of specific computer programs might help with the primer design.

15. Because the number of target molecules used in this approach is high, 25–30 cycles should be sufficient. Typical denaturation conditions are 94°C for 30 s to 1 min. For G + C-rich targets, higher temperatures or longer denaturation times might be necessary. The extension time depends on the length of the target sequence and on temperature. About 1 min extension time/kb to be amplified is applicable.
16. UV light damages DNA. Use low UV light (~366 nm) to excise the DNA. It is preferable to use an aliquot of the PCR product to take a photo for documentation and a second aliquot for DNA isolation to minimize damage. We purified PCR products >400 bp with the GeneClean kit, and fragments <400 bp with the Mermaid kit from Bio 101. Low melt agarose or other standard methods can also be used.
17. The product amounts can be briefly calculated by comparison of the signal intensities with those of fragments with known concentrations, like marker bands.
18. Efficiency may be increased by running 6–10 cycles of PCR at low annealing temperature with the right and left half fragments without the outer primers to generate the full-length template first (Fig. 2, extension step). If the outer primers are added to the reaction right away, the first 6–10 cycles should be done at low annealing temperature to allow efficient binding in the region of overlap containing the mismatches, followed by 20–25 cycles at higher temperatures to amplify the full-sized product with the perfectly matching outer primers.
19. Random substitution rates of 1/840 to 1/4000 bp outside the region covered by the mutagenic oligonucleotides have been described *(1,2,5)*. These frequencies, as well as the fidelities of other thermostable polymerases, depend on the conditions used, and it is necessary to sequence the whole PCR-derived portion to exclude undesired mutations. For some applications (e.g., the amplification of larger fragments), it may be preferable to use themostable polymerases with higher fidelities than *Taq* DNA polymerase, like *Vent* (New England Biolabs, Beverly, MA) or *Pfu* polymerase (Stratagene), for amplification.

Acknowledgments

The authors thank Hilary G. Morrison and Dean Regier for their helpful advice. F. Kirchhoff is supported by a fellowship of the German BmFT AIDS program and by a grant of the Deutsche Forschungsgesellschaft.

References

1. Kirchhoff, F. W. and Desrosiers, R. C. (1993) A PCR-derived library of random point mutations within the V3 region of simian immunodeficiency virus. *PCR Methods Appl.* **2,** 301–304.

2. Morrison, H. G. and Desrosiers, R. C. (1993) A PCR-based stratagy for extensive' mutagenesis of a target DNA sequence. *BioTechniques* **14,** 454–457.
3. Hutchinson, C. A., Nordeen, S. K., Vogt, K., and Edgell, M. H. (1986) A complete library of point substitution mutations in the glucocorticoid response element of mouse mammary tumor virus. *Proc. Natl. Acad. Sci.* **83,** 710–714.
4. Hill, D. E., Oliphant, A. R., and Struhl, K. (1987) Mutagenesis with degenerate oligonucleotides: an efficient method for saturating a defined DNA region with base pair substitutions. *Methods Enzymol.* **155,** 558–568.
5. Ho, S. N., Hunt, H. D., Horton, R. M., Pullen, J. K., and Pease, L. R. (1989) Site directed mutagenesis by overlap extension using the polymerase chain reaction. *Gene* **77,** 51–59.
6. Horton, R. M., Hunt, H. D., Ho, S. N., Pullen, J. K., and Pease, L. R. (1989) Engineering hybrid genes without the use of restriction enzymes: gene splicing by overlap extension. *Gene* **77,** 61–68.
7. Hemsley, A., Arnheim, N., Toney, M. D., Cortopassi, G., and Galas, D. J. (1989) A simple method for site-directed mutagenesis using the polymerase chain reaction. *Nucleic Acids Res.* **17,** 6545–6551.
8. Jones, D. H., Skamoto, K., Vorce, R. L., and Howard, B. H. (1990) DNA mutagenesis and recombination. *Nature* **344,** 793,794.
9. Jones, D. H. and Howard, B. H. (1991) A rapid method for recombination and site-specific mutagenesis by placing homologous ends on DNA using polymerase chain reaction. *BioTechniques* **10,** 62–66.
10. Du, Z., Regier, D. A., and Desrosiers, R. C. (1995) An improved recombinant PCR mutagenesis procedure that uses alkaline-denatured plasmid template. *BioTechnques* **18,** 376–378.
11. Siderovski, D. P., Matsuyama, T., Frigerio, E., Chui, S., Min. X., Erfle, H., Sumner-Smith, M., Barnett, R. W., and Mak, T. W. (1992) Random mutagenesis of the human immunodeficiency virus type 1 trans-activator of transcription (HIV-1 Tat). *Nucleic Acids Res.* **20,** 5311–5320.

CHAPTER 30

Random Sequence Mutagenesis for the Generation of Active Enzymes

Margaret E. Black and Lawrence A. Loeb

1. Introduction

Classically, studies on the relationships between structure and function have focused on the synthesis of individual molecular species and then analyzed their functions in cells. Recently, an entirely different approach has become feasible. A series of techniques has made it possible to simultaneously synthesize enormous numbers of related species of molecules and to select from these libraries specific molecules encoding unique activities (Fig. 1). Vast libraries of proteins *(1,2)*, RNA *(3)*, DNA *(4)*, and small organic molecules *(5)* have been assembled. From these libraries molecules have been selected based on binding *(6)* and catalytic activities *(7)*.

Random sequence mutagenesis in concert with positive genetic selection is an incredibly powerful method to study the structure–function relationship in enzymes. One of the greatest strengths of this methodology is the possibility of creating enzymes with altered activities (altered substrate specificity) or even novel functions. It allows one to test all possible amino acid substitutions at any one position over a wide range of codons and to select functional enzymes from an enormous population of plasmids containing random nucleotide substitutions within genes. Sequence information of active clones can identify essential residues or positions depending on the number and type of amino acid able to functionally substitute for the wild-type residue. This technique allows one to rapidly identify important residues in a very short

From: *Methods in Molecular Biology, Vol. 57: In Vitro Mutagenesis Protocols*
Edited by: M. K. Trower Humana Press Inc., Totowa, NJ

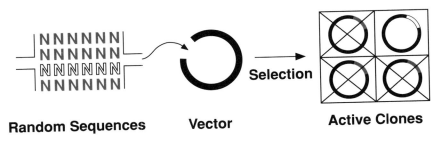

N N N N N N		
N N N N N N		
N N N N N N		
N N N N N N		

Random Sequences   **Vector**   **Active Clones**

Fig. 1. Overview of random sequence mutagenesis. Random sequences (NNN) are inserted into an expression vector. After transformation of the selection strain with a population of random sequence-containing plasmids, the active clones are selected on the basis of positive genetic selection.

period of time without protein purification or extensive biochemical or biophysical analysis.

Random sequence mutagenesis employs a plasmid backbone that encodes the gene of interest with restriction endonuclease sites flanking the segment to be replaced by an oligonucleotide containing the target randomized sequence *(4)*. In order to synthesize the insert, two overlapping complementary oligonucleotides (one or both) containing random sequences are hybridized, extended with DNA polymerase to produce a duplex, cut at restriction sites engineered into the ends of each oligonucleotide, and then ligated into a DNA vector. After ligation the recombinant molecules are used to transform *Escherichia coli*, and functional clones are identified on the basis of genetic complementation (Fig. 1). By sequencing the substituted segment of the plasmids obtained from bacteria that grow under selective conditions one obtains a catalog of all the amino acid changes at each position within the randomly mutagenized segment that encode an active enzyme. Any position that is permissive for a variety of amino acid residues suggests that the wild-type residue at that position is not essential or important for function *(7,8)*. Obversely, if no residues other than the wild-type residue are tolerated, then that position and particular residue are likely to be essential. Further analysis of such mutants will aid in identifying how particular residues are involved in catalysis or structural integrity. In this chapter, we describe and discuss the use of random sequence mutagenesis for the generation of random mutations in concert with selection of active recombinant molecules toward the identification of essential residues.

2. Materials
2.1. Purification of Oligonucleotides
Store at –20°C unless otherwise stated.

1. Random oligonucleotides (*see* Note 1).
2. 12–20% Urea-containing polyacrylamide gel *(9)*.
3. TBE (10X) buffer: 44.5 mM Tris base, 44.5 mM boric acid, 1 mM EDTA, pH 8.0. Store at room temperature.
4. DIF: Deionized formamide.
5. PEI cellulose TLC plate (EM Science, Gibbtown, NJ) or Parafilm (American National Can, Greenwich, CT): Store at 4°C.
6. Gel elution buffer: 0.5M NH$_4$Ac, 10 mM MgAc. Store at room temperature.
7. C18 SepPak (Waters, Milford, MA) or PolyPak (Glen Research, Herndon, VA): Store at room temperature.
8. T4 polynucleotide kinase (10 U/µL, New England Biolabs, Beverly, MA).
9. [γ^{32}P]ATP (10 pmol, 3000 Ci/mmol, DuPont New England Nuclear, Boston, MA).
10. Kinase buffer (10X): 0.5M Tris-HCl, pH 9.5, 0.1M MgCl$_2$, 50 mM dithiothreitol, 10 mM spermidine, 1 mM EDTA.

2.2. Preparation of Double-Stranded DNA from Oligonucleotides Containing Random Sequences
Store at –20°C unless otherwise stated.

1. Annealing buffer (10X): 70 mM Tris-HCl, pH 7.5, 60 mM MgCl$_2$, 200 mM Nacl.
2. 10 mM dNTPs: 10 mM of each dATP, dCTP, dGTP, and dTTP.
3. 0.1M Dithiothreitol. Filter sterilize.
4. *E. coli* DNA Polymerase I, Klenow fragment (5 U/µL).
5. Polymerase chain reaction (PCR) buffer (10X): 200 mM Tris-HCl, pH 8.3, 250 mM KCl, 15 mM MgCl 0.5% Tween-20.
6. 10 mg/mL Bovine serum albumin (BSA).
7. PCR primers (*see* Note 2).
8. *Taq* DNA polymerase: 5 U/µL (Perkin-Elmer Cetus, Norwalk, CT).
9. Mineral oil for PCR overlay. Store at room temperature.
10. Restriction endonucleases. These depend on the cloning sites used.

2.3. Ligation, Preparation of Competent Cells, and Transformation
1. Ligase buffer (10X): 0.5M Tris-HCl, pH 7.8, 0.1M MgCl$_2$, 10 mM dithiothreitol, 10 mM ATP, 250 µg/mL BSA. Store at –20°C.

2. *E. coli* strain (*see* Note 3).
3. 2X YT medium: 16 g tryptone, 10 g yeast extract, 5 g NaCl/L. For agar, add 15 g agar/L. Autoclave. Store at room temperature.
4. 10% Glycerol. Filter sterilize. Store at room temperature.
5. SOC: 2% Bactotryptone, 0.5% yeast extract, 10 m*M* NaCl, 2.5 m*M* KCl, 10 m*M* MgCl$_2$, 10 m*M* MgSO$_4$, 20 m*M* glucose. Filter sterilize. Store at 4°C.

3. Methods
3.1. Oligonucleotides
3.1.1. Purification of Oligonucleotides

Oligonucleotides can be purchased from a number of companies or can often be produced in house. It is important that the purity be high because the presence of incompletely elongated oligonucleotides will decrease hybridization and reduce the efficiency of subsequent processes. Purification of the full length oligonucleotide product is outlined in the following steps.

1. Add an equivalent volume of deionized formamide (DIF) to the oligonucleotide (20–50 µg) generally in a final volume of 100–200 µL.
2. Heat denature the mix at 95°C for 5 min to reduce secondary structure prior to loading onto 12–20% urea-containing polyacrylamide 1X TBE gels.
3. After electrophoresis, transfer the gel to Saran wrap and place it (gel side up) on a PEI cellulose TLC plate (EM Science) or on a piece of parafilm (American National Can). Using a hand-held UV lamp, the oligonucleotide bands can be visualized by UV shadowing. The PEI plate increases visualization of the UV adsorbing bands.
4. Excise and place the gel slice containing the full-length product in a 1.7-mL microfuge tube containing sufficient gel elution buffer to cover the excised gel slice. Wrap the tube lid with parafilm to prevent desiccation and incubate at 37°C overnight.
5. The next day aspirate the solution into a new tube and combine it with approx 200–500 µL of gel elution buffer used to rinse the gel slice.
6. Centrifuge the pooled supernatants several min to remove any acrylamide traces that may subsequently plug the column. Prepare either a C-18 SepPak (Waters) or PolyPak (Glen Research) reverse phase column and use it according to the manufacturer's instructions.
7. Dry each elution fraction completely in a Savant Spin Vac system or similar system.
8. Resuspend each fraction in 100 µL and take 1 µL for an OD$_{260}$ measurement. The majority of the oligonucleotide is eluted in the first fraction.

9. Calculate the concentration of purified oligonucleotides using extinction coefficients (*see* Note 4).

3.1.2. Visualization of Purified Oligonucleotides

For analysis of the purity of the oligonucleotides either before or after gel purification the following phosphorylation experiment can be performed with visualization of the products by autoradiography using 12–20% sequencing gels. Furthermore, the subsequent annealing and extension reactions can also be followed by using labeled oligonucleotides if desired.

1. Combine 3 μL [γ^{32}P]ATP, 1 μL 10X kinase buffer, 1 μL T4 polynucleotide kinase (10 U/μL), 2 μL purified oligonucleotide (10 pmol/μL), and 3 μL H$_2$O.
2. Incubate at 37°C for 30 min.
3. Heat denature the reaction at 95°C for 5 min prior to loading onto a denaturing 12–20% polyacrylamide-urea gel in 1X TBE buffer *(9)*. These samples should be run with radiolabeled molecular weight markers.
4. Cover the gel with Saran wrap and expose to X-ray film for 5–10 min. The major band should be the full-length oligonucleotide.

3.2. Preparation of Double-Stranded DNA from Oligonucleotides

3.2.1. Annealing

The next step involves hybridization of the two complementary, overlapping oligonucleotides (Fig. 2). In order to form stable hybrids, the overlapping area of complementarity should be at least 12–15 nucleotides in length.

1. Combine equimolar concentration of the oligonucleotides in a final volume of 40 μL (50 pmol of oligo #1, 50 pmol of oligo #2, 4 μL 10X annealing buffer).
2. Incubate the mixture at 95°C for 5 min.
3. Move the tube to a water bath or heating block at 65°C for 20 min.
4. Allow the reaction mixture to equilibrate to room temperature for a further 10 min.
5. Place the annealing reaction on ice.

3.2.2. Extension, Amplification, and Digestion

3.2.2.1. EXTENSION

By annealing the two oligonucleotides together the two 3' hydroxy termini are immediately upstream from a region of the oligonucleotide

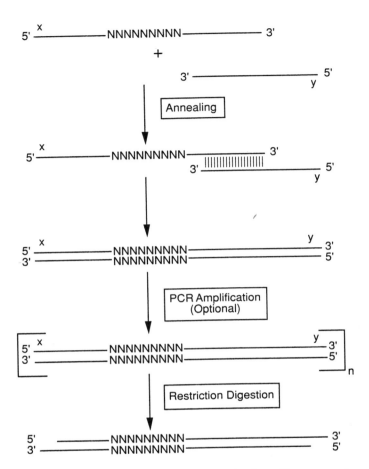

Fig. 2. Generation of random sequences for cloning. Two complementary, overlapping oligonucleotides with random sequences (NNN) on one or both strands are annealed together to form a duplex. Each oligonucleotide contains a restriction endonuclease site (X or Y) at the 5' end. A double-stranded fragment is created by extension of the two overlapping 3' ends with DNA polymerase (Klenow fragment). Amplification of the random double-stranded fragments is achieved by PCR. Prior to ligation with the restricted vector, the PCR products are digested with endonucleases X and Y and isolated from nondenaturing acrylamide gels.

that can serve as a template for chain elongation (Fig. 2). In this step, the Klenow fragment of *E. coli* DNA *Pol*I is used to elongate the primer strands and thus synthesize a complete double-stranded oligonucleotide. The result of such a synthesis is a double-stranded fragment with complete complementarity including the segments containing the random nucleotides. The entire library is random but each individual molecule contains two complementary DNA strands. If a large amount of random inserts will be needed, the double-stranded fragment is then amplified by PCR. The amplification step may be omitted if enough of the double-stranded fragment is produced. Restriction with the appropriate endonucleases at sites proximal to the ends of each oligonucleotide (now the ends of the dsDNA fragment) is done to aid in cloning efficiency. The doubly restricted fragment is then isolated and purified from nondenaturing 5–8% acrylamide gels.

1. For the extension reaction, add the following components to the 40 μL annealing reaction: 4 μL 10X annealing buffer, 5.6 μL 10 m*M* dNTPs, 1.6 μL 0.1*M* dithiothreitol, 4.8 μL Klenow (5 U/μL) in a final volume of 80 μL.
2. Incubate the extension reaction at 37°C for 30 min.
3. Inactivate the DNA polymerase (Klenow fragment) by incubation for at least 10 min at 65°C.
4. Incubate the reaction for 10 min at room temperature to allow rehybridization of denatured duplexes.
5. *See* Note 5.

3.2.2.2. AMPLIFICATION

Amplification of the extended products can be achieved by using PCR (Fig. 2). This is an optional step and can be omitted. We use a mixture of all the reagents except the extended products and aliquot the mixture into a number of small microfuge tubes containing the extended products or a control that lacks template DNA. In this fashion, the same concentration level of all the reagents in relation to the template DNA is maintained (*see* Note 6).

1. Combine the following ingredients: 50 μL 10X PCR buffer, 200 pmol of each PCR primer, 2 μL 10 mg/mL BSA, 2.5 μL 10 m*M* dNTPs, 2 μL *Taq* polymerase (5 U/μL), and H$_2$O in a final volume of 69.5 μL.
2. To each reaction tube add 13.9 μL of the mixture, 1–10 pmol of the extended product, and H$_2$O to a final volume of 100 μL.
3. Overlay the final reaction mixture with one drop of mineral oil.
4. Run 30 cycles of amplification in a DNA Thermal Cycler (Perkin-Elmer Cetus) using cycles of 94°C for 1 min, 34°C for 2 min, with a 7 min incubation at 72°C and left at 4°C (*see* Note 7).
5. Monitor the degree of amplification by running 1/10 the PCR on a 2–3% agarose gel (1X TBE), a MetaPhor gel (*see* Note 8), or a 5–8% nonde-

naturing acrylamide (1X TBE) gel depending on the size of the expected product.

3.2.2.3. DIGESTION

Restriction endonucleases are used to digest at sites engineered into the 5' ends of the mutagenic oligonucleotides (Fig. 2). This creates sticky ends for ligation and allows directional cloning into the prepared vector (Fig. 3). At this stage the fragments can be digested directly from the PCR or precipitated with ethanol prior to digestion with restriction enzymes.

1. Use approx 3–5 U of each endonuclease per microgram DNA and incubate for 2–4 h at the appropriate temperature to ensure complete digestion.
2. To assess whether the digestion is complete, run a portion of the reaction mixture on an 8% acrylamide gel (nondenaturing) or 3–4% MetaPhor gel (1X TBE) alongside the uncut product and products digested with either one of the endonucleases.
3. Purify the doubly digested fragment from an 8% nondenaturing acrylamide 1X TBE gel as described in the Section 3.1.1., or remove the small end fragments by gel filtration or ultrafiltration (Centricon microconcentrator, Amicon, Beverly, MA).

3.4. Vector Preparation

The next step is to prepare the vector containing the gene of interest by removing the DNA sequences between the restriction sites into which the pool of random fragments will be ligated (Fig. 3). We use a "dummy" vector in place of a vector containing the full-length, functional gene in order to reduce the frequency of false positives owing to incomplete digestion and/or religation.

1. Vector considerations (*see* Note 9).
2. Create a "dummy" vector (Fig. 3) (*see* Note 10).
3. Purify DNA by CsCl density gradient ultracentrifugation or by column chromatography, such as the Qiagen tip-500 columns (Qiagen, Chatsworth, CA) (*see* Note 11).
4. We typically digest 10 μg of DNA in a 100-μL vol with 3–5 U of each enzyme per microgram of DNA at the appropriate temperature for 1–2 h.
5. Remove a small aliquot (2 μL) from the digestion mix and run it on a 1% agarose/1X TBE gel to confirm complete digestion.
6. When complete digestion is confirmed, pour a preparative agarose gel and electrophorese the remaining digested vector DNA.
7. Stain the gel in ethidium bromide **(Caution: Carcinogenic.)** and excise the correct fragment band using a razor blade or scalpel.

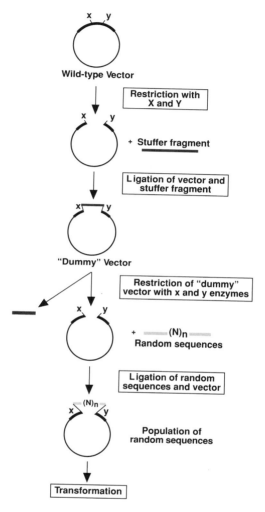

Fig. 3. Construction and use of a "dummy" vector. Creation of a "dummy" vector is achieved by replacement of the wild-type sequence in the region to be mutagenized with a larger, unrelated fragment (stuffer fragment). This is accomplished by restricting the wild-type vector with endonucleases X and Y, gel purification of the vector backbone, and ligation to a stuffer fragment. A large preparation of "dummy" vector DNA is then made and a portion restricted with X and Y. After gel purification of the plasmid backbone, random sequences are ligated to generate a library of plasmids containing a population of random sequences. The library is then used to transform *E. coli*, generally by electroporation.

8. Gel purify the excised band using GeneClean II (Bio 101, La Jolla, CA) according to their protocols (*see* Note 12).
9. Determine the efficiency and quality of gel purification by OD_{260} measurements and checking 0.2 μg of purified vector on a 1% agarose/1X TBE gel with the appropriate controls.

3.5. Ligation

Vector and insert DNAs are mixed and ligated together to create a pool of plasmids containing random sequences. This pool is then used to transform *E. coli* or other appropriate hosts that may be used for selection or screening.

1. Ligations are performed with roughly equimolar concentrations of insert and vector backbone in 1X ligase buffer and ligase (10 U/μL) in a 40-μL vol (*see* Note 13).
2. Incubate at 12–16°C overnight.
3. Check a small fraction (1/10) of the ligation on a 1% agarose/1X TBE gel. Also run ~0.2 μg of cut vector and insert in neighboring lanes to serve as markers. Instead of distinct vector and insert bands, the DNA should look smeared, usually increasing in size from the vector DNA band.

3.6. Competent Cells and Transformation

In the case where *E. coli* is the system used for selection or screening, preparation of highly competent cells (at least 10^8) is essential for creating very large libraries of random clones. Transformation is frequently the limiting step in the random mutagenesis procedure owing to the inefficiency of many transformation protocols (10^7–10^8 cfu/μg) *(10)*. In order to reduce the problems that arise from this limitation, we have found that electroporation is one way to achieve high transformation efficiencies (on the order of 10^9 cfu/μg DNA). A recent publication by Inoue et al. *(11)* reports similar levels of transformation efficiencies with their protocol. Because these transformation efficiencies are determined for particular strains of *E. coli*, it behooves the investigator to test the transformation efficiency of the particular strain used.

3.6.1. Preparation of Competent Cells for Electroporation

1. Inoculate 1 L of 2X YT (16 g tryptone, 10 g yeast extract, 5 g NaCl for 1 L) with a 1/200 dilution of an overnight culture.
2. Grow the culture at 37°C (permissive temperature) until an OD_{600} of 0.5–0.8 is attained.

3. Transfer the culture to centrifuge bottles and chill on ice for 15–30 min.
4. Pellet the cells by centrifugation for 15 min at 4°C at 4470g.
5. Decant the supernatant and resuspend the cells in 1 L of ice-cold sterile H₂O. Be cautious at this point as the cell pellets can be loose and easily discarded with the supernatant.
6. Respin 15 min at 4470g, 4°C to pellet the cells.
7. Decant the supernatant and resuspend the cells in 500 mL of ice-cold sterile H₂O.
8. Centrifuge the cells again for 15 min at 4470g and 4°C. Resuspend them in 20 mL of 10% glycerol (chilled).
9. Transfer the resuspended cells to a 50-mL conical centrifuge tube and centrifuge again.
10. Resuspend the pellets a final time in 2.5 mL 10% glycerol (chilled).
11. Aliquot 100–200 µL into 0.65-mL microfuge tubes on ice.
12. Quick-freeze the tubes in a dry ice/ethanol bath.
13. Store the cells at −70°C. Cells prepared in this manner are competent for at least 6 mo.

3.6.2. Transformation

1. Transform 50 µL electroporation competent cells with 1–15 µL or ligation mix using an electroporator according to the manufacturer's instructions (*see* Note 13).
2. After pulsing, immediately add 1 mL SOC (4°C) and transfer the transformation to a larger tube, such as a Falcon snap cap tube. Shake for 1 h at 37°C (permissive temperature).
3. Plate a small portion of the transformation on a nonselective medium to determine the total number of transformed cells. Plate the rest on a selective medium.
4. Incubate the plates at the appropriate temperature.

3.7. Selection

The strength of random sequence selection is positive genetic complementation. Active mutants can be identified easily by using a stringent selection protocol. For example, the use of a temperature sensitive strain able to grow efficiently at the permissive temperature but only marginally at the nonpermissive temperature, may not be adequate for selection, since it would be very difficult to distinguish a false positive (leaky wild-type) from a true positive and requires retransformation to establish a plasmid-derived phenotype. The time spent in fine-tuning a selection system minimizes problems associated with the frequent recovery of false positives. Clearly, the selection step is one that must be devised with a particular question in mind as well as a knowledge about the bacterial strain and requirements for the identification of positive clones. Alternatively, a negative selection can be used but requires that every potential mutant must be plated individually on both selective (death) and nonselective (growth) plates in order to retrieve any functional clones; a formidable task.

4. Notes

1. For each amino acid position there are 20 possible amino acid substitutions. At the nucleotide level the number of permutations for four amino acid residues (12 nucleotides) is 4^{12} or 1.7×10^7. Thus, a completely random library contains 20^4 or 1.6×10^5 different amino acid sequences. With six codons containing random nucleotide sequences, the number of clones with different nucleotide substitutions increases to 6.9×10^{10} and represents 6.4×10^7 different amino acid substitutions. Given a very efficient transformation protocol in concert with a strong selection system, it is feasible to examine this number of transformants and score for clones that contain inserts that code for active proteins. Stretches of larger numbers of random substitutions means that the total number of possible permutations cannot be analyzed, simply for the reason that there are too many to test. The major limitation to this procedure is the number of bacteria that can be transformed successfully. The number of codons randomized can be limited to a few residues *(1–6)* in order to generate all possibilities. Some investigators have mutagenized large regions of a polypeptide by creating many small libraries that span only two or three residues at a time *(12)*. Synthesis of the numbers of oligonucleotides required for such a study is very costly. One may want to consider constructing a 2–20% degenerative library initially and sequence a fair number of active clones. Although the absence of different amino acids does not necessarily mean that other residues are not permissible, it might also mean that not enough clones have been sequenced. In such a case, one may want to discern these two possibilities by generating a second library with 100% randomness. As a general approach, frequently it is advantageous to define the essentiality of different residues by utilizing a partially random sequence at specified positions.

   One way to reduce the complexity of possible permutations is to bias the mutagenesis toward the wild-type sequence (partially random). This slants the mutagenesis to favor single mutations and, also, toward a higher frequency of clones that encode enzymatically active proteins, since multiple mutations are more often nonfunctional than are single substitutions. For instance, if one desires single amino acid mutations at many residues one might maintain a high percentage of wild-type sequences with a low percentage of nonwild-type sequences at each position. For example, a partially random sequence might be comprised of 80% wild-type and 20% of all other three nucleotides at each nucleotide position. This biased ratio ensures that a greater proportion of positively selected sequences are owing to single amino acid substitutions within the random array. Completely random sequence mutagenesis leads to a higher frequency of multiple amino acid replacements. It seems likely that multiple amino acid replacements would not have been adequately screened during evolution and may provide a fertile field for the discovery of new enzymatic activities.

As with both random and partially random mutagenesis the introduction of stop codons can be of concern depending on the number of nucleotides to be mutagenized. Some investigators use NNG/C (where N denotes all four nucleotides) instead of NNN to avoid the potential insertion of two stop codons among the random inserts while still allowing all possible amino acid residues to be coded for *(13)*.

2. When designing the random oligonucleotides be sure to take into account that restriction endonucleases require a specified number of nucleotides on either side of the restriction site for recognition. Moreover, the ends of oligonucleotides may fray and not be tightly hybridized. Thus, it is advantageous to incorporate a few extra G-C pairs at the ends of the oligonucleotides that contain the random sequences or to incorporate additional terminal nucleotides at the ends of primers that may be used for PCR amplification.

3. The *E. coli* strain used will depend on the selection scheme. Use a *rec*A deficient cell line whenever possible to reduce nonhomologous recombination into the bacterial chromosome.

4. The use of an individual extinction coefficient in calculating oligonucleotide concentration provides a more accurate assessment than does a standard value for oligonucleotides. To determine the extinction coefficiency the number of each nucleotide species is multiplied by the values for the individual nucleotides (A = 15.4×10^3, C = 7.5×10^3, G = 11.7×10^3, T = 7.4×10^3) and the sum totaled. For each random position use the average of all four values ($N = 10.5 \times 10^3$). Division of the total OD_{260} reading by the oligonucleotide extinction coefficient gives mol/L and then multiply by 10^6 to give pmol/µL.

5. The efficacy of annealing can be monitored by using radiolabeled oligonucleotides in a parallel annealing reaction followed by electrophoresis in a nondenaturing gel. When visualizing annealed and extended labeled oligonucleotides, do not heat denature prior to running the reactions on a nondenaturing polyacrylamide gel. If annealing is not complete, a different (lower) temperatures and/or longer incubation times may be required.

6. At this point, if a scaled up reaction has been done, i.e., no PCR amplification, the DNA is ethanol precipitated and restricted with the appropriate endonucleases. Completion of fragment digestion can be monitored by subjecting the cut and uncut DNA to electrophoresis on a nondenaturing 5–8% acrylamide gel.
7. This has worked for different primer-template combinations but depending on the primers and template, the cycle times and/or temperatures may require modification.
8. As few as 4 bp differences can be resolved in a 3.5% MetaPhor (FMC Bio-Products, Rockland, ME) agarose (1X TBE) gel with a range from 70–300 bp.
9. There are several important considerations in choosing a vector for the cloning of random sequences. The copy number of the plasmid is worth noting especially if the gene product is slightly toxic. By keeping the number of copies low the toxic effects may be reduced. In the selection process, a low copy number plasmid might allow one to discern differential levels of mutant activities using selection plates containing a low concentration of substrates. A high copy number plasmid offers an additional advantage since sequencing is likely to involve double-stranded DNA and fair amounts of the DNA (2–3 µg) may be required. Furthermore, if a vector contains a single-stranded origin of replication then sequencing is greatly simplified.

Promoters are another consideration. For some situations it is important to maintain tight control on expression levels. In some instances, promoters may be the target for random mutagenesis *(4)*.
10. By exchanging a stuffer fragment of DNA that is longer that the native fragment, a nonfunctional "dummy" vector can be constructed (Fig. 3) *(1)*. The stuffer fragment replaces the wild-type sequences and occupies the same position that the random sequences will. There are two important reasons for using a "dummy" vector; first, one can discern between singly and doubly cut vector, and second, if the gel isolated vector (double cut) is contaminated with some uncut vector the selection would eliminate it as a nonfunctional clone whereas the vector containing a wild-type gene would register as a positive clone. The inclusion of an internal restriction site within the oligonucleotides described earlier, aids in discerning the wild-type gene containing vector from any recombinants. The use of a "dummy" vector removes the time-consuming step of performing restriction digests and running gels on all possible positives prior to sequencing. Generally, we only perform restriction analysis on the first 10–20 clones to confirm that the majority of the positive clones contain random sequence insertions.
11. Because the restricted vector DNA is gel purified, less clean DNA isolated from minipreparations can be used if only a small library is required and will not cause difficulties at subsequent steps.

12. Other kits and techniques are available and can be used in a similar fashion to purify the vector DNA.
13. Several ratios of insert to vector ligations should be tried in order to identify the best ligation conditions.
14. The volume of competent cells and ligation mix for maximal transformation efficiency needs to be determined for each strain and ligation. Furthermore, if arching occurs during electroporation, the ligation mix should be ethanol precipitated to remove excess salt.

References

1. Dube, D. K., Parker, J. D., French, D. C., Cahill, D. S., Dube, S., Horwitz, M. S., Munir, K. M., and Loeb, L. A. (1991) Artificial mutants generated by the insertion of random oligonucleotides into the putative nucleoside binding site of the HSV-1 thymidine kinase gene. *Biochemistry* **30,** 11,760–11,767.
2. Scott, J. K. and Smith, G. P. (1990) Searching for peptide ligands with an epitope library. *Science* **249,** 386–390.
3. Robertson, D. L. and Joyce, G. F. (1990) Selection *in vitro* of an RNA enzyme that specifically cleaves single-stranded DNA. *Nature* **344,** 467,468.
4. Horwitz, M. S. and Loeb, L. A. (1986) Promoters selected from random DNA sequences. *Proc. Natl. Acad. Sci. USA* **83,** 7405–7409.
5. Feng, Q., Park, T. K., and Rebek, J., Jr. (1992) Crossover reactions between synthetic replicators yield active and inactive recombinants. *Science* **256,** 1179,1180.
6. Ellington, A. D. and Szostak, J. W. (1990) *In vitro* selection of RNA molecules that bind specific ligands. *Nature* **346,** 818–822.
7. Black, M. E. and Loeb, L. A. (1993) Identification of important residues within the putative nucleoside binding site of HSV-1 thymidine kinase by random sequence selection: analysis of selected mutants *in vitro*. *Biochemistry* **32,** 11,618–11,626.
8. Bowie, J. U., Reidhaar-Olson, J. F., Lim, W. A., and Sauer, R. T. (1990) Deciphering the message in protein sequences: tolerance to amino acid substitutions. *Science* **247,** 1306–1310.
9. Sambrook, J., Fritsch, E. F. and Maniatis, T. (1989) *Molecular Cloning: A Laboratory Manual,* 2nd ed., Cold Spring Harbor Laboratory Press, Cold Spring Harbor, NY.
10. Hanahan, D. (1983) Studies on transformation of *Escherichia coli* with plasmids. *J. Mol. Biol.* **166,** 557–580.
11. Inoue, H., Nojima, H., and Okayama, H. (1990) High efficiency transformation of *Escherichia coli* with plasmids. *Gene* **96,** 23–28.
12. Reidhaar-Olson, J. F. and Sauer, R. T. (1988) Combinatorial cassette mutagenesis as a probe of the informational content of protein sequences. *Science* **241,** 53–57.
13. Reidhaar-Olson, J. F., Bowie, J. U., Breyer, R. M., Hu, J. C., Knight, K. L., Lim, W. A., Mossing, M. C., Parsell, D. A., Shoemaker, K. R., and Sauer, R. T. (1991) Random mutagenesis of protein sequences using oligonucleotide cassettes. *Methods Enzymol.* **208,** 564–586.

CHAPTER 31

Random Mutagenesis
by Using Mixtures of dNTP
and dITP in PCR

Oscar P. Kuipers

1. Introduction

Generating random mutations in a DNA fragment of a specific size is often the method of choice for changing specific properties of an encoded protein or for studying the functional properties of a specific DNA fragment. In all these cases it is helpful and in some cases essential to have a screening method available that allows for distinction between phenotypic changes brought about by one or more random mutations in the DNA fragment of interest.

Several methods have been described using mixed synthetic oligonucleotides for random mutagenesis, which work efficiently but can only be applied for mutagenesis of DNA fragments of limited size *(1–3)*. Alternative methods using polymerase chain reaction (PCR) with reduced fidelity have been described that offer an increased mutation frequency as well as the advantage of random mutations in relatively large DNA fragments and a random distribution of the types of mutation *(4–6)*. However, for many applications it is desirable to use a method that allows the modulation of the desired number of mutations in a DNA fragment of a specific size and the degree of randomness of the mutations. The method described here *(7)* offers the advantage of choosing preferred nucleotides being randomly incorporated as well as adjusting the mutation frequency to almost any desired level. This method is based on the following principles:

From: *Methods in Molecular Biology, Vol. 57: In Vitro Mutagenesis Protocols*
Edited by: M. K. Trower Humana Press Inc., Totowa, NJ

1. When one of the four nucleotides in a PCR reaction with the DNA fragment to be mutagenized as a template is present in a limiting amount, incorporation of any of the other three available nucleotides is favored. However, the efficiency of amplification will be reduced dramatically.

2. The limiting amount of one of the nucleotides (typically ranging between 5 and 10% of the usual concentration) can be replenished by dITP. This will restore to a large extent the efficiency of the PCR reaction and will force dITP to be incorporated at the sites of the depleted nucleotide. The efficiency of incorporation of dITP has been reported to be approximately fourfold lower, relative to that of the natural nucleotides *(8)*. The lower the concentration of the depleted nucleotide, the higher the mutation frequency will be.

3. In the next cycle, each of the three other nucleotides or dITP itself will be incorporated as a complement to dITP, giving rise to mutations.

4. To mutagenize a certain DNA fragment, routinely four PCR reactions are set up, each depleted in a different nucleotide and replenished by dITP.

5. Following PCR, the DNA fragments from each reaction are purified, pooled, digested, and ligated into an appropriate vector, which is then used to transform the microorganism of choice. Each colony will contain plasmids, harboring either wild-type DNA fragments or a fragments containing one or more point mutations. Occasionally, deletions and insertions may be found in the fragments.

6. Preferably, a screening method is available, for rapid distinction between wild-type and mutant phenotypes.

   This method will elevate the mutation frequency from approx 5×10^{-4} (owing to the intrinsic error frequency of *Taq* DNA-polymerase) to at least 40×10^{-4}. A cloned fragment of 1 kbp will thus contain an average of four point mutations. When one wishes to elevate the mutation frequency even more, 0.5 mM Mn^{2+} can be included in the PCR reactions *(4)*. The method described here is simple, flexible, fast, and low cost.

2. Materials

1. Standard mixture for preparing 30 PCR reactions (aliquoted in volumes of 40 µL): Total vol of 1200 µL containing 150 µL 10X *Taq*-buffer (500 mM NaCl, 100 mM Tris-HCl, pH 8.8, 50 mM MgCl$_2$), 6 µL *Taq*-polymerase (5 U/µL, Gibco-BRL, Gaithersburg MD), 12 µL dNTPs (stock solution containing 25 mM of each nucleotide), 75 µL stabilizer (1% W-1) (Gibco-BRL) and 957 µL distilled water. Each reaction mix is then covered with two drops of light mineral oil and may be stored at −20°C for several months if required. After adding primers and DNA template, the final volume of the reaction mix should be increased to 50 µL.

2. 100 mM dITP solution.

3. PCR primers, preferably containing restriction sites and, when appropriate 3 to 5 bp-sized clamps (*see* Note 1) at their 5' ends to allow for efficient digestion of the PCR products and subsequent cloning (10 pmol of each primer in a PCR reaction).
4. Template DNA (approx 10 ng plasmid or 100 ng chromosomal DNA for each PCR reaction).
5. Ethidium bromide (5 mg/mL stock solution).
6. TAE-agarose gels (0.8–2%).
7. GeneClean (Bio 101, La Jolla, CA).
8. Appropriate restriction endonucleases.
9. Appropriate cloning vector and *Escherichia coli* or any other host strain.
10. $1M$ MnCl$_2$ (stock solution).
11. Biomed Thermocycler 60 or any other thermocycler.

3. Methods
3.1. Standard PCR Reaction Conditions

It is difficult to define a single set of conditions to ensure successful PCR of a target sequence. However, the conditions described herein, which may be used for amplifying DNA fragments between 100 and 3000 bp, may be tested before attempting any variations

1. Prepare PCR reaction mixes using the solutions described in Section 2., item 1.
2. Program on the thermocycler: 30 cycles, each consisting of a denaturing step at 93°C for 1 min, a primer annealing step at a temperature depending on the T_m of the primers for 1.5 min (*see* Note 2), and an extension step at 72°C for 2.5 min *(9)*.

To achieve efficient amplification one might have to reduce the Mg^{2+} concentration, however, the highest Mg^{2+} concentration that generates the desired product is preferred (*see* Note 3).

3.2. PCR Mutagenesis Conditions

Once a set of conditions has been identified that produces the desired amplified DNA fragment, mutagenesis of the target sequence may be attempted.

1. Prepare four different sets of PCR reaction mixes using the solutions described in Section 2., item 1 with the alteration that 200 μM of dITP is added to each reaction and at the same time one of the four dNTP concentrations (200 μM) is reduced to 10–20 μM (corresponding to 1.25–2.5 mM in the dNTP stock solution mentioned in Section 2., item 1) (*see* Notes 4–8).

2. Following PCR, estimate the yield of each of the four depleted reactions by analyzing the samples by TAE-agarose gel electrophoresis and staining with ethidium bromide.

3. Recover the DNA fragments from the agarose gel by the Gene-Clean procedure (Bio 101). Pool the contents of the four depleted reactions in the desired ratio (*see* Note 9).

4. Digest the pool of PCR products with appropriate restriction enzymes, inactivate the restriction enzymes by either high temperature (only possible with some of the enzymes; *see* supplier's recommendation), phenol treatment and ethanol precipitation, or the Gene-Clean procedure (Bio 101).

5. Ligate the pool of restriction fragments into a digested cloning vector.

6. Transform the ligation mixture into a competent *E. coli* host strain.

The mutation frequency can be determined by picking individual colonies and sequencing the mutagenized fragments by established procedures. By sequencing, e.g., 24 clones of a 500-bp mutagenized fragment, one obtains a fairly good insight in the efficiency of the mutagenesis procedure. For example, a mutation frequency of 0.004, which is easily achievable, will cause an average total number of mutations in these sequenced fragments of 48, and will give insight in the distribution and randomness of the mutations. The frequency of occurrence of deletions and insertions does not seem to be greatly influenced by using this method and is always below 2.2×10^{-4} *(7)*. In my experience, the mutations will be distributed randomly over the full PCR fragment. However, the occurrence of cloned PCR fragments with a significant higher or lower number of mutations than the average number expected, is notable.

4. Notes

1. To facilitate later cloning of PCR fragments, one can use primers with internal restriction sites. This can be accomplished by choosing the primer sequence in such a way that the restriction sites are:
   a. Present in the template sequence;
   b. Introduced by one or more point mutations in the middle part of the primer; or
   c. Introduced as a 5' extension, including a clamp of three or more residues to ensure efficient digestion (for details on the minimal length of clamps, *see*, e.g., the New England Biolabs Catalog 1992, p. 182).

2. The primer annealing temperature can be estimated by adding 2°C for each A and T residue and 4°C for each G and C residue present in the primer,

which are complementary to the template, and subtraction of 4°C. For reasons of specificity, annealing temperatures between 50 and 65°C are recommended.

3. The maximal Mg^{2+} concentration tolerated can vary greatly depending on the nature of the primers and the template used, but usually will range between 2 and 10 mM.

4. For determining the concentration of the depleted nucleotide that will still yield a PCR product, one is advised to prepare only a limited number of PCR reaction mixes. Usually, the concentration of the depleted nucleotide will range between 10 and 20 µM. The protocol given in Section 2., item 1 can be adjusted by reducing the concentrations of all chemicals proportional to the desired total volume.

5. If one wishes, the GC content of the template can be taken into account in estimating the chance that the reaction will be depleted prematurely, giving rise to a low yield (or no yield at all!) of PCR product. For instance, when the template consists of 60% AT, one can consider making PCR reaction mixes containing 18 µM of either A or T nucleotides and 12 µM of G or C nucleotides. Another finding is that the yield of PCR product in T and C depleted reactions is sometimes lower than that of A and G depleted reactions at the same concentrations of limiting nucleotide, probably because of a lower pairing capacity of dITP with A or G residues (P. A. Franken and C. Martinez, personal communication, July 1994). Therefore, one might have to raise the concentrations of dTTP and dCTP in depleted reactions relative to the concentrations of dATP or dGTP in the other depleted reactions to obtain similar yields.

6. When the desired mutation frequency should be as high as possible, adjust the concentration of the depleted nucleotides to a level as low as possible, e.g., giving a yield between 5 and 20% of the yield using the standard PCR mix.

7. If a higher mutation frequency and increased randomization of the types of mutation (inversion, transition) is desired, the use of an additional 0.5 mM of $MnCl_2$ or more in each PCR reaction is recommended *(4)*. Furthermore, one can decrease the ratio between the concentrations of Mg^{2+} and Mn^{2+} to increase the mutation frequency and to obtain more randomly distributed mutations. However, if increased randomness is wanted, without a concomitant increase in mutation frequency, one should raise the concentration of the limiting nucleotide, while keeping the Mg^{2+}/Mn^{2+} ratio constant.

8. A general rule is: The lower the yield of PCR product in a depleted reaction is, the higher the mutation frequency will be. If the yield is too low, one might consider a second PCR using less stringent conditions, with the first purified PCR product as a template.

9. The fragments obtained from the four reactions can be pooled in any desired ratio that will give the preferred types of mutation. For example, when only changes in G and C bases are preferred, the products of the G and C depleted reactions are pooled and subsequently used in further experiments.

Acknowledgments

I am grateful to Johan Spee and Willem de Vos for their contributions to this work.

References

1. Matteucci, M. D. and Heyneker, H. L. (1983) Targeted random mutagenesis: the use of ambiguously synthesized oligonucleotides to mutagenize sequences immediately 5' of an ATG initiation codon. *Nucleic Acids Res.* **17**, 3113–3121.
2. Ner, S. S., Goodin D. B., and Smith, M. (1988) A simple and efficient procedure for generating random point mutations and for codon replacements using mixed oligodeoxynucleotides. *DNA* **7**, 127–134.
3. Wells, J. A., Vasser, M., and Powers, D. B. (1985) Cassette mutagenesis: an efficient method for generation of multiple mutations at defined sites. *Gene* **34**, 315–323.
4. Leung, D. W, Chen, E., and Goeddel, D. V. (1989) A method for random mutagenesis of a defined DNA segment using a modified polymerase chain reaction. *Technique* **1**, 11–15.
5. Zhou, Y., Zang, X., and Ebright, R. (1991) Random mutagenesis of gene-sized DNA molecules by use of PCR with *Taq* DNA polymerase. *Nucleic Acids Res.* **19**, 6052.
6. Cadwell, R. C. and Joyce, G. F. (1992) *PCR Methods Appl.* **2**, 28–33.
7. Spee, J., de Vos, W. M., and Kuipers, O. P. (1993) Efficient random mutagenesis method with adjustable mutation frequency using PCR and dITP. *Nucleic Acids Res.* **21**, 777,778.
8. Innis, M. A., Myambo, K. B., Gelfand, D. H., and Brow, M. A. (1988) DNA sequencing with *Thermus aquaticus* DNA polymerase and direct sequencing of polymerase chain reaction-amplified DNA. *Proc. Natl. Acad. Sci. USA* **85**, 9436–9440.
9. Kuipers, O. P., Boot, H. J., and de Vos, W. M. (1991) Improved site-directed mutagenesis method using PCR. *Nucleic Acids Res.* **16**, 4558.

CHAPTER 32

PCR-Mediated Chemical Mutagenesis

Donald J. Roufa

1. Introduction

Randomly induced point mutations provide an effective strategy to recognize and characterize functionally significant features of cloned DNAs. When coupled with sensitive assays for gene function, random mutagenesis permits one to resolve active DNA motifs within a gene's regulatory and protein-coding gene domains. When gene sequences of interest are short, it is efficient and cost-effective to generate comprehensive libraries of random point mutations by chemical synthesis of oligonucleotides from appropriately "doped" mixtures of DNA substrates *(1–5)*. However, when the target DNAs are long (>50 bp), chemical synthesis of randomly mutated sequences is expensive as well as time-consuming and depends on extensive use of costly instruments and reagents.

To overcome these limitations and provide an affordable, yet efficient and straightforward method for randomly mutagenizing large cloned DNAs, a protocol designated PCR-mediated chemical (PMC) mutagenesis *(6)* was devised. As its name implies, the procedure is based on random modification of cloned duplex DNAs by treatment with chemical mutagens with known reaction specificities on DNA (e.g., formic or nitrous acid, sodium bisulfite, hydrazine, dimethyl sulfate, etc.) and use of the PCR *(7,8)* to resolve and amplify mutated duplex DNAs for introduction into appropriate recombinant cloning vectors.

PMC mutagenesis requires relatively inexpensive chemical reagents and only the equipment necessary to PCR amplify mutagenized target

From: *Methods in Molecular Biology, Vol. 57: In Vitro Mutagenesis Protocols*
Edited by: M. K. Trower Humana Press Inc., Totowa, NJ

DNAs, i.e., a programmable thermocycler. It involves a single molecular cloning operation and may be used in conjunction with all cloning vectors that accept double-stranded DNA inserts, including customized shuttle and expression vectors. Most important, PMC mutagenesis can be applied conveniently to duplex DNA clones of any length.

A similar procedure based on denaturing gradient gel electrophoresis (DGGE) was described by Myers and his colleagues *(9,10)*. Unlike PMC mutagenesis, their protocol requires multiple subcloning operations, a specialized single-stranded DNA vector encoding a "GC-clamp," and a sophisticated electrophoretic procedure (DGGE) that limits the length of mutagenic DNA targets to 600 bp or less. In addition, DGGE must be optimized for each gene segment analyzed. In contrast, PMC mutagenesis requires only the oligonucleotide primers and PCR cycle conditions necessary to enzymatically amplify the target DNA. Indeed, a single pair of vector-specific PCR primers, such as the M13 forward and reverse sequencing primers *(11)*, can be used to amplify multiple mutagenized gene segments carried in standard, commercially available cloning vectors.

A representative protocol for PCR-mediated nitrous acid mutagenesis of a bacterial plasmid vector carrying a 200 bp segment of human ribosomal protein S14 cDNA *(12)* is described. Nitrous acid treatment deaminates cytosine, guanine, and adenine to yield uracil, xanthine, and hypoxanthine nucleotides within duplex DNA. Because DNA uridine replicates as thymine and DNA hypoxanthine, as guanine, nitrous acid induces both $dC \cdot dG \rightarrow dT \cdot dA$ and $dA \cdot dT \rightarrow dG \cdot dC$ transition mutations. Analogous protocols based on other chemical mutagens and recombinant DNA cloning vectors can be devised following the same general strategy, so long as the chemical modification used does not abrogate the target DNA's PCR template activity.

2. Materials

All solutions described in the following are prepared in glass-distilled water sterilized by boiling and/or ultrafiltration.

2.1. Standard Buffers

1. Tris-EDTA (TE): $0.01M$ Tris-HCl, $0.001M$ Na$_2$-EDTA, adjusted to pH 7.5 with HCl.
2. $0.3M$ Sodium acetate adjusted to pH 4.3 with acetic acid.
3. $2.5M$ Sodium acetate adjusted to pH 7.0 with acetic acid.

2.2. DNA Targets

Because the chemical mutagenesis reaction must be designed to yield a single, randomly located base substitution in each target DNA molecule, it is important to control conditions for base-specific DNA modification reactions carefully. To accomplish this, concentrations of target DNA and mutagen as well as reaction times and temperatures must be optimized systematically. It has been found that 60 nmol of target DNA nucleotide (i.e., 20 mg) in 100-µL modification reactions is experimentally convenient and yields a very large number of mutant target DNA clones. The maximum length DNA suitable for analysis is limited only by one's ability to PCR amplify the target DNA. Conventional PCR technology, therefore, sets an upper limit for target DNA length at ~2000 bp, although newer methods and reagents promise to extend this limit to 10–20 kbp (*see* Note 1). For a 200-bp cDNA target carried in a 2.8-kbp plasmid vector, 60 nmol of target DNA nucleotide contains ~6 × 10^{12} (i.e., ~10 pmol) of intact recombinant plasmid DNAs.

2.3. Chemical Mutagens

The recipes for the following mutagen solutions were taken from Myers, Lerman, and Maniatis *(9)*. When prepared within 1 wk of use, they have been shown to be effective in the PMC mutagenesis procedure:

1. Nitrous acid (modifies C, A, and G): $1.25M$ sodium nitrite in $0.3M$ sodium acetate buffer, pH 4.3.
2. Formic acid (modifies G and A): $15M$ formic acid in distilled water.
3. Hydrazine (modifies C and T): 75% (w/v) hydrazine in distilled water.

2.4. PCR Reagents

One should employ PCR components and conditions optimized for each particular target DNA and primer pairs analyzed. Routinely, PCR reactions are assembled in the author's laboratory from the following reagents:

1. 5X PCR buffer: 50 mM Tris-HCl, 5 mM $MgCl_2$, 250 mM KCl, 0.5% (w/v) porcine skin cell gelatin (Sigma, St. Louis, MO), 0.5% (v/v) Triton X-100 adjusted to pH 8.5 with HCl. Add 10 µL of this solution to each standard 50-µL PCR.
2. Deoxyribonucleoside triphosphates (2 mM) dissolved in 10 mM Tris-HCl, pH 7.5, containing 1 mM dithiothreitol. Store these solutions at –20°C and assemble them into a stock cocktail containing 0.5 mM each of dATP, dCTP, dGTP, and dTTP. Add 20 µL of the cocktail to each 50 µL PCR reaction.

3. Primer oligonucleotides are dissolved in 10 m*M* Tris-HCl, pH 7.5, at concentrations of 0.5 A$_{260}$/mL (i.e., 75 m*M* nucleotide). Add 1 μL of each primer (~3 μmol of a 20–25 nt primer) to the standard PCR reaction mixture.

4. *Taq* DNA polymerase at 2–5 U/μL, where a unit of activity is defined as the amount of enzyme that polymerizes 10 nmol of deoxyribonucleoside triphosphates in 30 min at 74°C. Add 1 μL of this stock solution to each PCR.

5. Paraffin oil sterilized either by autoclaving or microwave irradiation. Overlay PCR reactions assembled in 0.5 mL conical microcentrifuge tubes with ~25 μL of paraffin oil to preclude evaporation in the thermocycler.

6. PCR stop buffer: 10 m*M* Tris-HCl, pH 7.5, 12.5 m*M* Na$_2$-EDTA, 0.25% (w/v) sodium dodecylsulfate. Add 100 μL of PCR stop buffer with thorough mixing to terminate amplification reactions.

2.5. DNA Ligation Reagents

1. T4 DNA ligase (1–10 Weiss units *[13]*/μL).
2. 5X T4 ligase reaction buffer: 250 m*M* Tris-HCl, pH 7.6, 50 m*M* MgCl$_2$, 5 m*M* ATP, 5 m*M* dithiothreitol, 25% (w/v) PEG-8000 (Sigma).

3. Methods

PCR-mediated chemical mutagenesis is a three-step procedure (Fig. 1).

1. Treat a purified duplex target DNA (maintained in either a plasmid, viral, or episomal cloning vector, Fig. 1A) with a chemical mutagen that modifies DNA bases directly. This results in single-base alterations, usually transition mutations, that are randomly distributed throughout both the target and vector sequences (represented by * in Fig. 1).

2. Using synthetic oligonucleotide primers that encode segments of the cloned target DNA or flanking vector sequences (P$_1$ and P$_2$ in Fig. 1B), PCR amplify the heterogeneous population of mutagenized target molecules. This step resolves modified nucleotides into standard DNA basepairs (depicted as **o**s in Fig. 1) and facilitates construction of mutant gene libraries.

3. Purify the amplified DNAs by standard methods, i.e., electrophoresis, phenol:chloroform extraction, or chromatograpy.

4. Subclone the mutagenized target DNAs into an acceptor test vector (Fig. 2) in the biologically functional molecular orientation. This can be accomplished conveniently using a pair of restriction endonuclease cleavage site termini (represented as a and b in Figs. 1 and 2) either within the amplified

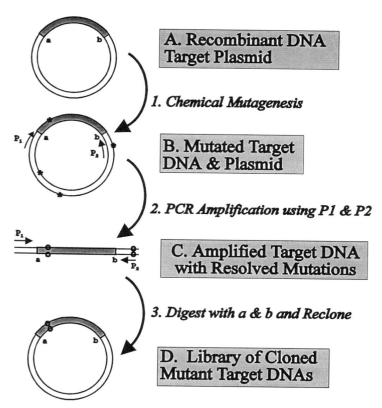

Fig. 1. The PMC mutagenesis strategy. A target DNA sequence bounded by restriction endonuclease cleavage sites a and b (shaded segment) is carried in a conventional plasmid cloning vector. As illustrated, PCR primer oligonucleotides (P_1 and P_2) have been designed from vector sequences that flank the target DNA insert. Chemical mutagenesis randomly generates modified DNA bases (*) throughout the target and vector sequences. Subsequently, modified bases in the target DNA are replicated as standard base pairs (o) during PCR amplification, and amplified target molecules are cloned into an acceptor vector for analysis.

target DNA, in flanking vector sequences, or prepended to the 5' ends of the PCR primers.

5. Use DNA sequence analysis and/or functional tests for the DNA's biological activity to recognize individual target DNA subclones carrying precisely defined, single-base mutations.

Each of these steps are discussed in greater detail in the following.

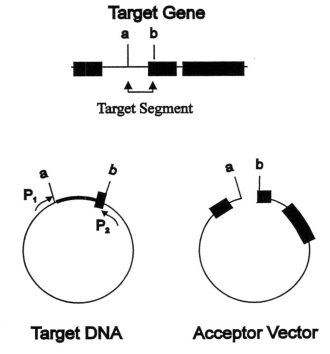

Target DNA   **Acceptor Vector**

Fig. 2. Cloned DNA constructs required for PMC mutagenesis. A mutagenesis target DNA segment bounded by restriction endonuclease cleavage sites a and b is cloned into a recombinant vector for which a pair of flanking PCR primers (P_1 and P_2) is available. Target gene exons are illustrated as shaded rectangles and introns, as thinner lines. The acceptor vector contains the entire gene sequence but for the target segment. Individual molecules (alleles) of the mutagenized target are introduced into the acceptor vector in the biologically functional orientation by ligation at a and b to test their biological activities.

3.1. Chemical Mutagenesis

The experimental goal is to randomly modify a cloned DNA target sequence with single-base substitutions and to generate a library of DNA clones whose members carry point mutations evenly distributed throughout the target sequence. The reaction conditions necessary to achieve these goals must be set empirically for each target DNA, primer pair, and chemical mutagen used. In order to obtain approx one modification per kbp of target sequence, 60 nmol of target DNA in 100 µL mutagenesis reactions are used. To establish these reaction conditions:

1. Add 20 µg of the target DNA to 80 µL of the mutagen solutions described in Section 2.3.
2. Adjust reaction volumes to 100 µL with sterile distilled water.
3. Incubate mutagenesis reaction mixtures at 22°C for 60 min, withdrawing 20-µL samples (i.e., 12 nmol of target nt) at 15-min intervals.
4. Quench each sample by addition to 100 µL of 2.5*M* sodium acetate, pH 7.0, with thorough mixing. For a 200-bp cDNA carried in a 2.8-kbp plasmid cloning vector, each quenched sample contains ~2 pmol (1.2 × 10^{12} molecules) of recombinant plasmid.
5. Add 5 vol (600 µL) of 95% ice-cold ethanol to each DNA sample and precipitate modified DNAs at −20°C for at least 1 h.
6. Finally, harvest the DNAs by centrifugation (12,000*g* for 15 min) at 4°C and wash pelleted precipitates in ice cold 70% ethanol (*see* Note 2).

3.2. PCR Amplification

The user must select PCR primers and reaction cycle conditions that are optimal for amplification of the target DNA sequence. This choice depends on:

1. The base composition (and, therefore, thermal denaturation properties) of candidate primer pairs as well as the target DNA sequence between them;
2. The total length of the target DNA;
3. The potential for primer:primer interactions; and
4. The location of restriction endonuclease cleavage sites within the amplified target sequence.

In order to ensure uniform distribution of point mutations throughout a DNA target and facilitate analysis of mutated molecules in single DNA sequence ladders, it is useful to clone long target sequences as overlapping 50–300-bp segments. This can be accomplished using a single pair of flanking PCR primers (*see* Note 3) and multiple restriction endonuclease cleavage sites within the amplified DNA (*see* Note 4), or with a battery of PCR primer pairs that define adjacent, overlapping amplicons within a long target DNA. In the latter case, prepend 6-bp restriction endonuclease cleavage sites (*Eco*RI, *Bam*HI, or *Hin*dIII) to the 5' ends of PCR primers to facilitate subcloning of amplified mutant DNA sequences (*see* Note 5 and Section 3.3.).

Mutagenized DNA samples are amplified >1000-fold using a protocol optimized for each test DNA and primer pair. The standard 50-µL PCR reaction protocol is as follows:

1. Add ~2 pmol of the mutagenized target vector, 3 μmol each of two PCR primers, all four deoxyribonucleoside triphosphates (10 nmol each), and 2–5 U of *Taq* DNA polymerase to 1.5-mL conical microcentrifuge tubes (*see* Sections 2.4. and 3.1. as well as Note 6).
2. PCR amplify the mutagenized target DNA using a protocol whose conditions of time and temperature are optimized for target DNA denaturation, primer annealing, and target DNA synthesis. A thermocycle program optimized for amplification of mutagenized mammalian ribosomal protein S14 cDNAs consists of 30 iterations of denaturation for 30 s at 92°C followed by 2 min of primer annealing and DNA synthesis at 70°C *(6,14)*. Using this protocol, it has been observed that nitrous acid treatments as long as 120 min do not interfere with PCR amplification of target S14 cDNA fragments *(6)*.
3. Terminate amplification reactions by addition of 2 vol (100 μL) PCR stop buffer (*see* Section 2.4.) with thorough mixing.
4. Purify amplified DNA products by extraction in phenol:chlorofom:isoamyl alcohol (25:24:1) and precipitation from 70% ice-cold ethanol.

3.3. DNA Purification and Subcloning

1. Redissolve the amplified target DNAs in TE buffer (*see* Section 2.1.) or a buffer optimal for digestion with a necessary restriction endonuclease *(see the following)*.
2. If required by the subcloning strategy used, digest the DNAs with appropriate restriction endonucleases (*see* Note 7) and:
   a. Purify the digestion product by agarose gel electrophoresis;
   b. Recover the DNA fragment by electroelution or chromatography in a chaotropic buffer system.
3. Ligate the amplified DNA fragments into an appropriate acceptor vector (Fig. 2). For details, *see* Note 8.
4. Introduce recombinant acceptor vectors into a transformation-competent bacterial host strain to generate minilibraries of modified DNAs from each mutagenesis time point (*see* Section 3.1.).

3.4. Analysis of Mutated DNA Sequences

To determine the modification reaction time point that yielded the highest fraction of useful base substitution mutations, approx 10 independent target molecules are clone purified from each mutagenesis time point's minilibrary (*see* Section 3.1.) and surveyed for mutated DNA molecules. These clones can be screened for alterations in nucleic acid sequence or in biological function. As indicated earlier, when testing for altered DNA sequences, it is convenient to clone target DNA molecules as short segments (<300 bp) so that each clone can be evaluated by a single DNA sequence ladder. Alternatively, when screening for altered biological function, subclone amplified target DNAs into specially engineered "acceptor" vectors (Fig. 2) to reconstruct biologically active transcription units *(6,14)*. Of course, functional "acceptor" vectors and PCR amplification primers (P$_1$ and P$_2$, Figs. 1 and 2) also can be used to survey the mutants for altered DNA sequence.

When cloned target DNAs are treated with nitrous acid, the great majority (~90%) of mutated DNAs carry transition mutations *(6,14)*. The remainder of the molecules (~10%) harbor both transversion and deletion frameshift mutations *(14)*. The chemical action of nitrous acid on DNA does not account for transversion and deletion mutations in a straightforward manner. Nonetheless, their strict localization within amplified target DNA segments suggests that the deletion and transversion mutations isolated result from *Taq* polymerase-mediated replication of chemically modified DNAs without a stringent DNA proofreading and repair process *(6,14)*. It is likely that deaminated DNA bases generated by nitrous acid treatment are prone to misreplication in vitro and that uncorrected replication errors account for the transversions and deletions observed in PMC mutant DNAs. Although the mechanism that produces the relatively small number of nitrous acid induced transversion and deletion mutations is not well understood, it is useful in that it enhances the spectrum of random mutations obtained using the PMC mutagenesis strategy.

4. Notes

1. Several protocols and reagents that appear to extend the size limitation of DNAs amenable to PCR amplification recently have been described *(15)* and now are available commercially. These include the TaqStart reagent marketed by Clontech Laboratories, Inc. (Palo Alto, CA) and Taq Extender, a product of Stratagene (La Jolla, CA).
2. Ideally, one would like to obtain a population of mutagenized DNAs in which each target sequence carries a single base substitution mutation. Under the reaction conditions described, DNA aliquots taken between 20 and 45 min of nitrous acid treatment yield clones in which approximately half of the target cDNAs lack mutations and the other half contain between one and three single base substitutions each *(6,14)*.
3. Outside PCR primer pairs can be designed from the terminal sequences of the target DNA itself or, alternatively, from flanking vector sequences.

Primer pairs complementary to vector DNAs permit one to isolate point mutations throughout the entire target DNA clone and can be used to amplify multiple target DNAs cloned into a single vector site (usually within a vector polylinker). The M13 forward and reverse sequencing primers have been used successfully in conjunction with the pUC and pGEM series of plasmid vectors as well as the λGEM series of bacteriophage vectors obtained from Promega Corp. (Madison, WI).

4. When restriction endonuclease cleavage sites within a long target sequence are used to generate PMC-mutagenized DNAs as cloned target segments, it is not possible to recover mutations that affect the restriction sites themselves. To avoid this limitation, one should use cleavage sites that define overlapping segments of the target sequence.

5. As indicated in Note 4, use of PCR primer pairs that define *overlapping segments* of a target DNA permits one to obtain point mutations within target DNA sequences complementary to the primer oligonucleotides.

6. For longer recombinant target DNAs, one should use a proportionally lower concentration of oligonucleotide primers. Conversely, for shorter DNA targets, proportionally higher primer concentrations are optimal. The goal is to maintain a primer:target DNA ratio of approx $1–2 \times 10^3{:}1$.

7. To ensure that the target DNA's molecular orientation within a test vector is biologically functional, it is desirable to employ two different restriction endonuclease cleavage sites as the target DNA's termini.

8. Standard 20-μL ligation reactions are assembled using 4 μL of 5X T4 DNA ligase reaction buffer (*see* Section 2.4.), 25 ng of amplified target DNA, 300 ng of linear acceptor vector, and 1 Weiss unit *(13)* of T4 DNA ligase. Under these conditions, the molar ratio of target to vector DNAs is approx 1:1. Ligation reactions are incubated for 30 min at 22°C and then at 15°C overnight. The reactions are terminated by fivefold dilution with 80 μL of ice-cold TE buffer. Ligated DNAs can be efficiently introduced into transfection-competent bacteria without further purification. Generally, use *E. coli* TB1 (Life Technologies, Gaithersburg, MD) rendered competent for transfection by treatment with $1 M$ $CaCl_2$ *(16)* as the bacterial host strain.

References

1. Hutchinson, C. A., III, Nordeen, S. K., Vogt, K., and Edgall, M. H. (1986) A complete library of point substitution mutations in the glucocorticoid response element of mouse mammary tumor virus. *Proc. Natl. Acad. Sci. USA* **83,** 710–714.
2. Fritz, H.-J., Hohlmaier, J., Kramer, W., Ohmayer, A., and Wippler, J. (1988) Oligonucleotide-directed construction of mutations: a gapped duplex DNA procedure without enzymatic reactions *in vitro. Nucleic Acids Res.* **16,** 6987–6999.

3. Higuchi, R., Krummel, B., and Saiki, R. K. (1988) A general method of *in vitro* preparation and specific mutagenesis of DNA fragments: study of protein and DNA interactions. *Nucleic Acids Res.* **15,** 7351–7367.

4. Kramer, W., Ohmayer, A., and Fritz, H.-J. (1988) Improved enzymatic *in vitro* reactions in the gapped duplex DNA approach to oligonucleotide-directed construction of mutations. *Nucleic Acids Res.* **16,** 7207.

5. Murray, R., Pederson, K., Prosser, H., Muller, D., Hutchison, C. A. I., and Frelinger, J. A. (1988) Random oligonucleotide mutagenesis: application to a large protein coding sequence of a major histocompatibility complex class I gene, *H-2DP*. *Nucleic Acids Res.* **16,** 9761–9773.

6. Diaz, J.-J., Rhoads, D. D., and Roufa, D. J. (1991) PCR-mediated chemical (PMC) mutagenesis of cloned duplex DNAs. *BioTechniques* **11,** 204–211.

7. Saiki, R. K., Scharf, S., Faloona, F., Mullis, K. B., Horn, G. T., Erlich, H. A., and Arnheim, N. (1985) Enzymatic amplification of β-globin genomic sequences and restriction site analysis for diagnosis of sickle cell anemia. *Science* **230,** 1350–1354.

8. Mullis, K. B. and Faloona, F. A. (1987) Specific synthesis of DNA *in vitro* via a polymerase-catalyzed chain reaction. *Methods Enzymol.* **155,** 335–350.

9. Myers, R. M., Lerman, L. S., and Maniatis, T. (1985) A general method for saturation mutagenesis of cloned DNA fragments. *Science* **229,** 242–247.

10. Myers, R. M., Fischer, S. G., Maniatis, T., and Lerman, L. S. (1985) Modification of the melting properties of duplex DNA by attachment of a GC-rich DNA sequence as determined by denaturing gradient gel electrophoresis. *Nucleic Acids Res.* **13,** 3111–3129.

11. Messing, J. and Vieira, J. (1982) A new pair of M13 vectors for selecting either DNA strand of double-digest restriction fragments. *Gene* **19,** 269–276.

12. Rhoads, D. D., Dixit, A., and Roufa, D. J. (1986) Primary structure of human ribosomal protein S14 and the gene that encodes it. *Mol. Cell. Biol.* **6,** 2774–2783.

13. Weiss, B., Jacquemin-Sablon, A., Live, T. R., Fareed, G. C., and Richardson, C. C. (1968) Enzymatic breakage and joining of deoxyribonucleic acid. VI. Further purification and properties of polynucleotide ligase from *Escherichia coli* infected with bacteriophage T4. *J. Biol. Chem.* **243,** 4543–4555.

14. Diaz, J.-J. and Roufa, D. J. (1992) Fine structure map of the human ribosomal protein gene *RPS14*. *Mol. Cell. Biol.* **12,** 1680–1686.

15. Barnes, W. M. (1994) PCR amplification of up to 35-kb DNA with high fidelity and high yield from lambda bacteriophage templates. *Proc. Natl. Acad. Sci. USA* **6,** 2216–2220.

16. Dagert, M. and Ehrlich, S. D. (1979) Prolonged incubation in calcium chloride improves the competence of *Escherichia coli* cells. *Gene* **6,** 23–28.

CHAPTER 33

Oligonucleotide-Directed Random Mutagenesis Using the Phosphorothioate Method

Susan J. Dale and Maxine Belfield

1. Introduction

Oligonucleotide-directed mutagenesis has become the primary method for testing theories of protein structure/function and control of gene expression by specifically altering DNA sequences. Random oligonucleotides can be used to extend this approach to genes where less structural information is available. These can be prepared by spiking each of the phosphoramidites used in oligonucleotide synthesis with a mixture of the other three bases. The spiked oligonucleotides are then used for in vitro mutagenesis to produce a library of random mutants (Fig. 1).

Hermes et al. *(1)* used this approach to mutate the whole coding region of the triose phosphate isomerase gene using 10 spiked oligonucleotides and the original phosphorothioate method. We have performed similar experiments on the β galactosidase gene using the improved phosphorothioate method described in Chapter 5 *(2)*.

Random mutagenesis using spiked oligonucleotides has several advantages over traditional methods, such as exposure to ultraviolet radiation or chemicals *(3)*. Spiking produces truly random mutations with no mutational "hotspots." The region of mutagenesis can be defined and the average number of mutations introduced per clone can be predetermined. The library of random mutants can be screened functionally for altered properties. The selected mutants can be sequenced to localize various activities within the gene. Screening for gene products with altered

From: *Methods in Molecular Biology, Vol. 57: In Vitro Mutagenesis Protocols*
Edited by: M. K. Trower Humana Press Inc., Totowa, NJ

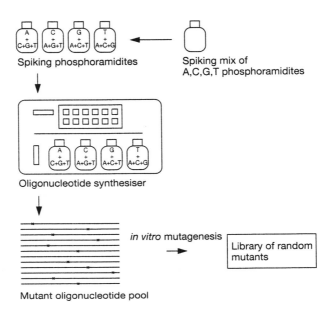

Fig. 1. Diagram of the steps involved in oligonucleotide-directed random mutagenesis.

activities also allows protein engineering to be performed without prior knowledge of protein structure or function.

2. Materials

The list of materials given in Chapter 5 also applies here. Additional materials required are:

1. An automated DNA synthesizer (Applied Biosystems Inc., Foster City, CA).
2. Lyophilized phosphoramidites of A, C, G, and T bases (Applied Biosystems Inc.) dissolved to a final concentration of 100 mM in anhydrous acetonitrile. The phosphoramite solutions should be freshly prepared, as all four bases should have equal reactivity to generate a truly random distribution of mutations.

3. Methods
3.1. Design of Spiked Oligonucleotides

The advice on oligonucleotide design given in Note 1 of Chapter 5 should also be applied when preparing spiked oligonucleotides. In addition, consider the three points that follow.

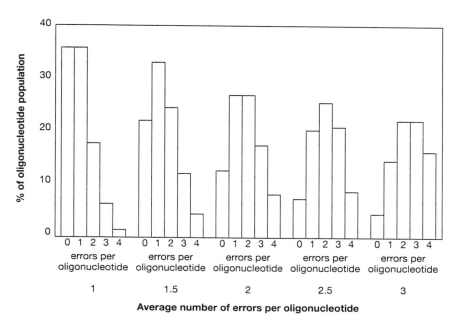

Fig. 2. Distribution of mutations in oligonucleotide populations. From the histograms it can be seen that as the average number of mutations per oligonucleotide is increased, the distribution of the number of errors per oligonucleotide shifts, so that the number of oligonucleotides with no mutations decreases and the number of oligonucleotides which carry multiple mutations increases. The histograms can be used to decide the optimal number of mutations per oligonucleotide for each application.

1. The length of the oligonucleotide should be between a minimum of about 20 bases and a maximum of 100 bases. Shorter oligonucleotides will not anneal to the template efficiently, and longer ones cannot be made at a suitable yield because of the limitations of automated DNA synthesis. A series of overlapping oligonucleotides can be used to mutate a region larger than 100 bases long.

2. A binomial distribution is observed for the number of mutations per oligonucleotide depending on the degree of spiking (Fig. 2). The ideal mutation rate depends on the application. A single base substitution per oligonucleotide may be appropriate for the mutational analysis of a DNA control region. This will be achieved by choosing an average number of errors of one per oligonucleotide. However, a single base change in a coding region may be silent because of the degenerative nature of the genetic code. Two errors per oligonucleotide would yield more mutants

with altered sequences and a greater possibility of detecting altered properties in the gene product.

3. Random mutations in the last few bases at either end prevent efficient annealing and may not be detected. Therefore the oligonucleotide sequence should be up to 10 bases longer at either end than the target region for mutagenesis.

3.2. Preparation of Spiked Oligonucleotides

1. Calculate the error rate required.

    Error rate = (average number of mistakes per oligonucleotide/length of oligonucleotide)

2. Calculate the volume of spiking mix to remove from each 100 m*M* phosphoramidite solution, using the following equation.

    Volume of spiking mix (mL) = Error rate × 1.33 × volume of pure phosphoramidite (mL)

    The figure of 1.33 corrects for the spiking mix being made of all four phosphoramidites, rather than just the three needed for spiking. An example of these calculations is given in Note 1.

3. Remove the calculated volume from each phosphoramidite and combine in a fresh vial. This is the spiking mix. Add a quarter of the spiking mix back to each pure phosphoramidite. The phosphoramidite solutions are now spiked to give the desired error rate.

4. Load the spiked phosphoramidites onto the oligonucleotide synthesizer and program in the wild-type sequence. A silent base change can be introduced as a marker to check the efficiency of mutagenesis.

5. Purify oligonucleotides <30 bases long by desalting, e.g., using an OPC column. Longer oligonucleotides should be purified by electrophoresis through a 12–20% acrylamide gel *(4)* *(see* Note 2).

6. Follow the protocol for phosphorylation of oligonucleotides in Chapter 5.

7. The phosphorylated spiked oligonucleotide should be used in the protocols for the mutagenesis reaction in Chapter 5.

8. The affect of mutagenesis can be assessed by a functional assay for the expressed product, or by sequencing DNA extracted from the transformants. The number of A, C, G, and T bases introduced should be approximately equal, showing that mutagenesis is truly random. The distribution of the number of mutations per clone should follow that predicted in Fig. 2.

4. Notes

1. The calculation of the volume of spiking mix is best illustrated by an example. To make an oligonucleotide 74 bases long containing two errors per oligonucleotide, the error rate would be 2/74 = 0.027. The volume of spiking mix required would therefore be 0.027 × 1.33 × 5 = 0.18 mL. A volume of 180 μL from each 5 mL 100 m*M* phosphoramidite would be taken and placed in a fresh vial to give a total of 720 μL spiking mix. One hundred eighty microliters of this would be added back to each pure phosphoramidite to give the desired level of spiking.

2. Frameshift mutations owing to single base deletions are more frequently created when spiked oligonucleotides are used in mutagenesis than standard oligonucleotides *(5)*. We detected 15% point deletions when 45 random mutants were analyzed by sequencing *(2)*. These deletions are created during oligonucleotide synthesis, as addition of each base is not 100% efficient. Automated synthesizers use a capping step to prevent oligonucleotides that have not had a base added during a round of synthesis from extending. A few molecules will also escape the capping reaction, allowing DNA synthesis to continue, even though a base has been missed out. Purification of longer oligonucleotides by acrylamide gel electrophoresis would normally remove truncated byproducts. Owing to the sequence variation within a random primer, oligonucleotides of different lengths can migrate similarly and will be copurified. Frameshift mutants produced from these primers also give information about the functional domains of the protein products and will be detected during sequencing.

3. As each transformant is a clone with particular random mutations, it is important to generate a large library so that a high proportion of the possible mutations are represented. A higher efficiency of transformation can be achieved by using electroporation than with chemically competent cells *(4)*.

4. The method described for making random mutations has the drawback that once the phosphoramidites have been spiked, they can only be used to make oligonucleotides of the same length and error rate. This can be overcome by a DNA synthesizer that allows protocol editing and accurate delivery of phosphoramidite solutions for on line mixing. The synthesizer simultaneously takes up an accurate volume of pure phosphoramidite and an aliquot of an equimolar phosphoramidite mix from a separate vial. It can be programmed to randomize only a specific segment of the sequence leaving the rest unmodified, for example the ends of the oligonucleotide.

References

1. Hermes, J. D., Parekh, S. M., Blacklow, S. C., Koster, H., and Knowles, J. R. (1989) A reliable method for random mutagenesis: the generation of mutant libraries using spiked oligodeoxyribonucleotide primers. *Gene* **84,** 143–151.
2. Dale, S. J., Belfield, M., and Richardson, T. C. (1991) Oligonucleotide-directed random mutagenesis using a high-efficiency procedure. *Methods* **3,** 145–153.
3. Myers, R. M., Lerman, L. S., and Maniatis, T. (1985) A general method for saturation mutagenesis of cloned DNA fragments. *Science* **229,** 242–247.
4. Sambrook, J., Fritsch, E. F., and Maniatis, T. (1989) *Molecular Cloning: A Laboratory Manual*, 2nd ed, Cold Spring Harbor Laboratory Press, Cold Spring Harbor, NY.
5. Carter, P., Garrard, L., and Henner, D. (1991) Antibody engineering using very long template-assembled oligonucleotides. *Methods* **3,** 183–192.

CHAPTER 34

An Efficient Random
Mutagenesis Technique
Using an *E. coli* Mutator Strain

Alan Greener, Marie Callahan,
and Bruce Jerpseth

1. Introduction

Site-directed mutagenesis has become an extremely powerful means by which the nature and function of critical amino acids within a protein can be assessed and altered. However, the ability to exploit this technique requires that detailed structural information about the protein (or related proteins) is available. For many gene products of interest, this information does not yet exist. In addition, variants that have particular qualities can be missed if one relies solely on the introduction of specific predetermined mutations.

In these and many other situations, having a method to efficiently generate a library of single (or double) point mutations scattered randomly throughout a gene would make it possible to locate and define the important amino acids involved in a particular biological process. A number of polymerase chain reaction (PCR)-related procedures designed to accomplish this have been developed; however, each of them require that the mutated gene be recloned into the vector. Relying on PCR to generate random mutations has obvious advantages in that a specific region within a gene can be targeted. However, the rate at which mutations accumulate often can be difficult to control. Therefore, PCR-directed random mutagenesis must be continuously tested empirically to monitor the relative number of mutations introduced. Moreover, many cloning opera-

From: *Methods in Molecular Biology, Vol. 57: In Vitro Mutagenesis Protocols*
Edited by: M. K. Trower Humana Press Inc., Totowa, NJ

tions must be performed to reconstitute the plasmid containing the mutated segment of interest.

Escherichia coli strains that contain mutations in various DNA repair pathways have long been known to exhibit an increase in the spontaneous mutation rate (*see* ref. *1* for a recent review). This increase, measured by a number of in vivo tests, was observed to be from 5- to 100-fold higher than a wild-type strain depending on the repair pathway that was eliminated. Initially, it was thought that propagating a plasmid containing a gene of interest in a strain of this type could yield a family of randomly mutated molecules. However, as shown in Table 1, the mutation frequency within a cloned gene would require that the plasmid be propagated for 1200 generations (if mutation frequency were 100-fold higher) to achieve a saturation level where every clone would carry a mutation. This lengthy growth requirement makes this approach impractical.

We have developed a new strain of *E. coli* called XL1-Red that was engineered to contain mutations that inactivate three independent DNA repair pathways *(2)*. We have estimated that the spontaneous mutation rate of this strain is approx 5000-fold greater than the wild-type parent (*see* Note 1). As a result, generation of a family of single-point mutations randomly within a cloned gene of interest becomes possible with just overnight growth (*see* Table 1). Propagation of plasmids through this strain results in a high frequency of single point mutations within a cloned gene (*see* Note 2). Furthermore, if a selection or a screen for phenotypic variants of a gene is possible, one can rapidly isolate the desired variant without being encumbered by the need to subclone or otherwise manipulate the gene or target of interest.

2. Materials
2.1. E. coli *Strains*

1. XL1-Red (Δ*[mcrA]*183, Δ*[mcrCB-hsdSMR-mrr]*173, *endA1, supE44, thi-1, gyrA96, relA1, mutS, mutT, mutD5, lac*) is a derivative of XL1-MRA (Stratagene, La Jolla, CA) that contains mutations in the mismatch repair pathway (*mutS; 3*), the oxo-dGTP repair pathway (*mutT; 4*), and the 3'–5'exonuclease subunit of DNA polymerase III (*mutD; 5*). Competent cells of this strain are available from Stratagene (*see* Note 3).
2. XL1-Blue: A nonmutator host is necessary into which to introduce the mutant pool of plasmids. We have routinely used XL1-Blue (Stratagene) for this purpose; if the plasmid of interest is tetracycline resistant, we then use XL1-Blue MRF'Kan (Stratagene, La Jolla, CA), a kanamycin-resis-

Table 1
Predicted Spontaneous Mutation Frequency/Gene[a]

Host	Sp. mut. freq.[b]	Mutations/gene	Generations of growth[c]
Wild type	10^{-10}	1/4000	120,000
muts	10^{-8}	1/40	1200
XL1-Red	5×10^{-6}	1.2	24

[a]The predicted spontaneous mutation frequency/gene is calculated based on the size of the *E. coli* genome (5×10^6 bp), the copy number and size of a common colE1 cloning vector (copy number = 100; total size = 4 kb), and the number of basepairs comprising the target of interest (1 kb). The actual spontaneous mutation frequency in XL1-Red has been empirically determined to be 0.5 mutations/kb *(2)*.
[b]The spontaneous mutation frequency for the wild-type and *muts* E. coli strains can be found in ref. *1*.
[c]Generations of growth are the number of cell doublings required to result in one point mutation/1 kb target DNA cloned on a colE1 origin plasmid.

tant tetracycline-sensitive derivative of XL1-Blue. However, most *E. coli* strains are suitable for this purpose.

3. SOC medium: 2% tryptone, 0.5% yeast extract, 10 m*M* NaCl, 10 m*M* MgCl$_2$, 10 m*M* MgSO$_4$, 0.4% glucose.
4. LB broth (per liter): 10 g tryptone, 5 g yeast extract, 10 g NaCl. Adjust to pH 7.0 with NaOH and then make up to a final volume of 1 L with distilled water. Autoclave.
5. LB agar: As for LB broth except for the addition of 15 g bactoagar.
6. Falcon 2059 tubes.

3. Methods
3.1. Transformation into XL1-Red

Because of the multiple mutations inactivating key repair pathways, the growth rate and transformation efficiency of XL1-Red are greatly reduced compared with most *E. coli* strains. The doubling time of XL1-Red in LB media at 37°C is approx 90 min; the transformation efficiency is 1×10^6 transformants/μg of DNA. A standard transformation protocol is performed with 1–10 ng of the plasmid of interest using competent cells prepared by the method of Hanahan *(6)*.

1. Thaw the competent XL1-Red cells on ice and aliquot 100 μL into a prechilled Falcon 2059 tube.
2. Add 1–10 ng of plasmid DNA to the cells and incubate on ice for 20–60 min.
3. Subject the cells to a 45-s heat pulse at 42°C, and directly return the tube to ice.

4. Add 0.9 mL of SOC medium and grow the cells at 37°C for 1 h with aeration.
5. Select transformants by plating 100 µL of the reaction on LB agar plates with the appropriate antibiotic selection.
6. If more transformants are desired, then concentrate the entire 1 mL volume by centrifugation, resuspend the pellet in 100 µL of SOC medium and plate directly.

3.2. Starter Culture Preparation

The aformentioned transformation experiment will yield 100–1000 colonies depending on the amount of DNA added and the volume plated. To ensure optimal random representation of mutations, we recommend pooling all transformants obtained to form a starter culture.

1. Add 2–4 mL of sterile LB broth to the transformation plates and scrape the colonies from the agar using the end of a sterile pipet.
2. Form a starter culture by transferring the cell mass to a sterile culture tube and allow to incubate at 37°C for 1 h with aeration.

3.3. Recovery of Pooled Mutated Plasmid DNA

This starter culture, which represents approx 20 generations of growth in the mutator strain, can be used directly to isolate plasmid DNA. Alternatively, it may be diluted for continued growth until stationary phase is reached, at which stage the dilution/growth cycle is repeated or the plasmid DNA is recovered. (*See* Notes 1 and 4 for further guidance on the number of growth cycles required to achieve the desired level of random mutagenesis.)

1. Isolate plasmid DNA directly from the starter culture using standard miniprep protocols (*see* Note 5).
2. Alternatively, make a 1:1000 dilution of the starter culture into LB broth with appropriate antibiotic selection. Grow overnight until the culture is in stationary phase, and then prepare plasmid miniprep DNA.
3. Repeat step 2 as required.

3.4. Retransformation into a Nonmutator Strain

Once the DNA of interest has been propagated for the requisite time in XL1-Red and isolated by miniprep, the plasmid pool is then transformed into any standard *E. coli* host.

1. Transform 1–10 ng of plasmid DNA prepared from each cycle of growth (*see* Note 5) into competent cells of any standard *E. coli* strain using the protocol outlined in Section 3.1.

2. Plate transformed cells on LB medium containing the appropriate antibiotic selection.

The transformed cells may be then subjected to analysis/selection/ screening to isolate mutant clones associated with altered biological activity. (*See* Notes 6–9 for various types of screens/selections that have been used with XL1-Red.)

4. Notes

1. It has been reported that the spontaneous mutation rate in wild-type *E. coli* is approx 1 mutation/10^{10} bp/generation/cell *(1)*. Given that the *E. coli* genome consists of 5×10^6 bp and that it takes approx 30 cell doublings for a single *E. coli* cell to reach stationary phase, the calculated spontaneous mutation frequency is about 1.5×10^{-2} mutations/bp/cell/30 generations. One would have to sequence 66 entire bacterial genomes to find one that carried a single mutation. Furthermore, if the goal is to generate random mutations within a discrete segment, this number is proportionally lower. For example, if a 1-kb gene is cloned into pBluescript (copy number = 100; 4 kb), the likelihood of finding a spontaneous mutation within that 1-kb segment becomes 1/4000.

XL1-Red has been observed to have a spontaneous mutation rate of approx 5000-fold higher than wild type *(2)*. If this increase directly translated into mutations per basepair, then by the aforementioned calculations, there should arise approx 1 mutation/1 kb DNA that is propagated on a pBluescript-like plasmid (after 30 generations of growth). We have evaluated the random mutation rate after 30 generations by sequence analysis of a pBluescript derivative. The experimental data (based on a limited sample of 12,000 bases sequenced) suggests that the spontaneous mutation rate on a pBluescript plasmid is 1 mutation/2 kb cloned DNA after 30 generations of growth.

This result can be used as a guide for the researcher to determine prior to the experiment how many generations of growth are optimal for their gene and their plasmid. If the target is a 2-kb gene on a pBluescript-like vector, then 30 generations should be sufficient for finding one mutation per target. If the gene of interest is smaller (or if only mutations within a part of the gene are desired), then the number of generations that the plasmid must be propagated to achieve the level of 1 mutation per target can be varied proportionally. In addition, the copy number of the plasmid vector must be considered since the relative gene dosage of the target will be lower if the plasmid is at a lower copy number. Therefore, if a 2-kb segment is being propagated on a vector-like pBR322 that has a copy number 1/4 that of pBluescript, then a fourfold increase in the number of generations will be necessary to yield the same relative saturation of random mutations. If the gene is cloned on a non-colE1 replicon (i.e., pACYC, R6K, F, RK2, etc.) that exists at a significantly lower copy number, the predicted number of cell doublings required for generating a sufficient number of mutations would be proportionally higher than pBluescript-like plasmids. However, because these lower copy number plasmids utilize *E. coli* DNA polymerase III as their replication enzyme (colE1 plasmids use DNA polymerase I), the *mut*D mutation will enhance the spontaneous mutation rate compared with colE1-based plasmids. Therefore, shorter than predicted propagation times are necessary. Although we have not empirically determined these parameters, it is likely that the required number of generations that the clones must be propagated is approximately the same.

It is important to note that the mutations induced by XL1-Red that have been sequenced were transitions, transversions, and 1-bp insertions.

2. There are some limitations to random mutagenesis using XL1-Red. If the target of interest is very small (<100 bp) or if multiple changes are desired, the number of generations that would be required to propagate the target become large and impractical. In these cases, a PCR-based method is recommended.

3. Because of the mutations in these three repair pathways, the spontaneous mutation rate of DNA propagated in this strain has been determined to be approx 5000-fold higher than the XL1-MRA parent strain *(2)*. Users are cautioned not to propagate the strain for prolonged periods on Petri dishes since the rapid accumulation of mutations will affect the host itself and the specific genotype cannot be guaranteed. Toward that end, we have evaluated the essential features of the strain prior to and on completion of large-scale fermentation preparations to ensure the competent cells exhibit the elevated mutagenesis phenotype. A detailed description of the genetic construction of the strain can be found in Greener and Callahan *(2)*.

4. The rate of spontaneous mutagenesis in XL1-Red is directly proportional to the number of generations the DNA of interest is propagated in the host. Depending on the size and the approximate number of mutations per target that is desired, the number of generations can be varied by repeating the 1:1000 dilutions (approx 10 generations), when the culture reaches stationary phase (*see* Note 1). When the desired number of generations has been attained, the DNA is retrieved by miniprep. If the relative saturation of mutations desired is not known, DNA can be retrieved from each cycle of growth, and material representing 20, 30, 40, and so on, generations can be prepared and each pool analyzed separately.

5. The XL1-Red mutator strain contains the *endA1* mutation which has been shown to improve the quality and quantity of DNA retrieved using both standard alkaline lysis or boiling miniprep procedures.

6. The most powerful method to find mutants of interest is to have available a positive genetic selection for the desired activity. pBR322 is a standard *E. coli* cloning vector containing the colE1 origin of replication that is used for pBluescript, pUC, pGEM, pET, and so on. The copy number of pBR322, however, is approx 1/4 to 1/5 that of the pUC-like plasmids presumably because of the presence of the *rop* gene that produces a small protein effectively reducing plasmid copy number *(7,8)*. We wished to test whether the XL1-Red strain could produce mutations within pBR322 that increased the plasmid copy number. It has been demonstrated by Uhlin et al. *(9)* that ampicillin resistance expressed by an *E. coli* cell is directly proportional to the number of copies of the gene (assuming all other genetic signals are the same). Therefore, copy up mutations of pBR322 should result in an *E. coli* cell exhibiting greater resistance to ampicillin. We empirically determined that when pBR322 DNA was transformed into *E. coli* (XL1-Blue), colonies were obtained if selected on LB plates with 100 or 1000 µg/mL ampicillin, but none were apparent on plates containing 7500 µg/mL ampicillin.

pBR322 DNA was transformed into XL1-RED, and ampicillin-resistant transformants (100 µg/mL selection) were pooled and grown for an additional 10 generations (total of 30 generations). The mutant pool was isolated by miniprep, transformed into SCS-1 (Stratagene), and colonies selected on LB plates containing either 100 or 7500 µg/mL ampicillin. Approximately 10,000 transformants were obtained on the low ampicillin plate and there were 42 colonies present on the high ampicillin plate. These colonies represent either:

a. Copy up mutants that have a higher gene dosage of the native ampicillin resistance gene;

b. Structural gene mutants of the ampicillin resistance protein that have a greater specific activity; or

c. Mutants in the gene regulatory signals for ampicillin resistance that result in a greater quantity of the normal resistance protein.

To distinguish among these possibilities, the potential mutants were restreaked and their DNA content analyzed by whole cell lysis (*see* Fig. 1). If the high ampicillin resistance were owing to a copy up mutation, there would be a correspondingly increased plasmid DNA band compared with the parental pBR322 cells. If the mutation resulted in an enhanced expression of native ampicillin resistance protein or in a variant that had a greater specific activity, then the plasmid DNA content should remain unchanged.

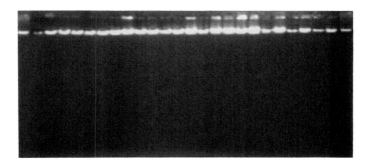

Fig. 1. Miniprep analysis of potential pBR322 copy mutants. Whole cell lysates from XL1-Blue cells containing either wild-type pBR322 or mutants expressing increased resistance to ampicillin. The two outside lanes are the native pBR322 controls and the inner 24 are the potential mutants. For many of the colonies tested, the plasmid DNA band is distinctly more intense than the control and we presume that these represent copy up mutations. For those lanes that do not exhibit an increased plasmid intensity, we infer that the increased level of ampicillin resistance is owing to a mutation within either the structural gene or the genetic control region that results in the overexpression of the native protein.

As seen in Fig. 1, for 14–18 of the 24 plasmids tested, the pBR322 plasmid DNA band was substantially greater, suggesting that they were copy up mutants. For the remaining plasmids, the similar intensities of the DNA bands suggest they are of the increased expression/activity class. The preponderance of copy number mutants compared with increased activity/ expression mutations may be a reflection of the number of potential sites and changes required to give rise to these phenotypes. Copy up mutations can arise if any mutation in *rop* occurs that abolishes its activity, whereas increased expression/activity mutants will arise only if specific bases are altered.

These copy up mutants were analyzed by restriction enzyme digestion and observed to be identical to that of the parent pBR322 vector. When they were retransformed into SCS-1, the total number of colonies obtained on LB plates with either 100 or 7500 µg/mL ampicillin were equivalent. This indicated that the mutation causing the elevated drug resistance was carried on the plasmid and not a result of a spontaneous host mutation.

Large-scale plasmid DNA preparations from two of these mutants yielded 2.0 mg/L plasmid DNA compared with 500 mg/L for the native pBR322, an expected outcome if the mutations resulted in a higher copy number.

7. A second method for mutant screening often involves isolating variants having reduced expression/activity of a gene or complete loss of activity. To test the mutator strain for the ability to give rise to these types of variants, the following experiment was performed. pGC10, a pBluescript derivative that contained the Cam^R gene in addition to the ampicillin resistance gene, was transformed into XL1-Red and propagated for 30 generations. The pool of mutant plasmid DNA was then isolated and transformed into XL1-Blue, selecting for Amp^R transformants. 500 Amp^R colonies were then patched onto LB amp plates containing either 34 or 300 μg/mL chloramphenicol. XL1-Blue cells containing the wild-type pGC10 grew well on both the CAM plates. Of the 500 transformants containing pGC10 plasmids that had been propagated through XL1-Red, 16 (3.2%) were unable to grow on either of the CAM plates, indicating they had become CAM sensitive. Furthermore, a total of 89 colonies (17.8%) were able to grow on the 34 μg/mL CAM plate but unable to grow on 300 μg/mL. These data indicate that a high percentage incurred a mutation(s) that either reduced the activity of the Cam^R protein, reduced the level of CAM expression, or lowered the copy number of the pGC10 plasmid.

8. A third type of mutant screening often performed is searching for variants of proteins, which have increased (or decreased) activity, that can be assayed directly. One such example that we have attempted is to introduce mutations in a cloned alkaline phosphatase gene. The gene of interest was isolated from a hyperthermophilic archebacterium, *P. furiosus* (Cline et al., unpublished). The cloned alkaline phosphatase gene was observed to have very low activity at 37°C in an *E. coli* host that carried a deletion for its endogenous alkaline phosphatase gene (strain HB3). This observation was based on the inability to hydrolyze the chromophore BCIP (5-chloro-4-bromo-3-indolyl phosphate) when present in LB plates at 125 mg/mL. By comparison, when the *E. coli* alkaline phosphatase gene cloned onto an identical vector was transformed into HB3 cells, intensely blue colonies on the same plates appeared. We wished to determine if variants of the *P. furiosus* alkaline phosphatase that had greater activity at 37°C could be isolated. We performed the standard XL1-Red mutagenesis on the alkaline phosphatase containing plasmid and transformed the pool into the alkaline phosphatase deleted host HB3 and screened for blue colonies at 37°C. Of approx 10,000 transformants, 6 were observed to be dark blue. These 6 were purified by miniprep and retransformed to confirm that the mutation was carried on the plasmid and not a result of a spontaneous host mutation. All 6 were observed to be owing to plasmid mutations.

We then remutagenized each of these 6 plasmids in XL1-Red (standard conditions) and retransformed HB3, selecting for blue colonies at 37°C with 1/3 less BCIP substrate in the selection plates (40 μg/mL). Each of the original 6 mutants were very light blue on these plates. A total of approx 10,000 transformants for each mutant were screened; for 2 of the 6, variants that were more intensely blue were observed. For the remaining 4, there were none exhibiting this phenotype. We chose to focus our analysis on one "family" of mutants. The initial first round mutant (called *Pfu*-5) and the two second round mutants (*Pfu* 5-1 and *Pfu* 5-2) were isolated and their DNA sequences determined. We found that the *Pfu*-5 mutant contained a 1-bp insertion of a G residue upstream of the coding region in the area that constitutes its presumed promoter. The mutation altered the −35 hexamer (TTCCAA) to (TTGCCA) that is closer to the consensus *E. coli* promoter sequence and concomitantly changed the spacing of the −35 and −10 hexamers to the more conserved distance of 17 bp *(10)*. The mutations in *Pfu* 5-1 and 5-2 were base substitutions within the 494 amino acid coding region. *Pfu* 5-1 resulted in a leu → pro change at amino acid 224 and *Pfu* 5-2 was a gly → arg mutation at amino acid 241. Presumably, these structural gene mutations result in a variant having higher specific activity at 37°C or higher specific activity at all temperatures. These data confirm the utility of random mutagenesis when screening for variants of this type.

9. Notes 6–8 describe methods for utilizing the XL1-Red mutator strain for introducing random mutations in a cloned gene when a genetic selection or screen for the variants is available. However, in many instances, this will not be the case. The advantage in using XL1-Red for random mutagenesis (over, e.g., chemical mutagenesis or a PCR-based protocol) is that the mutation rate can be carefully controlled. By propagating the target DNA of interest in XL1-Red for the requisite number of generations prior to miniprep and retransformation into the nonmutator strain, random colonies can be analyzed by DNA sequence analysis to search for the random mutations.

Acknowledgments

We thank Alison Fowler, David Cotton, and Patty Evans for media preparation; Randy Carver for preparation of the figure; and K. Carine for critical reading of the manuscript.

References

1. Miller, J. H. (1992) *A Short Course in Bacterial Genetics,* Cold Spring Harbor Laboratory Press, Cold Spring Harbor, NY.
2. Greener, A. and Callahan, M. (1994) XL1-RED: a highly efficient random mutagenesis strain. *Strategies* **7,** 32–34.

3. Radman, M., Wagner, R. E., Glickman, B. W., and Meselson, M. (1980) DNA methylation, mismatch correction, and genetic stability, in *Progress in Environmental Mutagenesis* (Alevic, M., ed.), Elsevier, Amsterdam, pp. 121–130.

4. Cox, E. C. (1976) Bacterial mutator genes and the control of spontaneous mutation. *Ann. Rev. Genet.* **10,** 135–156.

5. Scheueurmann, R., Tam, S., Burgers, P. M. J., Lu, C., and Echols, H. (1983) Identification of the ε-subunit of *Escherichia coli* DNA polymerase III holoenzyme as the *dnaQ* gene product: a fidelity subunit for DNA replication. *Proc. Natl. Acad. Sci. USA* **80,** 7085–7089.

6. Hanahan, D. (1983) Studies on transformation of Escherichia coli with plasmids. *J. Mol. Biol.* **166,** 557–580.

7. Tomizawa, J. and Som, T. (1984) Control of ColE1 plasmid replication: enhancement of binding of RNA 1 to the primer transcript by the rom protein. *Cell* **38,** 871–878.

8. Lacatena, R. M., Banner, D. W., Castagnoli, L., and Cesareni, G. (1984) Control of initiation of pMB1 replication: purified rop protein and RNA 1 affect primer formation *in vitro*. *Cell* **37,** 1009–1014.

9. Uhlin, B. E., Molin, S., Gustafsson, P., and Nordstrom, K. (1979) Plasmids with temperature dependent copy numbers for amplification of cloned genes and their products. *Gene* **6,** 91–103.

10. Harley, C. B. and Reynolds, R. P. (1987) Analysis of *E. coli* promotor sequences. *Nucleic Acids Res.* **15,** 2343–2361.

Index

A

Agarose gel electrophoresis, 61, 144,
 199, 207, 208

B

Biotin-16-dUTP, 101, 297–310
Biotin–streptavidin interaction
 (*see* Streptavidin–biotin
 interaction)

C

Cassette mutagenesis, 229
Chemical mutagens, 357
 formic acid, 359
 hydrazine, 359
 nitrous acid, 359
Chemical mutagenesis, 362, 363
Competent *E. coli* cell
 preparation,
 CaCl$_2$ method, 60, 68, 69, 94, 95
 electrocompetent, 344, 345
 Hanahan method, 8, 9

D

dam gene, 246
Double-stranded DNA preparation
 (*see* Plasmid/phagemid DNA
 preparation)
DNA amplification (*see* PCR)
DNA ligase,
 T4 DNA ligase, 24, 89, 243
 thermostable, 149

DNA polymerases,
 Klenow DNA polymerase,
  63, 89
 blunt-ending, 144, 302–304
 double-stranded DNA preparation, 339–341
 strand-displacement activity,
  23, 24, 54, 133
 pfu DNA polymerase, 150, 201
 blunt-ending, 242
 proofreading (*see pfu* and *vent*
  DNA polymerases)
 T4 DNA polymerase, 24, 31, 54,
  133, 140
 T7 DNA polymerase,
  33, 54, 63
 Taq DNA polymerase, 97, 154
 fidelity, 174, 187, 200, 201,
  351, 355
 nontemplated A addition, 175,
  210–213
 Taqplus DNA polymerase, 240
 Vent DNA polymerase, 182, 187,
  201, 332
DNA purification,
 DE-81 paper, 182, 183
 electroelution, 208, 253
 gel purification, 173, 198, 199
 squeeze freeze, 199, 208
 membrane filtration, 207
 phenol/chloroform extraction,
  ethanol/salt precipitation, 6,
  92, 143, 233, 253, 254, 264,
  273, 304
DNA sequencing, 305, 306

387

E

Escherichia coli strains,
    amber suppressor strains, 65
    DH5α, 16
    dut⁻ ung⁻ strain, 48, 230
    JM109, 9
    mismatch repair-deficient (*mut*S)
        strains, 2, 14, 83, 122
    BMH71-18, 2, 16, 83, 124
    ES1301, 2
    XL*mut*S, 33
    TG1, 58
    XL1-Blue, 34, 376, 377
    XL1-Blue MRF'Kan, 376, 377
    XL1-Red mutator strain, 376
Exonuclease III, 57, 139
    digestion, 59, 144

G

Gapped heteroduplex methods,
    75–85, 87–95, 97–107

H

Helper phage, 46
    M13K07, 2, 233
    R408, 2, 50
    stock preparation, 49, 50

K

Kunkel method, 45, 233, 275

L

LCR conditions (*see* Ligase chain
    reaction conditions)
Ligase chain reaction conditions,
    153
Ligase (*see* DNA ligase)
Ligation,
    in melted agarose, 317
    standard, 344, 366

M

Magnetic beads, 97
Megaprimer method, 177,
    203–215
Miniprep DNA preparation (*see*
    Double-stranded DNA
    preparation)
Mutagenesis (*see* chemical mutagen-
    esis, cassette mutagenesis,
    site-directed mutagenesis,
    and random mutagenesis)
Mutant DNA strand selection by,
    phosphorothioate incorporation,
        55–64
    positive antibiotic selection,
        1–12
    restriction enzyme digestion,
        13–29, 31–44, 119–137
    uracil incorporation, 45–54
Mutant DNA strand synthesis, 7, 8,
    19, 20
Mutant screening, 9, 94, 116, 130,
    131, 222, 223, 225, 226
    restriction digestion, 225
    colony hybridisation, 225, 226,
        306, 307
    rapid insert PCR screen, 189, 190
*mut*D, 380

N

Nested deletions, 119–137,
    139–147

O

Oligodeoxyribonucleotide cassettes,
    297
Oligonucleotides (*see* Primers)
Ordered deletions (*see* Nested
    deletions)
Overlap extension mutagenesis,
    167–176, 177–191, 193–202,
    323–333

P

PCR, 149, 193, 375, 375
  asymmetric, 229
  denaturation/reannealing of
    product, 221, 222
  dITP incorporation, 352
  mutagenic conditions, 353–356
  Mn^{2+}, 352, 355
  standard conditions, 102, 152,
    153 172, 173, 198, 206, 207,
    210–213, 241, 242, 251–253,
    263, 274, 290, 291, 316, 317,
    327–329, 341, 342, 353, 364
Phosphatase, alkaline calf-intestinal,
  79, 92
Plasmid/phagemid,
  biotinylation, 101
  DNA denaturation/annealing, 7,
    19, 27, 28, 79–81, 89, 93,
    126, 135, 136
  DNA, nicking, 59, 140, 144, 146
  DNA preparation,
    bacterial cultures, 6, 7, 66–68,
      129, 272, 273,
    bacterial colonies, 130, 305
    COS cells, 115
  uracil-containing, 275
  vectors,
    pALTER series, 4
    pBR322, 125, 381, 382
    pSP189 (*see* shuttle vector)
    pUC, 157
    pUC19M, 24, 25
Polymerases (*see* DNA polymerases)
Polymerase chain reaction (*see* PCR)
Primer(s),
  annealing, 7, 8, 19, 36, 37, 51, 52,
    59, 79, 126, 339
  biotinylated, 102
  degenerate oligonucleotide
    synthesis, 315, 325, 326
  extension, 7, 8, 19, 20, 37, 59, 81,
    126, 127, 339–341

  megaprimer, 206, 207,
    209, 210,
  MUT primers, 159
  mutagenic design,
    random, 346, 347, 370, 371
    site-directed, 10, 25, 26, 35, 36,
      164
    triple helix-targeted, 113, 114
  PCR, 169–172, 184–186, 242, 292,
    318, 325, 354, 355
  phosphorylation, 19, 27, 51, 92,
    106, 126, 234, 282
  psoralen, 111
  purification, 234, 338, 339
  quantitation, 186
  spiked, 369
  triplex formation, 109
  visualization, 339
Psoralen photoactivation, 113

R

Random mutagenesis, 119, 139, 279,
  287, 311, 323, 335, 351, 357,
  369, 375
Restriction enzymes,
  *Bsp*MI, 260
  *Dpn*I, 242
  *Nci*I, 56, 63
  *Sau*3AI, 269
  *Sap*I, 298
  *Tsp*509I, 259
Restriction enzyme digestion, 37, 38,
  42, 91, 92, 129, 163, 342

S

S1 nuclease, 144
Sequencing (*see* DNA sequencing)
Shuttle vector,
  pSP189, 112
Single-stranded DNA template
  preparation, 4–6
  uracil-containing, 49–51, 223, 224

Site-directed mutagenesis, 1, 13, 31
  45, 55, 65, 75, 87, 97, 109, 149,
  157, 167, 177, 193, 203, 217,
  229, 239, 249, 259, 269, 297
SOE (*see* Overlap extension)
Streptavidin–biotin interaction,
  97
SV40-based shuttle vector (*see*
  pSP189)

T

T4 DNA ligase (*see* Ligation)
T4 gene 32, 235
T4 polynucleotide kinase (*see* primer
  phosphorylation)

T5 exonuclease, 55
Transfection, 114, 115
Transformation,
  M13, 60, 61
  plasmids/ phagemids,
  chemical, 9, 21, 38–40, 61, 128,
    145, 377, 378
  electroporation, 21, 115, 128,
    222, 345
Transversions, 111
Triple helix formation, 114

U

Unique restriction site elimination,
  13–29, 31–34, 120

Methods in Molecular Biology™

Methods in Molecular Biology™ manuals are available at all medical bookstores. You may also order copies directly from Humana by filling in and mailing or faxing this form to: Humana Press, 999 Riverview Drive, Suite 208, Totowa, NJ 07512 USA, Phone: 201-256-1699/Fax: 201-256-8341.

60. **Protein NMR Protocols,** edited by *David G. Reid, 1996* • 0-89603-309-0 • Comb $69.50 (T)

59. **Protein Purification Protocols,** edited by *Shawn Doonan, 1996* • 0-89603-336-8 • Comb $64.50 (T)

58. **Basic DNA and RNA Protocols,** edited by *Adrian J. Harwood, 1996* • 0-89603-331-7 • Comb $69.50 • 0-89603-402-X • Hardcover $99.50

57. **In Vitro Mutagenesis Protocols,** edited by *Michael K. Trower, 1996* • 0-89603-332-5 • Comb $69.50

56. **Crystallographic Methods and Protocols,** edited by *Christopher Jones, Barbara Mulloy, and Mark Sanderson, 1996* • 0-89603-259-0 • Comb $69.50 (T)

55. **Plant Cell Electroporation and Electrofusion Protocols,** edited by *Jac A. Nickoloff, 1995* • 0-89603-328-7 • Comb $49.50

54. **YAC Protocols,** edited by *David Markie, 1995* • 0-89603-313-9 • Comb $69.50

53. **Yeast Protocols:** *Methods in Cell and Molecular Biology,* edited by *Ivor H. Evans, 1996* • 0-89603-319-8 • Comb $74.50

52. **Capillary Electrophoresis:** *Principles, Instrumentation, and Applications,* edited by *Kevin D. Altria, 1996* • 0-89603-315-5 • Comb $74.50

51. **Antibody Engineering Protocols,** edited by *Sudhir Paul, 1995* • 0-89603-275-2 • Comb $69.50

50. **Species Diagnostics Protocols:** *PCR and Other Nucleic Acid Methods,* edited by *Justin P. Clapp, 1996* • 0-89603-323-6 • Comb $69.50

49. **Plant Gene Transfer and Expression Protocols,** edited by *Heddwyn Jones, 1995* • 0-89603-321-X • Comb $69.50

48. **Animal Cell Electroporation and Electrofusion Protocols,** edited by *Jac A. Nickoloff, 1995* • 0-89603-304-X • Comb $64.50

47. **Electroporation Protocols for Microorganisms,** edited by *Jac A. Nickoloff, 1995* • 0-89603-310-4 • Comb $69.50

46. **Diagnostic Bacteriology Protocols,** edited by *Jenny Howard and David M. Whitcombe, 1995* • 0-89603-297-3 • Comb $69.50

45. **Monoclonal Antibody Protocols,** edited by *William C. Davis, 1995* • 0-89603-308-2 • Comb $64.50

44. **Agrobacterium Protocols,** edited by *Kevan M. A. Gartland and Michael R. Davey, 1995* • 0-89603-302-3 • Comb $69.50

43. **In Vitro Toxicity Testing Protocols,** edited by *Sheila O'Hare and Chris K. Atterwill, 1995* • 0-89603-282-5 • Comb $69.50

42. **ELISA:** *Theory and Practice,* by *John R. Crowther, 1995* • 0-89603-279-5 • Comb $59.50

41. **Signal Transduction Protocols,** edited by *David A. Kendall and Stephen J. Hill, 1995* • 0-89603-298-1 • Comb $64.50

40. **Protein Stability and Folding:** *Theory and Practice,* edited by *Bret A. Shirley, 1995* • 0-89603-301-5 • Comb $69.50

39. **Baculovirus Expression Protocols,** edited by *Christopher D. Richardson, 1995* • 0-89603-272-8 • Comb $64.50

38. **Cryopreservation and Freeze-Drying Protocols,** edited by *John G. Day and Mark R. McLellan, 1995* • 0-89603-296-5 • Comb $79.50

37. **In Vitro Transcription and Translation Protocols,** edited by *Martin J. Tymms, 1995* • 0-89603-288-4 • Comb $69.50

36. **Peptide Analysis Protocols,** edited by *Ben M. Dunn and Michael W. Pennington, 1994* • 0-89603-274-4 • Comb $64.50

35. **Peptide Synthesis Protocols,** edited by *Michael W. Pennington and Ben M. Dunn, 1994* • 0-89603-273-6 • Comb $64.50

34. **Immunocytochemical Methods and Protocols,** edited by *Lorette C. Javois, 1994* • 0-89603-285-X • Comb $64.50

33. **In Situ Hybridization Protocols,** edited by *K. H. Andy Choo, 1994* • 0-89603-280-9 • Comb $69.50

32. **Basic Protein and Peptide Protocols,** edited by *John M. Walker, 1994* • 0-89603-269-8 • Comb $59.50 • 0-89603-268-X • Hardcover $89.50

☐ 31. **Protocols for Gene Analysis,** edited by *Adrian J. Harwood, 1994* • 0-89603-258-2 • Comb $69.50

☐ 30. **DNA–Protein Interactions,** edited by *G. Geoff Kneale, 1994* • 0-89603-256-6 • Paper $64.50

☐ 29. **Chromosome Analysis Protocols,** edited by *John R. Gosden, 1994* • 0-89603-243-4 • Comb $69.50 • 0-89603-289-2 • Hardcover $94.50

☐ 28. **Protocols for Nucleic Acid Analysis by Nonradioactive Probes,** edited by *Peter G. Isaac, 1994* • 0-89603-254-X • Comb $69.50

☐ 27. **Biomembrane Protocols:** *II. Architecture and Function,* edited by *John M. Graham and Joan A. Higgins, 1994* • 0-89603-250-7 • Comb $64.50

☐ 26. **Protocols for Oligonucleotide Conjugates:** *Synthesis and Analytical Techniques,* edited by *Sudhir Agrawal, 1994* • 0-89603-252-3 • Comb $64.50

☐ 25. **Computer Analysis of Sequence Data:** *Part II,* edited by *Annette M. Griffin and Hugh G. Griffin, 1994* • 0-89603-276-0 • Comb $59.50

☐ 24. **Computer Analysis of Sequence Data:** *Part I,* edited by *Annette M. Griffin and Hugh G. Griffin, 1994* • 0-89603-246-9 • Comb $59.50

☐ 23. **DNA Sequencing Protocols,** edited by *Hugh G. Griffin and Annette M. Griffin, 1993* • 0-89603-248-5 • Comb $59.50

☐ 22. **Microscopy, Optical Spectroscopy, and Macroscopic Techniques,** edited by *Christopher Jones, Barbara Mulloy, and Adrian H. Thomas, 1993* • 0-89603-232-9 • Comb $69.50

☐ 21. **Protocols in Molecular Parasitology,** edited by *John E. Hyde, 1993* • 0-89603-239-6 • Comb $69.50

☐ 20. **Protocols for Oligonucleotides and Analogs:** *Synthesis and Properties,* edited by *Sudhir Agrawal, 1993* • 0-89603-247-7 • Comb $69.50 • 0-89603-281-7 • Hardcover $89.50

☐ 19. **Biomembrane Protocols:** *I. Isolation and Analysis,* edited by *John M. Graham and Joan A. Higgins, 1993* • 0-89603-236-1 • Comb $69.50

☐ 18. **Transgenesis Techniques:** *Principles and Protocols,* edited by *David Murphy and David A. Carter, 1993* • 0-89603-245-0 • Comb $69.50

☐ 17. **Spectroscopic Methods and Analyses:** *NMR, Mass Spectrometry, and Metalloprotein Techniques,* edited by *Christopher Jones, Barbara Mulloy, and Adrian H. Thomas, 1993* • 0-89603-215-9 • Comb $69.50

☐ 16. **Enzymes of Molecular Biology,** edited by *Michael M. Burrell, 1993* • 0-89603-322-8 • Paper $59.50

☐ 15. **PCR Protocols:** *Current Methods and Applications,* edited by *Bruce A. White, 1993* • 0-89603-244-2 • Paper $54.50

☐ 14. **Glycoprotein Analysis in Biomedicine,** edited by *Elizabeth F. Hounsell, 1993* • 0-89603-226-4 • Comb $64.50

☐ 13. **Protocols in Molecular Neurobiology,** edited by *Alan Longstaff and Patricia Revest, 1992* • 0-89603-199-3 • Comb $59.50

☐ 12. **Pulsed-Field Gel Electrophoresis:** *Protocols, Methods, and Theories,* edited by *Margit Burmeister and Levy Ulanovsky, 1992* • 0-89603-229-9 • Hardcover $69.50

☐ 11. **Practical Protein Chromatography,** edited by *Andrew Kenney and Susan Fowell, 1992* • 0-89603-213-2 • Hardcover $59.50

☐ 10. **Immunochemical Protocols,** edited by *Margaret M. Manson, 1992* • 0-89603-270-1 • Comb $69.50

☐ 9. **Protocols in Human Molecular Genetics,** edited by *Christopher G. Mathew, 1991* • 0-89603-205-1 • Hardcover $69.50

☐ 8. **Practical Molecular Virology:** *Viral Vectors for Gene Expression,* edited by *Mary K. L. Collins, 1991* • 0-89603-191-8 • Paper $54.50

☐ 7. **Gene Transfer and Expression Protocols,** edited by *Edward J. Murray, 1991* • 0-89603-178-0 • Hardcover $79.50

☐ 6. **Plant Cell and Tissue Culture,** edited by *Jeffrey W. Pollard and John M. Walker, 1990* • 0-89603-161-6 • Comb $69.50

☐ 5. **Animal Cell Culture,** edited by *Jeffrey W. Pollard and John M. Walker, 1990* • 0-89603-150-0 • Comb $69.50

---

ne _____

artment _____

itution _____

ress _____

/State/Zip _____

ntry _____

ne # _____ Fax # _____

notes a tentative price. Prices listed are Humana Press prices, current as of October 1995, and do
flect the prices at which books will be sold to you by suppliers other than Humana Press. All
subject to change without notice.

rope, Middle East, and Africa: Order directly from Chapman & Hall by faxing to: +44-171-522-9623.

Postage & Handling: *USA Prepaid (UPS):* Add $4.00 for the first book and $1.00 for each additional book. *Outside USA* (Surface): Add $5.00 for the first book and $1.50 for each additional book.

☐ **My check for $_____ is enclosed**
 (Drawn on US funds from a US bank).

☐ Visa   ☐ MasterCard   ☐ American Express

Card # _____

Exp. date _____

Signature _____